Surgery for Epilepsy

Contemporary Issues in Neurological Surgery

GENERAL SERIES EDITORS

Harold J. Hoffman MD, FRCSC
Professor of Surgery, University of Toronto;
Neurosurgeon-in-Chief, Hospital for Sick Children,
Toronto, Ontario, Canada

Julian T. Hoff MD
Professor of Surgery;
Chief, Section of Neurosurgery,
University of Michigan,
Ann Arbor, Michigan

PREVIOUS TITLES IN THE SERIES

Mild to Moderate Head Injury
Julian T. Hoff, Thomas E. Anderson, and Theodore M. Cole

Contemporary Issues in Neurological Surgery

Surgery for Epilepsy

EDITED BY

Susan S. Spencer MD
Associate Professor of Neurology;
Director, Clinical Epilepsy Service,
Department of Neurology,
Yale University School of Medicine,
New Haven, Connecticut

AND

Dennis D. Spencer MD
Section Chief, Section of Neurological Surgery,
Yale University School of Medicine,
New Haven, Connecticut

FOREWORD BY

Robert G. Grossman MD
Baylor College of Medicine
Houston, Texas

BOSTON

BLACKWELL SCIENTIFIC PUBLICATIONS

OXFORD LONDON EDINBURGH

MELBOURNE PARIS BERLIN VIENNA

Editorial offices:
3 Cambridge Center, Cambridge
Massachusetts 02142 , USA
Osney Mead, Oxford OX2 0EL, England
25 John Street, London WC1N 2BL
England
23 Ainslie Place, Edinburgh EH3 6AJ
Scotland
54 University Street, Carlton
Victoria 3053, Australia

First published 1991

Set by Best-Set Typesetter, Hong Kong
Printed and bound in the
United States of America by
Hamilton Printing Company,
Rensselaer, New York
91 92 93 94 5 4 3 2 1

DISTRIBUTORS

USA and Canada
Mosby-Year Book, Inc.
11830 Westline Industrial Drive
St Louise, Missouri 63146
(*Orders:* Tel: 800 633 6699)

Australia
Blackwell Scientific Publications
(Australia) Pty Ltd
54 University Street
Carlton, Victoria 3053
(*Orders:* Tel: 03 347 0300)

Outside North America and Australia
Marston Book Services Ltd
PO Box 87
Oxford OX2 0DT
(*Orders:* Tel: 0865 791155
Fax: 0865 791927
Telex: 837515)

Library of Congress
Cataloging-in-Publication Data

Surgery for epilepsy/edited by Susan S. Spencer, Dennis D. Spencer.
p. cm. — (Contemporary issues in neurological surgery)
Includes bibliographical references.
Includes index.
ISBN 0–86542–089–0 (case)
1. Epilepsy—Surgery. 2. Temporal lobectomy. 3. Brain — Surgery.
I. Spencer, Susan S. II. Spencer, Dennis D.
III. Series.
[DNLM: 1. Epilepsy — Surgery. W1 CO769MRB v. 2/WL 385 89615]
RD594.S89 1990
616.8′53 — dc20

To our parents and children,
for teaching us what's important

Contents

Part II: Surgery

Part III: Outcome

List of Contributors

Frederick Andermann MD FRCP(C)
Professor of Neurology, McGill University; Director of Epilepsy Service, Montreal Neurological Hospital and Institute

Richard A. Bronen MD
Assistant Professor, Radiology, Yale University School of Medicine

Paul H. Crandall MD
Professor Emeritus, Division of Neurosurgery and Department of Neurology, UCLA School of Medicine

Hans Lüders MD PhD
Head, Section of Epilepsy and Clinical Neurophysiology, Cleveland Clinic Foundation

George A. Ojemann MD
Professor of Neurological Surgery, University of Washington; Director of Epilepsy Center, Harborview Medical Center

André Olivier MD, PhD, FRCS(C), DABNS
Professor of Neurosurgery, McGill University; Neurosurgeon, Montreal Neurological Institute and Hospital

Sherrill J. Purves BA, MD, PhD, FRCP(C)
Director of Epilepsy Unit and Director of EEG, Vancouver General Hospital; Clinical Associate Professor, University of British Columbia

David W. Roberts MD
Associate Professor of Surgery (Neurosurgery), Dartmouth–Hitchcock Medical Center, Dartmouth Medical School

A. David Rothner MD
Head, Section of Pediatric Neurology, Cleveland Clinic Foundation

Dennis D. Spencer MD
Nixdorff-German Professor of Neurosurgery and Chief, Section of Neurosurgery, Yale University School of Medicine

Susan S. Spencer MD
Associate Professor of Neurology and Director, Clinical Epilepsy Service, Yale University School of Medicine

William H. Theodore MD
Chief, Clinical Epilepsy Section, Medical Neurology Branch, National Institute of Neurological Disorders and Stroke

Peter D. Williamson MD
Associate Professor of Neurology, Yale University School of Medicine; Assistant Chief, Neurology Service and Director, Epilepsy Center, VA Medical Center

Allen R. Wyler MD
Professor of Neurosurgery, University of Tennessee; Director, Epicare Center

Elaine Wyllie MD
Coordinator, Pediatric Epilepsy Monitoring Unit, Cleveland Clinic Foundation

Foreword

The surgical treatment of epilepsy has developed rapidly in the past decade. At the present time, epilepsy surgery is performed at about one-third of the approximately 140 medical schools in North America and at additional hospital-based programs. In the previous decade there were less than a dozen centers with programs in epilepsy surgery in the United States and Canada, and a similarly small number overseas. The rapid growth of epilepsy surgery has been due to the dedicated work of a number of epilepsy research programs, in which the indications for surgery, the methods of localization of seizure onset, the techniques of surgery and the outcome of surgery have been meticulously documented. The recent findings of these centers provide the basis for this monograph. The excellent outcome of surgical treatment obtained at these centers has spurred the growth of epilepsy surgery. An additional impetus has been provided by the advances that have been made in the technology of intensive monitoring, electrode design, imaging of the brain and microneurosurgical technique. These advances have provided a degree of precision of localization of seizures and an improvement in the ease and safety of surgery that was not available to the pioneers of this field.

The first operation for the treatment of epilepsy was performed by Victor Horsley more than 100 years go. However, the modern era of epilepsy surgery began approximately 50 years ago when Wilder Penfield and Herbert Jasper began the systematic application of the disciplines of electrophysiology, radiology, and neuropsychology to the localization of seizures. The literature of the past 50 years concerning the indications for surgery, methods of localization, techniques of surgery and evaluation of outcome can be found in the specialty journals of a wide range of scientific disciplines. It would be a daunting task for an individual entering the field today to access this literature and to master it.

The authors of the present volume have recognized the need for a current and comprehensive presentation of epilepsy surgery.

In addition, they have also appreciated the diverse methods used at different centers for preoperative investigation and surgical treatment. The following subjects have therefore received particular attention in this volume: the definition of uncontrolled epilepsy, the proper extent of temporal lobectomy, the optimal age for operation in children, the indications for section of the corpus callosum, the role of intraoperative electrocorticography, the role of brain stimulation in localizing eloquent cortex, the factors determining outcome, and its analysis. Both the experienced clinician and the clinician entering the field of epilepsy surgery can benefit from this lucid and detailed presentation of the current practice of epilepsy surgery by the neurologists and surgeons who have played major roles in its development.

ROBERT G. GROSSMAN MD
Baylor College of Medicine
Houston, Texas

Preface

Practical knowledge placed in perspective is the goal of this newest monograph on the treatment of uncontrolled epilepsy with surgery. The past two decades have seen a remarkable increase in the interest and practice of epilepsy surgery, with a suitable number of publications in manuscript and book form to correspond with this resurgence of interest. This volume is of somewhat more limited scope than some others that have appeared recently. It is meant to provide a basis of practical knowledge for centers, neurologists, and neurosurgeons interested in developing epilepsy surgery programs and/or interested in learning more about the diversity that exists in other programs. In particular, we have attempted to place many of the issues in perspective by having one authority write each chapter, and the editor or another authority comment afterwards.

The comments reflect opinions in the context of what has been written in each chapter. Overall, the editors and authors tried not to present a unilateral viewpoint but to enable the reader to make his own decisions based upon objective and subjective information, and to recognize that controversies exist. With respect particularly to the percentage of patients undergoing intracranial monitoring, the techniques of intracranial monitoring, and the techniques of temporal lobectomy, this approach will hopefully provide a more scholarly background than is usually presented. We have restricted chapter length somewhat so that the volume is not overwhelming and can be read easily by most individuals with these interests. We have also enjoyed placing this information in a single accessible form and hope that it will fulfill our purposes.

Acknowledgments

We wish to acknowledge with sincere appreciation the invaluable assistance of Josephine Early, Deborah Barnes, Kathy Malinconico, and Lisa Miller. Their attention to detail, tireless handling of telephone calls and correspondence, and consistent good humor have been primarily responsible for our completing this project. Additionally, our sincere thanks are extended to the authors of this volume, who worked with us in an expedient, accurate, and cooperative manner. These individuals have been the reason for the timeliness and intellectual sophistication of the chapters in this volume, which we believe make it a resource to be used for many years.

Disclaimer. The indications and dosages of all drugs in this book have been recommended in the medical literature and conform to the practices of the general medical community. The medications described do not necessarily have specific approval by the Food and Drug Administration for use in the diseases and dosages for which they are recommended. The package insert for each drug should be consulted for use and dosage as approved by the FDA. Because standards for usage change, it is advisable to keep abreast of revised recommendations, particularly those concerning new drugs.

part I

Selection

chapter 1

What is Uncontrolled Epilepsy, and Who Should be Referred for Surgery?

William H. Theodore

Although as many as 1% of the population of the United States may suffer a seizure at some time in their lives, the number who will develop "intractable epilepsy" is smaller. A subset of that population, patients with uncontrolled partial seizures, are most likely to be considered for surgery. In 1975, Hauser and Kurland reported that the prevalence of partial seizures in Rochester, Minnesota was 4/1000, and of epilepsy in general 6.5/1000 [1]. In an English study, the lifetime prevalence of seizures was 20.2/1000, but only 5.3/1000 had "active epilepsy" — a seizure in the last 5 years, or were currently taking antiepileptic drugs (AEDs) [2]. Similar prevalence figures have been reported from other countries, including Japan (2.8/1000), and Finland (5.4/1000) [3, 4]. Fifty-six percent of patients reported by Keranen *et al.* had partial seizures; 7.5% had simple partial seizures alone [4].

These numbers partly reflect lifetime prevalence figures, rather than the number of active patients with frequent seizures. Few who have had a single seizure in the last 5 years or are seizure-free on medication would be considered surgical candidates. It has been suggested that approximately 45% of patients with partial seizures may be "uncontrolled" by current medications, but accurate statistics are difficult to obtain [5]. Hauser has suggested that of the approximately 160 000 patients in the United States presenting with a first unprovoked seizure each year, 5–10% may prove eventually to have "non-remittent" epilepsy, but this estimate may include patients who are seizure-free or have rare seizures as long as therapeutic AED levels are maintained [6]. Based on the same figures, a more conservative estimate suggests that there may be only 1500–3000 new intractable cases per year.

Not all will be appropriate "epilepsy surgery" candidates. Some of the patients with partial seizures, perhaps 3–5%, will have brain tumors, altering the emphasis of their care [7]. Not all have partial seizures. Myoclonic, atonic and "minor motor" seizures have a particularly poor prognosis for medical therapy [8, 9]. But the surgery most often performed for these patients, corpus callosotomy, is more complex and has a higher complication rate than the focal resections carried out in patients with partial seizures (see Chapter 4).

Differential diagnosis

The first step in identifying patients for possible surgical therapy is to confirm the diagnosis of epilepsy and establish that the seizures cannot be controlled by medication. Prolonged video-EEG monitoring, combined with frequent measurement of AED blood levels is essential. The following case histories illustrate several aspects of the differential diagnosis of uncontrolled seizures.

An 18-year-old woman was admitted for a history of seizures beginning at the age of 2, characterized by a sudden fall, and 1–3 minutes of unresponsiveness, followed by 30 minutes of grogginess and headache. After several episodes she was treated with phenobarbital until the age of 6. The spells recurred at age 10, when while sitting she suddenly lost tone and fell to the floor. Her arms went up, and she made a fist. After the attack she was confused and complained of headache. Barbiturates were restarted. Episodes (four to six per year) continued to be characterized by tonic extension of the arms at the shoulders with flexion at the elbows, occasionally accompanied by a few low amplitude jerks of the legs, and loss of consciousness lasting 30–60 seconds, followed by headache and confusion. At the age of 17 the episodes increased in frequency to between two and four per month, and tonic–clonic activity in the arms was noted. Blurred vision preceded some of the spells. A maternal aunt had seizures and mental retardation attributed to perinatal hypoxia. A paternal first cousin had seizures controlled by phenytoin. Neurologic examination was normal. The initial diagnostic impression was tonic seizures, but simultaneous EEG and ECG recording during videotelemetry showed that the episodes were preceded by periods of prolonged sinus arrest lasting up to 6 seconds, with a decrease in systolic blood pressure to as low as 50 mm of mercury. Further study led to a diagnosis of vasodepressor syncope with inhibition of sympathetic neural responsiveness. Fitted elastic stockings relieved the attacks [10].

A 41-year-old man was well until 3 years before admission when he woke up in the middle of the night and told his wife that he smelt gas in the house. He went outside in the snow, then came back into the house and got into bed, spoke incoherently about Texas and haircuts, and went to sleep. Several months later while driving, he smelt fumes in the car, lost consciousness, and was found at the side of the road slumped over the steering wheel. Similar episodes occurred approximately monthly, leading to one car accident. On one occasion he was found sitting on the toilet in the middle of the night with his arms extended straight out ahead, his lips shaking, his head turned to the right banging rhythmically against the wall. The episode lasted 1–2 minutes and was followed by sleep. More recently, episodes of confused speech and staring, deep breathing, blinking of the right eye and jerking of the right leg were noted two to three times per week, lasting several minutes. He had experienced a personality change, difficulty controlling his temper, and an addiction to violent television programs. He had been treated with phenytoin 400 mg, carbamazepine 1200 mg, primidone 1000 mg, and methsuximide 300 mg/day, with good blood levels. On admission, the patient was thought to have complex partial seizures. However no abnormalities were detected on more than a dozen interictal EEGs, as well as over 100 hours of video-EEG recording. Recurrent episodes of violent, agitated behavior were recorded, lasting up to 50 minutes, unaccompanied by any EEG changes. No clinical features suggestive of seizures were observed. After extensive psychiatric evaluation, a diagnosis of multiple personality was made. AED withdrawal and psychiatric treatment over several years led to a decrease in the frequency of the episodes and improved impulse control.

These two cases illustrate some of the pitfalls in evaluating patients with seizures. Nonepileptic attacks are diagnosed in as many as 22% of patients admitted to monitoring units for uncontrolled epilepsy. Psychiatric episodes are most common, but cardiovascular and sleep disorders may be misdiagnosed as epilepsy as well [11–13]. A minority of patients may have both pseudoseizures and real epilepsy [14]. In these cases it is essential, before considering surgical therapy, to try to determine the frequency of each type of episode and their relation to the patient's overall function. The presence of even a few documented nonepileptic events would deter many centers from considering a patient for surgery. Occasional patients considered to have pseudoseizures by referring physicians may be found to have epilepsy after video-EEG monitoring [11].

Although no single criterion unequivocally differentiates pseudoseizures from epilepsy, several factors may be helpful (Table 1.1). Pseudoseizures do not conform to the clinical patterns of recognized seizure types. True seizures are disabling, impairing normal neurologic function, especially acts involving high degrees of coordination. Suspicious events include elaborate behavioral patterns which could not be performed without normal control over motor function. Pseudoseizure frequency is not related to AED levels. Even patients with severe uncontrolled com-

TABLE 1.1 Criteria for differential diagnosis of seizure types and distinction from pseudoseizures

	GTCS	CPS	SPS	Absence	Pseudoseizure
Aura	Short	Short	Short	None	May be complex, prolonged
Ictal duration	1–2 min	1–2 min	<1 min	<30 sec	Variable, often long
Behavior	Little variation Stereotyped events Tonic, clonic, phases Autonomic changes	Most common features well described 'Disenabled' motor activity Stereotyped automatisms	Sensory-motor symptoms Psychic, autonomic No loss of conscious	Staring Eyeblinking Clonic jerks Automatisms may occur if prolonged	Wide range of behavior May include coordinated motor activity, or prolonged unresponsiveness
Postictal stage	Exhaustion	Confusion May sleep	Mild, if at all "Todd's paralysis" if focal motor	None	Difficult to differentiate clear postictal stage
Ictal EEG	Usually abnormal	Usually abnormal	May be abnormal	Always 3/ spike-wave	Usually normal Should not be clearly epileptic
Response to AEDs	Often good Seizures increase on withdrawal	Variable Usually at least transient help Seizures increase on withdrawal	Less responsive Focal motor seizures may be helped	Usually excellent (Myoclonic–atonic have poor prognosis)	None, except placebo

plex partial seizures (CPS) are helped by AEDs to some extent; when drugs are withdrawn, frequency increases and secondary generalized tonic–clonic seizures (GTCS) often appear [15]. EEG recordings should show neither epileptiform discharges during, nor slow activity after, pseudoseizures.

Cardiogenic syncope may be mistaken for seizures. Unfortunately, there are no physical or historical findings which exclude this diagnosis, and seizures themselves may evoke arrhythmias capable of producing loss of consciousness [16]. In order to be implicated as the cause of a neurologic event, the arrhythmia must be shown reliably to precede clinical and electrographic signs of "seizure onset." History and physical examination, as well as routine EEG, may suggest the diagnosis in about 50% of patients with cardiogenic syncope. If a cardiac etiology is suspected when these tests are negative, 24–72 hours of ambulatory EEG monitoring should be enough to detect an arrhythmia [16]. ECG and video-EEG recording can easily be combined in an epilepsy monitoring unit. Echocardiography is not indicated unless valvular or coronary disease is suspected; rare occult atrial myxomas may be detected [16].

Once the diagnosis of epilepsy is established, it is important to review the clinical seizure classification of patients considered for surgery (Table 1.1). CPS are often confused with absence or petit mal seizures. In addition to EEG patterns, they may be distinguished by clinical characteristics. The mean duration of CPS is longer, 128 vs. 10.5 seconds for absence [17, 18]. Absence seizures are not preceded by an aura, and begin and end abruptly. Forty-seven percent of absence, but only 14% of CPS have clonic components. Automatisms occur in nearly all CPS, usually involving trunk and legs [17]. While automatisms are frequent in absence, they are restricted to face and arms in 89% [18]. CPS, but not absence, are followed by postictal confusion.

Other seizure types which have a good prognosis need to be identified. Perhaps the most important of these is benign rolandic epilepsy, which may be confused with partial seizures of temporal origin [19]. Clinical features of benign rolandic epilepsy also distinguish them from CPS. These seizures spontaneously disappear at puberty in almost all cases [9,20]. Seizure frequency is usually lower than in patients with partial seizures of frontal or temporal origin who will be considered for surgery. Distinctive clinical and electrographic features may be detected by video-EEG monitoring. Seizures are common during sleep, but impairment of consciousness occurs in <50% of those occurring during wakefulness [21]. Hemifacial jerks, speech arrest despite preserved consciousness, oropharnygeal automatisms such as salivation, guttural sounds, perioral movements such as trembling of the chin, are common. Clonic jerking may extend to ipsilateral arm. Characteristic EEG discharges occur at F8–T4, or C4–T4, and are often bilateral [21].

In addition to video-EEG monitoring, neuroimaging tests are part of the presurgical evaluation of uncontrolled seizures. Computed tomography (CT) and magnetic resonance imaging (MRI) are usually performed; the former, although helping to exclude a tumor, is of less value. Single photon emission computed tomography (SPECT) and positron emission tomography (PET) have been used at some centers. At present, these are research procedures, and not of proven clinical value. The presence of an MRI lesion or PET hypometabolism is not an indication of intractable epilepsy, since both may occur in patients with well-controlled seizures, and be absent in patients with frequent ones [22–24].

Definition of intractability

Definitions of uncontrolled epilepsy are fluid. Seizure frequency (probably the most important, although not the only, factor to be considered) is usually very high in patients referred to "intensive monitoring" units for uncontrolled epilepsy. CPS frequencies range from one per week to five per day, although GTCS in the same patients may be very rare [12]. Sutula *et al.* reported that on admission, nearly 40% of patients had more than one seizure per day, and 60% more than one per week, although these rates were less than reported by the patients before admission, a well-described phenomenon [11–12]. These seizure frequencies are much higher than those used to define epilepsy in epidemiologic studies, making it more difficult to relate the latter to choice of patients for surgery.

Forty percent of children who underwent temporal lobectomy had a mean preoperative seizure frequency of 20 or more per month, but 5% had only one to five seizures per month [25]. Patients considered for corpus callosotomy may have 0–33 GTCS, but up to 500 simple partial seizures (SPC) per month [26]. Typical seizure frequencies in adults with uncontrolled CPS admitted to experimental AED trials are two to four per month, although two per week may be required for randomization in some studies [27].

However, patients with much rarer seizures may be considered to be, or regard themselves as, uncontrolled. The severity of the episodes is an important factor. Some CPS may be barely apparent to anyone except the patient, while others may cause marked disruption of daily activities and create severe social embarrassment. Significant injuries can occur as a result of infrequent seizures. Some patients may recover from seizures within minutes and return to normal function, while others may suffer prolonged postictal lassitude. In our society, the ability to drive is important, especially in the many regions of the United States with only rudimentary public transportation facilities. Even one seizure a year will preclude obtaining a driver's license in many jurisdictions. Thus a truck driver or trial lawyer or surgeon who suffers a seizure every 12 months may be uncontrolled in a significant sense of the word, even though few neurologists would consider such a patient a surgical candidate.

The reaction of family members and employers may influence a patient's concept of the severity of his or her seizures, and interest in surgery; it is important to understand where the idea originated. In some cases families may be more enthusiastic about surgery than the patients themselves. Ordinarily, a patient must tell the doctor that he or she is suffering from uncontrolled seizures and wishes to be considered for surgery. When children or patients with diminished intellectual capacity are considered for surgery, ethical and legal issues, the question of who is competent to decide, may have to be addressed. It may sometimes be legitimate to ask whether families of children with uncontrolled seizures have conflicting motives or unannounced agendas.

Medical therapy

How many drugs should be tried before a patient is considered "intractable"? A number of recent studies have advocated the use of "monotherapy" for epilepsy [28–29]. Schmidt reported decreased seizure frequency in 36%, and increased seizures in 17%, of patients changed from a multiple to a single drug regimen [28]. Not all studies have included controls for the drugs withdrawn, and fluctuations in blood levels; in some, substitution of a more effective agent was a clear factor [30]. It has been suggested that 10–15% of patients may become seizure-free when a second drug is added [31]. Most of these were performed in outpatient clinics, and included patients who had infrequent seizures. In a recent report, combination therapy with carbamazepine (CBZ) and phenytoin (PHT) was superior to results with either drug alone in the treatment of patients with frequent complex partial and secondary generalized seizures admitted to a monitoring unit [32]. Toxicity was not measurably increased on combination therapy.

It seems reasonable to treat either children or adults with uncontrolled partial seizures with at least two drugs, preferably CBZ and PHT in combination, before considering surgery. Phenobarbital (PB) and primidone (PRM) are only marginally less effective, and, although associated with greater neuropsychologic toxicity, are useful alternatives [31]. The role of valproic acid (VPA) in the treatment of CPS is uncertain. The management of patients, often children, with atonic and myoclonic seizures may be more difficult. VPA appears to be the most effective drug, although only 20% of patients are well controlled [33]. CBZ often is used in addition. Anecdotal reports of exacerbation of atonic seizures in children by CBZ have not been evaluated by a formal study.

It is important to make sure patients have had an adequate AED trial (Table 1.2). Blood levels should be measured in the morning before the patient has had any doses for the day. By increasing doses at intervals over several weeks, side effects can often be minimized. Patients with uncontrolled epilepsy should have blood levels maintained at the upper end of the therapeutic range or beyond; many patients can tolerate PHT levels above 20 mg/l, for example. VPA blood levels of 75–100 mg/l should be maintained. Drugs should be given often enough during the day to maintain steady levels and avoid fluctuations that could contribute to toxicity and endanger seizure control. CBZ and VPA should be given in at least three, and preferably four divided doses; PHT in at least two. The long half-life of barbiturates and benzodiazepines may also allow greater flexibility, but fluctuations in plasma levels will still occur when these drugs are given in a single dose.

Benzodiazepines have been used as adjunctive therapy for uncontrolled partial as well as atonic seizures. Unfortunately, the drugs produce side effects, including sedation and intellectual impairment which are similar to those occurring with barbiturates [34]. A new benzodiazepine, clobazam, has been reported to improve frequency in patients with intractable CPS, and has fewer cognitive side effects [35]. This drug is not yet available in the United States. Moreover, initial good results with all benzodiazepines have been reported to disappear over several weeks to months as tolerance develops. Benzodiazepine withdrawal is difficult, may be protracted, and often leads to increased seizures. Alternate-day benzodiazepine therapy has been suggested [36].

When more than one drug is used, pharmacologic interactions, although not necessarily significant in each case, need to be considered. VPA, for example, markedly impairs the metabolism of PB [37]. PHT increases conversion of primidone to phenobarbital and impairs metabolism of the latter; the PB : PRM ratio is markedly increased [38]. CBZ and PHT each speed clearance of the other, and higher doses must be given to maintain therapeutic plasma levels [39]. But CBZ has an active metabolite, carbamazepine-10,11-epoxide (CBZ-E), the proportion of which is usually increased by comedication [40]. In selected cases it may be

TABLE 1.2 Adult maintenance therapy for generalized tonic–clonic and partial seizures

Drug	Usual dose (mg/kg per day)	Therapeutic level (mg/l)	Comments
Carbamazepine	10–20	6–12	$t_{1/2}$ 8–12 hours No parenteral form Fewer reported drug interactions Less neuropsychological toxicity than PHT, PB
Phenytoin	4–6	10–20	Oral loading dose 5–10 mg/kg Nonlinear kinetics Slow approach to steady-state level Concentration-dependent $t_{1/2}$ (15–51 hours) Important drug interactions (e.g. coumadin, theophylline) Less neuropsychologic toxicity than PB Can be given IV
Phenobarbital	2–3	15–25	Oral loading dose 4–6 mg/kg Can be given IV Mean adult $t_{1/2}$ 96 hours Drug interactions
Valproic Acid	40–75	50–100	$t_{1/2}$ 8–15 hours No parenteral form Displaces other drugs from plasma protein Inhibits PB metabolism Significant dose-related toxicity Hepatic toxicity rare in adults

appropriate to measure CBZ-E as well as CBZ levels, although the extent to which the metabolite contributes to the therapeutic effect and toxicity of CBZ itself is uncertain. VPA increases PHT free fraction while lowering total plasma levels; the free PHT concentration may be unchanged. Although free PHT levels may be measured, their relation to drug efficacy and toxicity is not understood completely, and doses high enough to maintain therapeutic total plasma levels should be given [41–42]. The addition of a second agent may produce side effects due to alteration of the metabolism of the first.

Addition of second-line drugs is often of doubtful benefit. Dashieff *et al.* studied methsuximide, VPA and clorazepate in 66 patients with uncontrolled CPS who had not responded to PHT, CBZ, and PB [43]. Seven patients became seizure-free, but remissions lasted only for 1–6 months. Patients who do not respond to monotherapy or a combination of two among PHT, CBZ, PB, and perhaps VPA should consider other options.

Experimental drug trials are an alternative to surgery. Complete freedom from seizures is rarely obtained, and patients are often considered for drug trials if they do not wish to have an operation, or are thought to be ineligible for one. Since patients must be categorized according to seizure type in order to enter a drug trial, video-EEG monitoring is often performed before the patients are randomized. Many units which perform surgery enter patients into drug trials as well. Often, patients referred to an epilepsy center are monitored before being offered either participation in a drug trial or surgical evaluation.

Patients with partial seizures are particularly appropriate for clinical trials since these are frequent in adults, and most of the experimental drugs available have been developed through testing in animal models relevant to CPS [44]. There are no proven pharmacologic models of atonic seizures for preclinical drug development, and regulatory considerations complicate administration of experimental agents to children. For example, fewer alternatives are available for children with the Lennox–Gastaut syndrome, who might be considered for corpus callosotomy.

In order to obtain statistically significant results in clinical trials, patients with frequent seizures (i.e. four per month), and a high sample size (50–60 subjects) may be needed [44]. Studies are long, and patients must be highly motivated to comply with the protocol. Experimental drug studies have medical exclusion criteria, such as the need to take other drugs, which may disqualify some patients [44]. Moreover, frequent secondary GTCS may preclude participation for some, since even in an add-on study some active agents may have to be discontinued, and patients will spend periods on a placebo.

Prediction of medical intractability

Is it possible to predict the prognosis of patients with seizures accurately enough to decide who should be considered for surgery? There have been a series of studies of limited relevance to uncontrolled epilepsy, reporting the prognosis of patients with one or a small number of seizures. Several investigators have reported that AEDs may be tapered without recurrence in 60–70% of seizure-free children and adults [45–48]. Annegers *et al.* found that recurrence risk after a single unprovoked seizure was 36% at 1 year, and 56% at 5 years; initial partial seizures, EEG abnormalities, and abnormal neurologic examination, were associated with increased risk [49]. Elwes *et al.* reported that 35% of patients treated with CBZ or PHT who had had two or more generalized tonic–clonic seizures could be expected to enter a 2-year seizure-free period at the start of treatment, and 73% at the end of 2 years. Fifty-one out of 79 patients who had a seizure-free period lasting at least 2 years remained seizure-free for the median 66 month follow-up period of the study [50]. Adverse prognostic factors included the presence of partial seizures, high (more than two per month) pretreatment generalized tonic–clonic seizure frequency, neurologic, psychiatric, or social problems (which may have affected compliance) and a family history of epilepsy. Control became less likely the longer seizures persisted after treatment began; most treatment failures occurred within the first 2 years [51].

Similar data were obtained from Rochester, Minnesota. Seventy-six percent of patients who had experienced at least two seizures attained a 5-year remission, and 70% remained in remission 20 years after diagnosis [52]. Most remissions occurred within the first few years (51% in 2 years after eligibility, which began 5 years after diagnosis). The probability of attaining remission dropped to 33% by 10 years after diagnosis. The presence of partial seizures lowered a patient's chance of entering remission [52]. A Japanese study, including patients with single as well as multiple seizures, found a remission rate of 58%, favorably influenced by factors including low seizure-frequency, and absence of neurologic, social, or psychiatric abnormalities [53].

A number of studies have attempted to

assess risk factors for "intractable" epilepsy. Schmidt *et al.* reported that 63% of patients with three or more complex partial and secondary generalized seizures achieved a 2-year remission, but seizures control occurred in only 44% with more than one generalized tonic–clonic seizure per month [54]. Satischandra *et al.* compared patients who had had at least four complex partial seizures per month on AED therapy with patients who had been in remission for at least 2 years [54]. Development of secondary generalization during the first 2 years after seizure onset, a history of head trauma, prolonged labor, febrile seizures, family history of epilepsy, CPS clusters, psychiatric abnormalities, and multifocal or bilateral EEG discharges were adverse risk factors (the last appearing only in intractable cases) [55]. In a case-control study, Rocca *et al.* found that a history of maternal epilepsy, neonatal or febrile seizures, cerebral palsy and head trauma were more common in patients with complex partial seizures [7].

The absence of evidence of "early" brain damage, as well as the presence of generalized EEG discharges and generalized tonic–clonic seizures were associated with a higher probability of entering a 5 year remission in the Rochester study [56]. This report, surveying a geographically selected population, included patients with all types of epilepsy; those with generalized EEG discharges and generalized tonic–clonic seizures probably had primary generalized epilepsy, which often carries a good prognosis. This may account for the contrast with the results of studies confined to patients with partial seizures, in which evidence of secondary generalization or multifocal epileptogenic regions were adverse prognostic factors [50, 55, 57].

Prognostic factors have been identified in children with uncontrolled seizures as well. Lindsay *et al.* found that the absence of behavioral abnormalities commencing after age 2.4, and the ability to remain in normal classes, were associated with a good outcome for social adaptation as well as seizure control [58]. Low IQ, high seizure frequency, a history of status epilepticus, and a clear etiology such as meningitis or a structural lesion were adverse prognostic factors. One-third of children eventually became seizure-free; 79% of the remissions occurred by the age of 14 [58]. Similar factors were identified in a Swedish study; only 11% of children with normal neurologic and neuropsychologic examination, and with less than four seizures per year, had persistent attacks [8]. Although the study included patients with absence, significant differences in prognosis between different seizure types were not detected. Sofijanov reported that mental retardation and neurologic deficits were adverse prognostic factors in children with partial seizures [51].

An interesting aspect of epilepsy in children is the "silent interval" reported in 30 out of 50 patients who eventually had surgery for uncontrolled seizures [59]. The mean duration was 36 months for girls, and 57 for boys. This suggests that even prolonged remissions in children may only be temporary, a phenomenon observed by Rodin, who felt that about 80% of patients would eventually prove to have a chronic seizure disorder with periodic relapses and remissions [60]. However, in the Oxford pediatric series the course of the seizure disorder appeared to reveal itself over 4–5 years; moreover, this group had a high incidence of structural lesions, abnormal neurologic examinations, psychiatric and social problems; and mean seizure frequency was six episodes per day [59]. Bilateral or generalized EEG abnormalities were common. A poor response to medical therapy could have been predicted.

High pretreatment seizure frequency, abnormal neurologic examination, structural lesions (excluding the regions of focal gliosis now identified by increased signal intensity on MRI), a history of febrile convulsions, frequent generalized tonic–clonic seizures, generalized EEG abnormalities, family history of epilepsy, and psychiatric, or social problems are predictive factors for a poor response to AED therapy [8,50,51,57–62]. The *ca.* 5–10% of patients who experience a single seizure and who will become "intractable" can probably be identified within several years after onset. Unfortunately, some of the factors associated with poor medical prognosis may be predictors for an unfavorable surgical outcome as well [61]. This is not surprising, since they appear collectively to represent more severe underlying brain pathology, or a greater extent of "epileptogenic" tissue. Nevertheless, improved seizure frequency after focal resections has been reported in similar patients [59]. But the presence of severe preoperative neurologic or psychiatric impairment may make it much more difficult for the reduction in seizure frequency which surgery can reasonably expect to procure to make a significant overall difference in a patient's life.

The risks of persistent seizures

Another reason to consider surgery in addition to seizure frequency is the possibility of progressive neurologic damage from repeated seizures which may not by themselves be frequent enough to make a patient desire surgery. This issue has entertained neurologists since the nineteenth century. Reynolds, for example, writing in 1861, reviewed the already impressive earlier literature on the "epileptic personality," but suggested, on the basis of his own data, that mental impairment or changes in "character" were not inevitable accompaniments of epilepsy, and were related to an underlying cause rather than seizure frequency or duration of illness [63]. It has been suggested that epilepsy is a progressive disease, and that neuropathologic damage or secondary epileptic foci may develop in patients with uncontrolled seizures [5,64].

Modern studies have shown that "intelligence" test results are lower in patients with epilepsy than normal controls, although the differences may be small [65,66]. Patients with more frequent seizures may have poorer performance on tests such as the Halstead–Reitan battery and the Wechsler Adult Intelligence Scale than those whose seizures are well controlled [65]. Some of the subjects in these studies may have had absence attacks, and the results represent the effect of frequent but transient periods of ictal impairment, rather than cumulative cerebral damage which would be present interictally as well. Although frequent seizures obviously impair performance, it is not certain that the impairment would persist if the seizures were brought under control. Bourgeois *et al.* performed serial intelligence tests in 72 children with seizures [66]. Initial scores were not significantly different from nonepileptic sibling controls. In the whole group IQ showed no change over a mean observation period of 4 years. Only 11% of the children had a consistent decrease in IQ of 10 points or more; 16% had a consistent increase. In a discriminant analysis, the combination of drug toxicity and early seizure onset were the best predictors of IQ decline; a significant association was observed with seizure frequency as well [66]. Ellenberg *et al.* reported no difference in IQ at the age of 7 between children with one or more nonfebrile seizures and nonepileptic siblings when preseizure neurologic examination was normal [67].

Seizure frequency may be a factor in predicting intellectual decline in patients with epilepsy. However, would failure to control seizures except at high blood levels be an indication for surgery? What are the cognitive consequences of operation?

Global memory deficits, rarely reported after unilateral temporal lobectomy, have been attributed to resection of tissue contralateral to severely damaged hippocampus [68]. These devastating results can be avoided by careful preoperative evaluation, but more subtle effects may still occur. Memory deficits may be specific to the side operated on, verbal IQ (VIQ) declining more after left-sided lobectomies, and performance IQ (PIQ) after right-sided ones. Postoperative declines in global IQ of 5–15 points, have been greater with left than with right temporal lobe resection, perhaps because of the importance of verbal communication even in tests of nondominant hemisphere function [69–70]. If seizures are controlled, the memory deficits may be ameliorated or reversed over time [71–73]. Memory deficits have been reported after frontal resections and corpus callosotomy as well [74–75].

It is unlikely that systemic drug toxicity will be an indication for surgery in a large number of patients, but antiepileptic drugs may have significant adverse effects on learning and memory, especially in children [65]. Although toxicity may be reduced by a judicious choice of agents, and elimination of sedative hypnotic AEDs, no drug is completely benign [76]. Recent studies have shown, for example, that carbamazepine impairs choice-reaction time, and performance on card-sorting tasks [77]. However, if seizures are well controlled, adverse neuropsychologic effects of AEDs should not be an indication for surgery. The overall risks of surgery, although low, still seem greater than the risks of taking AEDs if seizures are well controlled. Most patients whose seizures are suppressed by AEDs respond to a single drug at well tolerated doses [31]. Moreover, drugs are usually continued for some time postoperatively even in patients who become seizure-free. There have been no studies of the effect of time of drug withdrawal on seizure recurrence, and prudence suggests maintenance of therapeutic levels of at least a single drug.

A variety of preoperative evaluation methods and modifications of surgical technique may reduce risks of memory loss, or specific functional deficits, but obviating them entirely may lead to sparing cortex which is critically involved in the epileptic process, and thereby reducing the chance of surgical success [78]. It seems reasonable to conclude that the neuropsychologic risks from surgery and AED treatment may be in the same order of magnitude, and that present data do not justify surgery with the goal of reducing the latter, as long as seizures are controlled.

Studies evaluating the social and vocational outcome of surgery have suggested that the limited postoperative improvement in employment and other measures observed is related to successful seizure control [79–80]. Surgery, even if successful, may not alleviate a preoperative psychosis; postoperative depression and the new onset of thought disorders may occur [81–82].

Persistent seizures are associated with additional risks. The standardized mortality ratio is increased for all patients with epilepsy (2.3 : 1), especially in the first 10 years after diagnosis [83]. Deaths occur in children as well as adults: 11 out of 194 over 12 years in a Swedish study, and 14 out of 100 over 15 years in the Oxford series [8,57]. Suicide, drowning, and sudden unexplained death have been identified in some series as increased, though not always to a statistically significant degree [81]. The mortality rate for temporal lobectomy and other focal cortical resections is <1%, and ranges from 2–4% for more extensive procedures such as corpus callosotomy or hemispherectomy [84]. Significant, though not necessarily permanent morbidity has been observed in 5% of patients after temporal lobectomy, and 11–17% in more complicated procedures [84]. Thus, the morbidity and mortality of surgery seem no greater than that of the natural course of the disease. The complications of invasive electrode recording do add significantly to the risk since they approximate those of the surgery itself [84].

"Uncontrolled epilepsy" is not a straightforward diagnosis. The particular circumstances of each patient need to be considered before a recommendation for surgical evaluation is made. The physician must assess the social, psychologic and medical features of the illness, offering advice as well as technical expertise. It may sometimes be necessary to restrain patients' enthusiasm; in our society surgery has an appeal which is peculiar to technologically complex and adventurous undertakings. Others have reasonable, but unwarranted, fears. Physicians should remember, and ensure that patients understand, what surgery for uncontrolled seizures can do — reduce the frequency of seizures.

References

1 Hauser WA, Kurland LT. The epidemiology of epilepsy in Rochester Minnesota from 1935 through 1967. *Epilepsia* 1975; **16**: 1–66.

2 Goodridge DMG, Shorvon DS. Epilepsy in a population of 6000. *Br Med J* 1983; **287**: 641–647.

3 Tsuboi T. Prevalence and incidence of epilepsy in Tokyo. *Epilepsia* 1988; **29**: 103–110.

4 Keranen T, Sillanpaa M, Riekkinen PJ. Distribution of seizure types in an epileptic population. *Epilepsia* 1988; **29**: 1–7.

5 Dreifuss FE. Goals of surgery for epilepsy. In Engel JP (ed) *Surgical Treatment of the Epilepsies.* Raven Press, New York, 1987, pp 31–50.

6 Hauser WA. Prognosis of seizures, efficacy of antiepileptic drugs. In Pritchard PB (ed) *Surgical Treatment of Epilepsy 1988* American Epilepsy Society Annual Course, Hartford CT, 1988, pp 6–14.

7 Rocca WA, Sharbrough FM, Hauser WA, Annegers JF, Schoenberg BS. Risk factors for complex partial epilepsy: a population-based case control study. *Ann Neurol* 1987; **21**: 22–31.

8 Brorson LO, Wranne L. Long-term prognosis in childhood epilepsy: survival and seizure prognosis. *Epilepsia* 1987; **28**: 424–430.

9 Loiseau P, Pestre M, Dartiques JF, Commenges D, Barberger-Gateau C, Cohadon S. Long-term prognosis in two forms of childhood epilepsy: typical absence seizure and epilepsy with rolandic (centro-temporal) EEG foci. *Ann Neurol* 1983; **13**: 642–648.

10 Goldstein DS, Spanarkel M, Pitterman A, *et al.* Circulatory control mechanisms in vasodepressor syncope. *Am Heart J.* 1982; **104**: 1071–1075.

11 Sutula TP, Sackellares JC, Miller JQ, Dreifuss FE. Intensive monitoring in intractable epilepsy. *Neurology* 1981; **31**: 243–247.

12 Theodore WH, Schulman EA, Porter RJ: Intractable seizures: long-term follow-up after prolonged inpatient treatment in an epilepsy unit. *Epilepsia* 1983; **24**: 336–343.

13 Mattson RH. Value of intensive monitoring. In Wada JA, Penry JK (eds) *Advances in Epileptology: 10th International Symposium.* Raven Press, New York, pp 43–51.

14 Trimble MR. Pseudoseizures. In Porter RJ, Theodore WH (eds) *Epilepsy* Neurological Clinics of North America. WB Saunders, Philadelphia, 1986, pp 531–548.

15 Desai BT, Porter RJ, Penry JK. Psychogenic seizures. *Arch Neurol* 1982; **39**: 202–209.

16 Dohrmann ML, Cheitlan MD. Cardiogenic syncope. In Porter RJ, Theodore WH (eds) *Epilepsy* Neurological Clinics of North America. WB Saunders, Philadelphia, 1986, pp 531–548.

17 Theodore WH, Porter RJ, Penry JK. Complex partial seizures: clinical characteristics and differential diagnosis. *Neurology* 1983; **33**: 1115–1121.

18 Penry JK, Porter RJ, Dreifuss FE. Simultaneous recording of absence seizures with videotape

and electroencephalography. *Brain* 1975; **98**: 427–440.
19 Loiseau P, Beaussart M. The seizures of benign childhood epilepsy with rolandic paroxysmal discharges. *Epilepsia* 1973; **14**: 381–389.
20 Ambrosetto G, Rossi P, Tassinari CA. Predictive factors of seizure frequency and duration of antiepileptic treatment in rolandic epilepsy: a retrospective study. *Brain Dev* 1987; **9**: 300–304.
21 Loiseau P, Beaussart M. The seizures of benign childhood epilepsy with rolandic paroxysmal discharges. *Epilepsia* 1973; **14**: 381–389.
22 Engel J Jr Kuhl DE, Phelps ME, *et al.* Interictal cerebral glucose metabolism in partial epilepsy and its relation to EEG changes. *Ann Neurol* 1982; **12**: 510–517.
23 Theodore WH, Newmark ME, Sato S, *et al.* ^{18}F Fluorodeoxyglucose positron emission tomography in refractory complex partial seizures. *Ann Neurol* 1983; **14**: 429–437.
24 Triulzi F, Franceschi M, Fazio F, Del Maschio A. Nonrefractory temporal lobe epilepsy: 1.5T MR imaging. *Radiology* 1988; **166**: 181–185.
25 Meyer FB, Marsh WR, Laws ER, Sharbrough FW. Temporal lobectomy in children with epilepsy. *J Neurosurg* 1986; **64**: 371–376.
26 Spencer SS, Spencer DD, Williamson PD, Sass K, Novelly RA, Mattson RH. Corpus callosotomy for epilepsy. 1. Seizure effects. *Neurology* 1989; **38**: 19–24.
27 Leppik IE, Dreifuss FE, Porter RJ *et al.* A controlled study of progabide in partial seizures: methodology and results. *Neurology* 1987; **37**: 963–968.
28 Schmidt D. Reduction of two-drug therapy in intractable epilepsy. *Epilepsia* 1983; **24**: 368–376.
29 Lesser RP, Pippenger CE, Luders H, Dinner DS. High-dose monotherapy in the treatment of intractable seizures. *Neurology* 1984; **34**: 707–711.
30 Callaghan N, O'Callaghan M, Duggan B, Feely M. Carbamazepine as a single drug in the treatment of epilepsy. *J Neurol Neurosurg Psychiatr* 1978; **41**: 907–912.
31 Mattson RH, Cramer JA, Collins JF, *et al.* Comparison of carbamazepine, phenobarbital, phenytoin and primidone in partial and secondarily generalized tonic–clonic seizures. *N Eng J Med* 1985; **313**: 145–151.
32 Lorenzo NY, Bromfield EB, Theodore WH. Phenytoin and carbamazepine: combination versus single-drug therapy for intractable partial seizures. *Ann Neurol* 1988; **24**: 136.
33 Covanis A, Gupta AK, Jeavons PM. Sodium valproate: monotherapy and polytherapy. *Epilepsia* 1982; **23**: 693–720.
34 Vining EPG. The use of barbiturates and benzodiazepines in the treatment of epilepsy. In Porter RJ, Theodore WH (eds) *Epilepsy.* Neurological Clinics of North America. WB Saunders, Philadelphia, 1986, pp 617–632.
35 Koeppen D, Baruzzi A, Capozza M, *et al.* Clobazam in therapy-resistant patients with partial epilepsy: a double-blind placebo controlled cross over study. *Epilepsia* 1987; **28**: 495–506.
36 Sher PK. Alternate day clonazepam treatment of intractable seizures. *Arch Neurol* 1985; **42**: 787–788.
37 Kapetanovic IM, Kupferberg HJ, Porter RJ, Theodore WH, Schulman E, Penry JK. Mechanisms of valproate–phenobarbital interaction in epileptic patients. *Clin Pharmacol Ther* 1981; **29**: 480–486.
38 Porro MG, Kupferberg HJ, Porter RJ, Theodore WH, Newmark ME. Phenytoin: an inhibitor and inducer of primidone metabolism in an epileptic patient. *Br J Clin Pharmacol* 1982; **14**: 294–297.
39 Ramsey RE. The use of phenytoin and carbamazepine in the treatment of epilepsy. In Porter RJ, Theodore WH (eds) *Epilepsy.* Neurological Clinics of North America. WB Saunders, Philadelphia, 1986, pp 586–600.
40 Theodore WH, Narang PK, Holmes MD, Reeves P, Nice FJ, Carbamazepine and its epoxide: relation of plasma levels to toxicity and clinical control. *Ann Neurol.* In press.
41 Theodore WH, Yu L, Price B, *et al.* The clinical value of free phenytoin levels. *Ann Neurol* 1985; **18**: 90–93.
42 Theodore WH. Should we measure free antiepileptic drug levels? *Clinical Neuropharmacol* 1987; **10**: 26–37.
43 Dashieff RM, McNamara D, Dickenson L. Efficacy of second-line antiepileptic drugs in the treatment of patients with medically refractive complex partial seizures. *Epilepsia* 1986; **27**: 124–127.
44 Porter RJ, While BG. Evaluation in man. In Meldrum BS, Porter RJ (eds) *New Anticonvulsant Drugs.* John Libbey, London, 1986, pp 49–61.

45 Thurston JH, Thurston DL, Hixon BB, Heller AJ Prognosis in childhood epilepsy. *N Eng J Med* 982; **306**: 831–836.
46 Emerson R, D'Souza BJ, Vining EP, Holden KR, Mellits ED, Freeman JM. Stopping medication in children with epilepsy. *New Eng J Med* 1981; **304**: 1125–1129.
47 Callaghan N, Garrett A, Goggin T. Withdrawal of anticonvulsant drugs in patients free of seizures for two years. *N Eng J Med* 1988; **318**: 942–946.
48 Shinnar S, Vining EPG, Mellits ED *et al.* Discontinuing antiepileptic medication in children with epilepsy after two years without seizures. *N Eng J Med* 1985; **313**: 976–980.
49 Annegers JF, Shirts SB, Hauser WA, Kurland LT. Risk of recurrence after an initial unprovoked seizure. *Epilepsia* 1986; **27**: 43–50.
50 Elwes RDC, Johnson AL, Shorvon SD, Reynolds EH. The prognosis for seizure control in newly diagnosed epilepsy. *N Eng J Med* 1984; **311**: 944–947.
51 Sofijanov NJ. Clinical evaluation and prognosis of childhood epilepsies. *Epilepsia* 1982; **23**: 61–69.
52 Annegers JF, Hauser WA, Elveback LR. Remission of seizures and relapse in patients with epilepsy. *Epilepsia* 1979; **20**: 727–737.
53 Group for the study of prognosis of epilepsy in Japan. Natural history and prognosis of epilepsy. *Epilepsia* 1981; **22**: 35–53.
54 Schmidt D, Tsai J-J, Janz D. Generalized tonic–clonic seizures in patients with complex partial seizures: natural history and prognostic relevance. *Epilepsia* 1983; **24**: 43–48.
55 Satischandra P, Lavine L, Theodore WH, Jabbari B, Dreifuss FE, Schoenberg BS. Risk factors associated with intractable complex partial seizures. *Epilepsia* 1987; **28**: 617.
56 Shafer SQ, Hauser WA, Annegers JF, Klass DW. EEG and other early predictors of seizure remission: a community study. *Epilepsia* 1988; **29**: 590–600.
57 Schmidt D. Prognosis of chronic epilepsy with complex partial seizures. *J Neurol Neurosurg Psychiatr* 1984; **47**: 1274–1278.
58 Lindsay J, Ounstead C, Richards P: Long-term outcome in children with temporal lobe seizures. 1: social outcome and childhood factors. *Dev Med Child Neurol* 1979; **21**: 285–298.
59 Lindsay J, Glaser G, Richards P, Ounstead C. Developmental aspects of focal epilepsies treated by neurosurgery. *Dev Med Child Neurol* 1984; **26**: 574–587.
60 Rodin EA. *The Prognosis of Patients with Epilepsy.* Charles Thomas, Springfield, 1968.
61 Dodrill CB, Wilkus RJ, Ojemann GA, *et al.* Multidisciplinary prediction of seizure relief from cortical resection surgery. *Ann Neurol* 1986; **20**: 2–12.
62 Reynolds EH. Early treatment and prognosis of epilepsy. *Epilepsia* 1987; **28**: 97–106.
63 Reynolds JR. *Epilepsy.* Churchill, London, 1861, pp 162–199.
64 Morell F. Secondary epileptogenesis in man. *Arch Neurol* 1985; **42**: 318–335.
65 Hirtz DG, Nelson KB. Cognitive effects of antiepileptic drugs. In Pedley TA, Meldrum BS (eds) *Recent Advances in Epilepsy 2.* Churchill Livingstone, Edinburgh, 1985, pp 161–182.
66 Bourgeois BFD, Prensky AL, Palkes HS, Talent BK, Busch SG. Intelligence in epilepsy: a prospective study in children. *Ann Neurol* 1983; **14**: 438–444.
67 Ellenberg JH, Hirtz DG, Nelson KB. Do seizures in children cause intellectual deterioration? *N Eng J Med* 1986; **314**: 1085–1088.
68 Jones-Gotman M. Commentary: Psychological evaluation, testing hippocampal function. In Engel J, Jr (ed) *Surgical Treatment of the Epilepsies.* Raven Press, New York, 1987, pp 203–211.
69 Milner B. Psychological aspects of focal epilepsy and its neurosurgical management. In Purpura DP, Penry JK, Walter RD (eds) *Neurosurgical Management of the Epilepsies.* Advances in Neurology No. 8. Raven Press, New York 1975, pp 299–322.
70 Powell G, Polkey C, McMillan T. The new Maudsley series of temporal lobectomy. 1. short term cognitive effects. *Br J Clin Psychol* 1985; **24**: 109–124.
71 Novelly R, Augustine E, Mattson RH, *et al.* Selective memory improvement and impairment in temporal lobectomy for epilepsy. *Ann Neurol* 1984; **15**: 64–67.
72 Ojemann GA, Dodrill C. Verbal memory deficits after left temporal lobectomy for epilepsy. *J Neurosurg* 1985; **62**: 101–107.
73 Rausch R, Crandall P. Psychological status related to surgical control of epileptic seizures. *Epilepsia* **23**: 191–202.
74 Sass KJ, Spencer DD, Spencer SS, Novelly RA, Williamson PD, Mattson RH. Corpus calloso-

tomy for epilepsy. 2. Neurologic and neuropsychological outcome. *Neurology* 1988; **38**: 24–28.

75 Jones-Gotman M, Milner B. Design fluency: the invention of nonsense drawings after focal cortical lesions. *Neuropsychologia* 1977; **15**: 643–652.

76 Theodore WH, Porter RJ. Removal of sedative–hypnotic antiepileptic drugs from the regimens of patients with intractable epilepsy. *Ann Neurol* 1983; **13**: 320–324.

77 Macphee GJA, Goldie C, Roulston D, *et al.* Effect of carbamazepine of psychomotor performance in naive subjects. *Eur J Clin Pharmacol* 1986; **31**: 195–199.

78 Ojemann GA. Surgical therapy for medically intractable epilepsy. *J Neurosurg* 1987; **66**: 489–499.

79 Dodrill CB. Commentary. Psychological evaluation. In Engel J, Jr (ed) *Surgical Treatment of the Epilepsies*. Raven Press, New York, 1987, pp 197–201.

80 Augustine E, Novelly RA, Mattson RH *et al.* Occupational adjustment following neurosurgical treatment of epilepsy. *Ann Neurol* 1984; **15**: 68–72.

81 Taylor DC. Mental state and temporal lobe epilepsy: a correlative account of 100 patients treated surgically. *Epilepsia* 1972; **13**: 727–765.

82 Jensen I, Larsen JK. Psychosis in drug-resistant temporal lobe epilepsy. *Neurol Neurosurg Psychiatr* 1979; **42**: 948–954.

83 Hauser WA, Annegers JF, Elveback LR. Mortality in patients with epilepsy. *Epilepsia* 1980; **21**: 399–412.

84 Van Buren J. Complications of surgical procedures. In Engel JP (ed) *Surgical Treatment of the Epilepsies*. Raven Press, New York, 1987, pp 465–475.

chapter 2

Approaches to Patient Selection for Resective Procedures

Selection of candidates for surgical resection in the treatment of epilepsy

Frederick Andermann

Early studies of focal epilepsy closely paralleled those on localization of function in the brain. McNaughton and Rasmussen [1] quoted Hughlings Jackson who wrote in 1873 [2]: "The mode of onset is the most important matter in the investigation of a case of epilepsy . . . No one can admit more fully than I do the difficulties in the localization of discharging lesions . . . ".

In the absence of other effective treatment at the time, an attempt to alleviate the problem by removing such discharging lesions seemed to be the logical next step. A hundred years ago, in 1886 Victor Horsley [3] pioneered cortical exploration based on clinical seizure patterns in patients with focal epilepsy, reproduced seizures by electrical stimulation, and showed that following excision of this area, the attacks usually ceased.

This work was continued by Ottfried Foerster and in 1928 Wilder Penfield went to Breslau (Wroclaw) to work with him. The subsequent experience at the Montreal Neurological Institute was summarized in 1954 by Penfield and Jasper [4]. Indications for consideration of surgical treatment at that time were outlined by McNaughton [5].

There has been a great improvement in the treatment of epilepsy during the last quarter-century. Better drugs have become available and the flowering of neuropharmacology and drug-level monitoring has brought about considerable advances in the utilization of antiepileptic drugs. Public awareness and understanding of epilepsy has improved and patients and their families are no longer willing to accept unquestioningly the continuing recurrence of uncontrolled epileptic attacks. There has been an increasing availability of neurologists specializing in the treatment of epilepsy in medical centers. These improvements have made patients whose epilepsy is uncontrolled by medical treatment much more conspicuous. This in turn, has led to greatly increased interest by physicians, patients and their families in surgical treatment as an alternative option.

In recent years, the indications for surgical treatment of epilepsy were reviewed by Falconer (1970) [6] Walker (1974) [7] McNaughton and Rasmussen (1975) [1] Green (1977) [8] Jensen (1977) [9] Glaser (1980) [10] Delgado-Escueta, Treiman and Walsh (1983) [11–13] and by Ward (1983) [14]. All agree that failure of a thorough trial of antiepileptic medication, and demonstration of focal origin of the attacks in an area of brain which can be removed without producing significant neurological deficit, are the fundamental criteria.

McNaughton and Rasmussen wrote: "Without doubt, the proper evaluation and selection of patients for surgical management of the symptom, epilepsy, is the most important single factor in determining the success or failure of this form of treatment in reducing the seizure tendency" [1].

Who should be studied, and why?

Patients with uncontrolled seizures

It was previously quite acceptable to perform only minimal investigation at the onset of the seizures and to reserve more searching studies for those people whose attacks proved impossible to control. Improved imaging, intensive monitoring, and increased demand for information have led to a trend for more searching investigations as soon as seizures start. A more definitive investigation is mandatory when seizures remain uncontrolled. In particular, a history suggestive of partial seizures or a focal component requires further investigation and clarification.

Importance of electroclinical correlation

Accurate identification of the type of epilepsy is essential for determining the optimal medical treatment. A satisfactory electroclinical correlation sometimes cannot be obtained while the patient is receiving antiepileptic medication, and admission to hospital followed by repeated EEG recordings while the medication is gradually diminished may be the only way of achieving this. An accurate correlation is, of course, an essential prerequisite for consideration of a surgical approach to the seizure problem.

Unexpected structural lesions and their prognostic significance

New imaging techniques have led to recognition of the otherwise unsuspected structural lesions such as small tumors, hamartomas, gangliogliomas or calcified cavernous hemangiomas. When epileptogenic, these lesions often lead to seizures which are medically uncontrollable. Surgical removal of the epileptogenic area, especially if the lesion can be included in the removal, usually results in excellent seizure control in the majority of patients.

Value of establishing a neuropsychologic baseline

Neuropsychologic study is an essential part of the baseline investigation. Parents and patients are very concerned by the possible deleterious effects of recurrent seizures and this question provides a ready subject for ongoing neurologic debate. There is no substitute however for careful early evaluation of various aspects of cognitive function including overall intelligence, verbal and visuospatial memory, and functions of specific brain regions relevant to the patient's type of seizure. Interference with these test results by antiepileptic drugs must be considered, but as long as drug levels are not toxic there appears to be little interference with the tests used to assess localized function. A study of intellectual deterioration provides useful guidance for evaluating whether or not a seizure problem is malignant from a cognitive point of view.

Clear formulation of treatment options to physician, patient, and family

The determination of a detailed baseline including clinical, imaging, electrographic, and neuropsychologic data, has many advantages. It permits clear, informed interpretation of the problem to the patient, the family, and the physician. It allows formulation of a treatment plan with sequential steps depending on the response. It leads to improved ability to establish a prognosis and to predict the likelihood that any particular mode of treatment will be effective. In some patients one can point out that, should antiepileptic medication be ineffective or insufficiently helpful, surgical treatment holds out hope for an alternative therapeutic option.

What constitutes an adequate trial of antiepileptic medication?

Onset of seizures is frightening, and adjustment to a new disability is difficult but, unless a lesion is detected which requires a surgical approach for its own sake, it is inadvisable to consider surgical treatment too early. The possibility of spontaneous improvement in the seizure tendency exists, and some patients with temporal lobe epilepsy have a benign and drug-responsive form of the disorder [15]. A thorough trial of major anticonvulsants such as carbamazepine and phenytoin at maximal tolerated levels should then be carried out despite the patient's inevitable complaints about medication side effects. The latter should be fully explained, preferably before they make themselves felt. Whether one major drug is more effective than another at high levels is questionable, but these substitutions are worth trying. The use of adjuvant drugs such as valproic acid, benzodiazepines, and succinimides in combinations of two or even three with the major drugs should be explored, again following thorough discussion of the potential benefits and side effects. Such combinations sometimes result in seizure control in patients who show little benefit in monotherapy. However, consideration of surgical therapy should not be delayed too long by experimenting with adjuvant drugs unless there is a definite response to these trials.

Compliance

Compliance may be a problem, and possible improvements should be discussed with the patient, family, referring neurologist, and psychiatric consultant. Experienced, perceptive, and observant patients, however, are often quite aware of the maximum benefit they can derive from antiepileptic medication and of the side effects they must expect in return. Patients and families must also be made aware of potential future progress in this field but, unfortunately, the hope for improved or rational treatment in the future is of little benefit in the present.

Likelihood of improved control

After at least 1, but not more than 4 years of careful observation, when the likelihood of spontaneous improvement has diminished, surgical treatment should be considered [1]. During this interval the educational and social adjustment should be scrutinized and the possibility of cognitive impairment and development of personality problems must be kept in mind. Many forms of epilepsy improve with age but it would be futile to spend a lifetime waiting for this to happen. Some patients whose epilepsy seemed quite mild and perhaps not too disabling are found after many years to have been affected much more than one would have expected. Their lives have been constricted, the side effects of medication are oppressive, and there is always the threat of more severe seizures when for reason of illness they are unable to take their regular medication. It is important to consider the patients' and families' perceptions of the disorder and its social impact rather than impose one's own views and judgements.

How bad does the epilepsy have to be?

Impairment of consciousness during seizures

There are several different modalities of response to antiepileptic medication in partial seizures, and complex partial attacks originating in the temporal lobe represent a good illustration of this range. In some patients, both major and minor attacks are fully controlled with medication, whereas in others, major seizures may be controlled but minor attacks persist. Attacks may at times be reduced in severity and frequency to the point of minor interference with awareness and responsivity. In others, the seizures do not respond at all, and some patients elect not to take any antiepileptic medication since it modifies the seizures but little.

The severity of seizures required to consider surgical therapy has changed greatly over the past half-century. Mortality and complications have progressively diminished and improvements in surgical technique and strategy have reduced the price the patient pays for improved seizure control. No longer are generalized seizures or falling attacks a necessary requirement — attacks with impairment of consciousness or awareness may now be considered to be severe enough to suggest a surgical option. It is unwise, however, to consider surgical treatment in patients who remain conscious or aware during their attacks.

Is expected reduction of medication alone sufficient to consider surgical therapy?

Occasionally patients or families inquire about the possibility of surgery when seizures are controlled but side effects of medication are troublesome; this situation does not at present justify serious consideration of operation.

Social disability resulting from attacks and from impact of attacks

The nature and circumstances of the attacks and their impact on the patients' lives are important. Some seizures are much more socially disabling than others. The person's aspirations and expectations, as well as intelligence, motivation, occupation, and environment must be considered in addition to the seizure pattern and frequency.

When asked what else they would do if their seizures ceased following operation, many young people now say "drive". At first this may seem frivolous; but there are a number of associated social considerations such as feelings of worthiness, acceptance, and esteem by their peers which may be subsumed under this heading. The hope to be able to obtain and keep employment is frequently expressed by people in their 20s and later.

Patients with infrequent attacks but recurrent status

Some seizure patterns, though occurring infrequently, may be life-threatening and represent an important indication for consideration of surgery; this is illustrated by patients with a tendency to recurrent status epilepticus or serial attacks.

Steps in initial investigation

Seizure history from patient and from witnesses

Much has been said in recent years, especially after the advent of video monitoring, about the unreliability of seizure histories and the inaccuracy of information provided by witnesses describing attacks that they repeatedly observed. Yet in many instances the description of the early components of his seizures by the patient remains invaluable. It may provide important evidence for the localization of seizure onset, for instance in temporal, occipital, or parietal structures. This localizing evidence, when confirmed by congruous findings from other investigations, is an important feature in leading one towards consideration of surgical therapy. A stable and unchanging habitual seizure pattern suggests a single and perhaps a circumscribed epileptogenic area. A repertory of progressively changing epileptic symptoms is not necessarily evidence for a tumor or for a progressive underlying disease, and such a pattern is not uncommon in patients with epilepsy arising in the temporal lobe. Discrepancies between the clinical symptoms and electrographic localization obtained by surface recording raise the suspicion that the seizures may not originate in the areas suggested by surface EEG. Such findings may be related to the presence of a gross structural lesion [16] or to the development of secondary epileptogenesis [17,18], complicating factors that can be resolved by the use of depth electrode studies.

Many patients with a long history of seizures have been repeatedly requestioned about possible symptoms at onset, and consequently have learned much about the symptomatology of seizures; this may colour the history they provide and may render it less reliable. The patients' perception of their own awareness during the attack and their ability to respond and remember what happens during seizures should be determined, and compared to the observations of family members and other witnesses. The presence of an aura may be inferred if the patient feels an attack coming which then does not occur.

When several types of seizures are described, one should try to determine whether they all start in the same way or represent increasingly severe manifestations or variations of the same pattern. By contrast, different seizure patterns may suggest the presence of qualitatively different epileptic mechanisms or indeed the presence of multifocal epileptogenic areas. Some patterns such as a sensation of familiarity or strangeness or an unformed visual hallucination have a very high correlation with a certain cerebral localization, whereas others such as turning, posturing, or motionless starting have less specific localizing significance.

Because awareness and recall are frequently impaired during seizures, a good description by witnesses is extremely important in the diagnosis of the different forms of epilepsy. The earliest visible manifestations of the seizure, type of automatisms, early or late occurrence of automatisms, postictal changes, and presence of precipitating factors are examples of pertinent observations. Descriptions of lateralization of increased tone, automatism, and even clonic movement are at times unreliable even though a parent may have been exposed to the seizures for many years. On the other hand, the family may have a better perception of the social significance of the seizures compared to the patient who is unaware of his appearance or behaviour during the attacks. Comparison of a patient's habitual seizures with those recorded during intensive video monitoring is important; the seizures occurring after reduction of medication are often more intense, and exceptionally they may be different from the usual attack [19].

Weighting of epileptic symptoms

Studies of cortical stimulation and recording from depth and subdural electrodes have expanded our knowledge of the degree of specificity of various epileptic symptoms and signs. It has become clear that all these are not of equal localizing or lateralizing value and that in this respect a veritable hierarchy of significance emerges. Though there seems to be general agreement that unforced turning from side to side is not of lateralizing value, there is currently a debate about the lateralizing value of forced adversion followed again by agreement on the significance of lateralized clonic movement [20,21]. Lateralized automatic movement may well prove to be ipsilateral to the clinically significant temporal focus, but this has not yet been conclusively demonstrated. Facial twitching may be contralateral or ipsilateral and thus is of no clear lateralizing value. Experiential or complex hallucinatory phenomena, uncinate symptoms, unformed visual hallucinations or a Jacksonian march have been confirmed to have a very high degree of localizing, and in some instances lateralizing, specificity and remain invaluable in identifying people with intractable epilepsy who may be helped by surgical therapy.

Medical record of early hospitalizations, previous EEGs and other studies

Recollection of significant early events in the patient's life is often sketchy and a review of a copy of pertinent hospital records may be important. Parents may, for instance, be unaware of the duration of febrile convulsions which are often proven in this way to have been prolonged and followed by a Todd's paresis. Such a finding is common in patients with hippocampal sclerosis and seizures arising in the temporal lobe and has both localizing and lateralizing value. Records of perinatal findings and of acquired illnesses may also provide pertinent and useful information about the etiology of the epilepsy.

All previous EEG studies should be reviewed. Early δ-foci or epileptic discharges may have lateralizing or localizing significance. Some patients continue to show lateralized or localized epileptic discharge even when receiving antiepileptic medication; knowledge of results of previous serial recordings in such persons are valuable, especially when bilateral independent epileptogenic foci are later found on searching investigation following reduction of antiepileptic medication.

Neurologic examination

Neurologic examination of candidates for surgical treatment is often described as normal. However, many patients with seizures arising in the temporal lobe have a facial asymmetry [22]. In 75% of these the face moves less and the corner of the mouth is lower opposite the side of the epileptogenic focus. Thus, this interesting physical finding is not of reliable lateralizing value. An unsuspected visual field defect, usually due to a vascular lesion, may also be found in patients with complex partial attacks [23]. The asymmetry of growth related to damage acquired at birth or in early life is most marked when the lesion involves or is near the postcentral gyrus. It may be found in the size of the hand or the foot or even in the width of the thumbnail, but it is more difficult to interpret when it involves the face. Such asymmetries of growth usually have lateralizing value.

Infantile hemiparesis may be associated with partial seizures, and from the neurologic examination itself it is impossible to determine from which area the seizures originate: frontal, temporal, parietal, or multilobe seizures may occur in this situation. Patients with a more severe hemiparesis may be candidates for a functionally complete but anatomically subtotal hemispherectomy [24,25]. When there are no useful fine finger movements, no additional motor deficit should result from surgery and, of course, the patient's ability to walk is not further impaired.

Radiologic studies

Since growth of the skull depends on brain growth, lesions acquired at birth or early in life may lead to the development of such radiologic signs as enlargement of the frontal sinuses, elevation of the mastoid pyramid, flattening of the vault or smallness of the middle fossa, depending on whether the whole hemisphere or only one lobe is involved. Focal thinning of the vault from craniocerebral cicatrix, intracranial calcifications, or old fractures may also be found. Arteriography demonstrates angiomas and may show old vascular occlusions or vascular narrowing.

That small foreign tissue or hamartomatous lesions are not uncommonly a cause of partial epilepsy has been shown by Penfield and Ward [26] and stressed by Falconer *et al.* [27]. The advent of the CT (computed tomography) scan has brought about a veritable explosion in the recognition and demonstration of such lesions. Gangliogliomas, hamartomas, calcified angiomas and areas of macrogyria associated with focal cortical dysplasia can be demonstrated in this manner. Multiple calcifications are not only an indication of tuberous sclerosis; familial cavernous hemangiomas, calcified parasitic granulomas or bioccipital calcified cortical angiomas without nevus flammeus [28] may present in this way. Though some atrophic changes can be seen in or around the temporal lobe, CT scanning has a relative blind spot in this area. Improved demonstration of atrophic changes has been obtained by using coronal sections and metrizamide [29], but visualization of this important area by CT remains inadequate.

Magnetic resonance imaging

The development of magnetic resonance imaging (MRI) has ushered in a new era of imaging in candidates for surgical treatment of epilepsy. Some of the initial reports were cautious, but atrophy can be shown better than with CT, lesions which cannot be seen with CT may be demonstrated, altered signals and smallness in the hippocampus suggesting Ammon's horn sclerosis can be seen, and widespread or extensive gliotic changes may be shown [30,31]. In addition to the presurgical evaluation, magnetic resonance imaging (MRI) may also be helpful in assessing postoperative changes such as gliosis or incompletely removed lesions which may explain some of the less successful outcomes following surgical treatment.

EEG recording on full medication

Initial electrographic studies are generally performed while the patient is receiving the full dosage of antiepileptic medication. Often the tracing is normal, particularly in patients with seizures originating in the temporal lobe. Background activity may be slow, and this may be related to long-term antiepileptic drug intake. At times however clear epileptogenic discharge and/or seizures may be recorded despite the presence of medication.

EEG studies on reduced medication

Because of the risks of status epilepticus, attempts to localize interictal and later ictal epileptiform abnormalities are usually carried out in hospital.

Antiepileptic drugs are gradually reduced starting with those least essential for seizure control or those used as adjuvants in the treatment of partial seizures. Benzodiazepines and valproic acid are withdrawn first, followed by phenobarbital and primidone. Phenytoin and carbamazepine are the last to be withdrawn. Drug reduction should be carried out slowly, and in particular, patients with a history of status epilepticus should be watched carefully. Drug-level determinations are obtained at regular intervals. Recently it has become clear that reduction of phenytoin and carbamazepine may lead to a withdrawal effect with a transient increase in seizures much like what is known to occur after cessation or reduction of phenobarbital and primidone [32]. Very gradual reduction of medication may avoid the flurries of minor or major attacks which may be followed by postictal psychotic reactions, particularly in patients with seizures originating in the temporal lobe.

When interictal epileptogenic abnormalities become clear-cut, and seizures arising in or involving mesial temporal structures are suspected, sphenoidal electrodes are inserted. These electrodes are well tolerated, though they may cause minor discomfort, and may be left in place for 2 weeks. In a large series we have encountered no infection and when the fine platinum wires break as they occasionally do, the internal fragments are left in place. The Teflon-coated, stranded, stainless steel sphenoidal wires used by Engel's group may be left in place longer without adverse effects [33].

Various interictal epileptogenic abnormalities may appear as the medication is reduced or removed. Some correlate well with the clinical attack pattern and others do not. Bilaterally synchronous, usually brief, bursts of spike and wave discharge may appear and at times are sensitive to hyperventilation. Generalized photosensitive abnormalities may also emerge. Generalized spike and wave discharges in patients with seizures originating in the temporal lobe have been studied by Sadler and Blume [34]. These generalized abnormalities most likely represent the expression of the genetic component of the patients' epilepsy. Only exceptionally are patients with complex partial seizures and this type of discharge aware of the brief spike and wave bursts which coexist with their focal discharges and complex partial attacks.

When the clinical seizure pattern is not clear-cut and not characteristic of localized onset, seizures should be recorded in order to assess more fully the possible clinical significance of these generalized epileptogenic discharges.

In patients with complex partial seizures whose clinical patterns suggest onset in the temporal lobe, interictal discharge should be recorded repeatedly in order to be certain that contralateral independent epileptogenic abnormality in clinically significant amounts does not eventually emerge. The number of records required to provide such information should be of the order of 10–12 over a 2–3 week period. When, despite repeated recording, there is no evidence for significant contralateral independent discharge and when the electrographic information correlates fully with the clinical, imaging, and neuropsychologic parameters, no further electrographic investigation may be required.

Recording of seizures

When the correlation between the clinical, electrographic, imaging, and neuropsychologic data is less than ideal, or when the amount of discharge from the less active side is >5–10%, recording of seizures becomes essential. This can rarely be achieved with prolonged recording but usually telemetry, if possible with video recording, is required. The montages are designed as a function of the particular clinical problem to be solved. When the area of onset of the seizures clearly coincides with the area of interictal discharge, this may provide sufficient electrographic information for a clinical decision. Sometimes, judging from other parameters, the localization is clear but the lateralization is in doubt. Seizures which are clearly lateralized but where the area of onset is unclear may be very helpful in clarifying this question. The number of seizures required in order to be reasonably certain of the localization of seizure onset varies; isolated attacks recorded on several different occasions are more meaningful than a large number of attacks recorded in one bout. For example, recording during status epilepticus where very frequent electrographic or minor clinical seizures occur from temporal structures on both sides may provide misleading information since this does not necessarily prove that the habitual and clinically significant seizures originate from both temporal lobes.

Recorded seizures do not always produce useful information. Artefact may obscure the tracing. In some cases muscle potentials may be filtered out using a computer program and underlying cerebral potentials can be more clearly visualized. The time of onset of the attack may not be obvious from surface EEG recording and many seconds may pass from the time the patient or the observer notes the clinical onset to the appearance of ictal discharges in the record. This suggests that the epileptogenic discharges in the depth are of insufficient amplitude to be recorded over the surface and such attacks are not very useful for localization of seizure onset. Seizure onset is frequently characterized electrographically by diffuse depression of ongoing background activity without any clearcut localization or lateralization. Some seizures do not permit lateralization at any time; others show lateralized discharges relatively late; and in some the seizure continues on the side opposite to where it started. Postictal slow activity however is usually a reliable lateralizing sign.

Consideration of intracranial recording

When the clinical pattern, electrographic information, imaging studies, and neuropsychologic findings do not provide the high degree of correlation which enables one to reach a clinical decision, further electrographic studies are necessary. These include investigations with depth or subdural strip electrodes. The advantage of such studies is the freedom from artefact and improved accuracy of localization. The procedures should be tailored to the specific clinical problem and the electrodes placed in a manner most likely to lead to clear answers to these questions.

Intracranial electrodes are specifically indicated in patients with temporal lobe seizures when bilateral independent temporal epileptic discharges are seen, and when the clinical pattern, EEG onset or other clinical findings make it impossible to distinguish between temporal and either frontal [35] or occipital [36] epileptic lesions.

Recording from depth electrodes can provide additional information in every patient but this may not be required for a clinical decision. The risks of using depth electrodes are similar to the risks of resective surgery in itself. Therefore these studies are performed only when necessary. In our center they are considered essential in only 15–20% of patients. Studies with invasive techniques are discussed by Spencer in Chapter 3.

Neuropsychologic testing

Many patients are surprised that psychologic investigation is part of the presurgical evaluation. They assume that such studies imply emotional disturbance and are not aware of the role of psychologic testing in determining cerebral localization and abnormalities of function.

Overall intelligence is determined by the Wechsler intelligence scales, and discrepancies between verbal and performance IQ point to dysfunction in the dominant or in the nondominant hemisphere. Among the battery of other tests used, are memory tests which are particularly sensitive to temporal lobe function, and offer good discrimination between dominant, nondominant, and bilateral temporal-lobe damage or dysfunction. In addition to yielding lateralizing and localizing information, memory test results provide a caveat as to the amount of mesial temporal structures that can safely be removed when there is any hint of contralateral dysfunction. Neuropsychologic tests are also sensitive to abnormal function of the convexity of the frontal cortex, and the card sorting test is particularly valuable in this respect [37].

Intracarotid Amytal tests for assessment of memory function and language lateralization

When more accurate information is required, the function of mesial temporal structures can be assessed by detailed testing while these structures are temporarily inactivated on one side and then on the other side by the intracarotid injection of Sodium Amytal. Test results reflect the functioning of the non-injected side. They are not invalidated by nonspecific systemic effects of the drug. Variations in the distribution of the cerebral circulation are assessed by arteriographic visualization using 3 cm^3 of contrast material.

Handedness and hemispheral dominance for language are initially assessed both clinically and with the use of specialized tests. If there is the suggestion that unusual cerebral organization such as bilateral or right-sided language localization may be present, the Sodium Amytal test will also be carried out to assess this further [38].

Positron emission tomography

The development of positron emission tomography (PET) has permitted study of cerebral blood flow, oxygen uptake and other aspects of cerebral metabolism in patients with epilepsy. Hypometabolic areas usually correlate with the epileptogenic area as determined electrographically [39–41], though the area of hypometabolism is usually more extensive than the electrographic abnormalities. PET scans have been helpful in lateralizing temporal lobe abnormalities when hypometabolism coincides with other evidence pointing to one or the other temporal lobe. Improved discrimination is required before intrahemispheric localization based on positron emission will be possible.

Interpretation of findings to patients and family

As the investigation progresses through these various and hopefully concurrent stages, the results of the last and the rationale of the next steps is explained to the patient and the family. Through these repeated discussions, their understanding of the possibilities and limitations of surgical and of medical therapy deepens, and their fears and hopes can be put into a realistic perspective. Misconceptions can be clarified and the prognosis interpreted. During these protracted and sometimes boring studies, which include waiting for the required electrographic evidence and last but not least the orchestration of a large team, the patient will require much support from his family, the referring physicians who usually know him well, and the staff. The aim is to determine whether a definitive approach to the epileptic problem is possible, and it is usually desirable to avoid the "revolving door syndrome" where patients are discharged before completion of the study to be repeatedly readmitted for successive steps of their investigation.

It is possible at this time to assess the patients' motivation to undergo irreversible brain surgery as well as their ability to cooperate in a lengthy procedure under local anesthesia. When the patient or the family are not fully convinced that surgical treatment holds out sufficient likelihood for reduction of the seizure tendency or they feel that the risks are too great, it is best to continue with medical treatment. At the same time they should be given the opportunity to rediscuss the problem periodically with the neurologist, the neurosurgeon, and the neuropsychologist.

Treatment strategies

The ideal aim of surgical treatment of epilepsy is to reduce the seizure tendency to the point where the person is free of attacks while either continuing to take medication or without the help of antiepileptic drugs. Though there is no routine in the study and plan of treatment for surgical candidates, similarities between certain groups of patients requiring a common treatment strategy emerge.

Indications for temporal lobectomy

The clinical symptomatology of some patients strongly suggests an onset in the temporal lobe; their early symptoms are specific to this area and are not known to arise from other brain regions. Amygdaloid symptoms such as fear or an epigastric rising sensation, experiential symptoms such as a feeling of strangeness or familiarity, complex visual hallucinations or gustatory and olfactory sensations are examples of this type. If the electrographic, imaging, PET and neuropsychologic studies are congruent as to localization and lateralization, such patients are excellent candidates for temporal lobectomy and the likelihood of a good result is very high.

Patients with "foreign tissue" lesions

Another group of patients who usually respond very well to surgical treatment are those who have small demonstrable "foreign tissue" lesions. Much depends on the location of both the lesion and the epileptogenic area. The latter is usually close to the lesion, but its extent cannot be predicted without demonstrating the EEG abnormalities and their field distribution. Anterior temporal lesions present no problem, especially if the EEG discharges are anterior and inferomesial temporal, and the clinical pattern suggests this as well. More posterior temporal lesions often also lead to anterior and inferomesial EEG discharges and the lesions themselves may be accessible even in the dominant hemisphere if sufficiently inferior. It may be justifiable to remove the most epileptogenic area even if the lesion itself is not surgically accessible, e.g. an anterior temporal lobectomy in patients whose lesion is deep in the posterior and mesial part of the temporal lobe. In such patients however the results are not as good, and palliation rather than complete seizure control is a more realistic goal. In other areas the approach depends both on the congruence of clinical, electrographic, imaging and other factors and on what is surgically accessible.

Suspected extratemporal involvement

Patients with predominantly temporal clinical and EEG patterns may also have extratemporal features such as clonic movement, lateralized abnormal sensations, and EEG abnormalities extending beyond the temporal lobe. In such cases, studies including recording from depth electrodes or subdural strips may be required in order to determine more clearly the area of onset and spread of discharge. In some of these patients, however, a temporal removal may convert an intractable epileptic problem into one which responds to currently available antiepileptic agents with resultant good seizure control.

Some patients have frontotemporal or occipitotemporal epileptogenic abnormalities where the lateralization of the abnormal process is clear, but more precise localization of seizure onset remains uncertain. Clarification in many of these patients still requires investigation with implanted electrodes or subdural strips. Patients with frontal or occipital structural lesions may show predominantly temporal epileptic discharges and a seizure pattern which does not permit more precise localization [18,35]. There too, as in the previous examples of inadequate correlation between the different parameters, studies with depth or subdural strip electrodes may be unavoidable.

Extensive glial scars following head injury or intracerebral hemorrhage may lead to large epileptogenic areas and patients with such lesions often respond well to surgical treatment. In patients with bifrontal lesions of this type, it may be possible to lateralize the maximal abnormality or the area of seizure onset and remove the epileptogenic tissue on that side.

Patients with hemiparesis

Patients with hemiparesis and seizures present more special problems. The epileptic abnormality and structural damage may be widespread within the damaged hemisphere and, in this situation, limited removals hold out little promise of rendering the patient seizure-free.

Hemispherectomy is effective in arresting the seizures but in a high percentage of patients eventually leads to cerebral hemosiderosis and hydrocephalus. This complication appears to be due to repeated small hemorrhages related to lack of support of the remaining hemisphere within the skull [24]. In an attempt to prevent this complication, Rasmussen devised the modified procedure of partial but functionally complete hemispherectomy where the frontal and/or occipital poles were disconnected from the rest of the brain but their blood supply remained intact [24]. This procedure has not led to cerebral hemosiderosis within a 10-year period and is effective in arresting the seizures. There is usually some improvement in overall intelligence (around 10 IQ points) and considerable improvement in both behaviour and social functioning. Bilateral, secondarily generalized epileptic discharges are not a contraindication for surgical treatment. In contrast, clearly independent epileptic discharges, or seizures originating in the better hemisphere, though associated with improvement in seizure tendency following hemispherectomy, usually lead to a less dramatic result. The latter patients are often more retarded and have evidence of greater dysfunction in the contralateral hemisphere.

Functional hemispherectomy does not lead to any loss of ability to walk. It is indicated when there is no useful fine-finger movement and when the arm is used as an assistor. There may be some improvement in spasticity but of course finger movement does not improve postoperatively. In such a patient, this procedure is preferable to callosotomy where complete cessation of attacks is uncommon, whereas following hemispherectomy over 80% of patients are seizure-free, many on reduced medication or without taking any drugs [25].

Where the epileptogenic discharges and cerebral damage are more localized, and where there is useful hand function, less extensive removals involving more than one lobe, mainly frontal and temporal, or temporal and occipital, may be considered. Results are more variable in this situation when compared with those obtained following functional hemispherectomy.

Some hemiparetic patients have seizures with symptoms pointing to onset in the temporal lobe. A temporal lobectomy may then be effective in reducing seizure tendency. Some of these patients have independent contralateral temporal epileptic abnormalities and these may be more striking than on the side of the lesion. With surface EEG, seizures may also appear to arise from the more normal hemisphere. Recording with depth electrodes has shown that the seizures actually do start on the side of the lesion, but the more damaged tissue is incapable of generating sufficient voltage on that side [16]. In view of the small number of cases studied, confirmation with depth recording is still required where such a situation is suspected.

Patients with much secondary generalized epileptic discharge

Candidates for resective surgery or callosotomy?

In the last several years there has been a cautious but rapidly spreading resurgence of interest in callosotomy for surgical treatment of patients whose seizure disorders are malignant and who would not be candidates for removal of epileptogenic brain tissue. Anterior callosotomy appears to be of benefit in abolishing or reducing drop attacks. This particularly disabling seizure pattern may be associated with either secondary generalized or frontal epileptic discharges and very often it is difficult to distinguish between the two. Thus patients with secondary generalized epileptic discharge and significant lateralization or structural evidence for lateralized damage are candidates for such a procedure. Other candidates are persons with multifocal discharge and those with secondary generalized epilepsy where cross-correlation studies [42] do not show evidence for lead-off in one hemisphere. In the latter group, results of this procedure seem slightly less encouraging.

Callosotomy remains a palliative procedure though it may lead to worthwhile improvement in desperate situations (see Chapter 4). Wherever clinical, imaging, electrographic and neuropsychologic criteria permit, removal of epileptogenic tissue remains preferable to callosotomy, since it holds out some promise of cessation of the attacks as well as the added benefit of improvement in intelligence and behavior, presumably through cessation of interference from the continuing epileptogenic discharge.

The patient with retardation

Practical and ethical considerations

Mental retardation is not a contraindication for surgical treatment, provided the usual criteria are met. McNaughton and Rasmussen [1] point out that care and supervision of the retarded and their quality of life can be greatly improved if their seizure disorder can be controlled or improved. Because of lack of cooperation, surgery must be performed under light general anesthesia which still permits localization of landmarks by cortical stimulation. At some centers because mental retardation constitutes evidence of diffuse brain damage, mentally retarded patients are usually not considered candidates for localized resective surgery. We have made no value judgements in selecting candidates for surgical treatment according to their intelligence. This approach corresponds to current views and thinking on social issues, particularly on the rights of the retarded.

The procedure is explained in detail to the patients at their level and care is taken to clarify for the parents and caretakers that the procedure is designed to improve seizure control, and additional benefits such as a rise in IQ or improved behavior should be considered as a bonus.

Psychosis and personality disorder

History of psychotic episodes

Psychotic episodes are not uncommon in epileptic patients, particularly those with temporal lobe seizures following bouts of recurrent major or minor seizures. These periods of psychosis, though frightening, are generally self-limited and benign [43] and do not constitute a contraindication to surgical treatment. It is wise to wait until these thought disorders have remitted before proceeding with surgery. According to Savard *et al.* and Jensen and Larsen [44,45], patients who have a good surgical result often show normalization or improvement of their psychiatric condition.

Presence of personality disorders

Personality disorders are not uncommon in patients with complex partial seizures. In younger individuals, when these disorders are relatively recent, there may be improvement following surgery, but where they are well established and of long standing they may persist despite improvement in the seizure tendency. In patients with severe personality disorders and seizures arising in both temporal lobes, surgery is sometimes carried out if the seizures are life-threatening or severely disabling. Seizure control can be greatly improved in these patients or they remain seizure-free; however, in some the personality disorder may be transiently aggravated and new behavioural patterns, mainly disinhibition, may appear. Only exceptionally are such changes long lasting [44].

The patient with ongoing psychosis

Patients who have a fixed or chronic schizophreniform psychosis which does not appear to fluctuate with the epileptic activity do not benefit from surgical treatment as far as their psychosis is concerned [1]. Such patients are generally not considered to be suitable candidates for surgical therapy, although one may still wonder whether the quality of their life would not improve if reduction in their seizure tendency could be achieved.

Patients and families commonly question whether the operation could lead to psychosis. It has been shown by Jensen and Larsen [45], Taylor and Falconer [46], and Taylor [47] that psychosis can develop in patients who have been surgically treated, often successfully, for temporal lobe epilepsy. Since the incidence of psychosis in patients treated or not treated surgically is uncertain, one can only answer this question by stating that there are risks either way. There is of course much less likelihood of a postictal psychosis in patients who have undergone operations; The mechanism of psychosis associated with temporal lobe dysfunction is multifactorial, and the link between schizophreniform behavior and limbic dysfunction is imperfectly understood.

Aims of surgery

Control or palliation?

Once the preoperative studies are completed, it is usually possible to plan the surgical approach. It will often be possible to anticipate whether there is a good likelihood of complete control of the attacks such as in persons with a well defined temporal abnormality where all parameters point to the same surgically accessible area. In other patients palliation is the most likely outcome as for instance in patients with macrogyria and focal cortical dysplasia or in patients with the "forme fruste" of tuberous sclerosis where postoperative suppression of all seizures is very unlikely. A surgical approach is valid in both situations.

Patients' and families' expectations

Although the best preoperative prognosis is made after the full evaluation is completed, valid impressions may be obtained early in the course and it is important to keep the patient and family informed, as well as assess their reactions and continued interest should a less than perfect result appear likely.

The risks, aims and possible outcomes of surgery should be discussed with patient and family and rediscussed as necessary. In particular the likelihood of control, improvement, and lack of change are explained, as are the risks of mortality and morbidity of the intended procedure. At this time the patients' and families' expectations should be reconsidered in the light of the results of the investigation and of the emerging prognosis. The extent of the procedure however depends also on the surgeon's findings and decisions at operation, and on the guidance which the electrocorticographer contributes.

The preoperative interpretation is extremely important and over the years we have repeatedly had the experience of obvious misunderstanding by patients and families of the test results, the possibilities of a surgical approach, and the prognosis.

All candidates for surgical treatment are not ideal: who should be deprived of the chance of being treated surgically?

It follows from the above that not all patients investigated are ideal candidates for surgical treatment, and that a considerable range of possible outcomes exists. The outcome, however, cannot be accurately assessed preoperatively, and can be better predicted only 1 or 2 years after operation [48–50]. If this form of therapy is only offered to patients who are very likely to have an excellent result, many patients who are likely to derive considerable benefit from surgical therapy will be deprived of it.

Expected improvements and the price one pays

Patients and their families often inquire about any possible loss of function following surgery. Such issues are best discussed early in the evaluation procedure to allow the patient and family to decide whether further investigation is appropriate for them. After anterior temporal lobectomy there is usually an increase in overall intelligence of about 10 points and this is attributed to a decrease in the interference which the epileptogenic activity creates [37,51]. A decrease in verbal (dominant hemisphere removals) or visuospatial (nondominant hemisphere removals) memory may, however, also result, and observant or introspective patients may be aware of this. Memory deficits of this nature are often also present preoperatively, and can be accentuated by the temporal lobe removal. The majority of patients consider such accentuation of their deficit a small price to pay for the improvement in their seizure tendency and develop mnemotechnic means of coping with it. It is important to discuss this aspect of the prognosis with the patient and family in detail. When the removal is extensive a partial upper quadrantonopsia may be found. The patients are usually not subjectively aware of this and are functionally unaffected. Ideally the neurologist, and the neurosurgeon as well as the neuropsychologist should be involved in the process of interpretation. The cost : benefit ratio of more restricted procedures such as amygdalohippocampectomy is now being considered by various groups [52,53].

Accentuation of a preexisting deficit may also be found following frontal removal in patients whose epilepsy originates in the frontal lobe. This too, particularly the possible loss of initiative and ability to plan which may make rehabilitation difficult, must be interpreted to patient and family.

Surgery in children

Awareness of the progressive development of personality changes, of psychosocial problems, and of downward social mobility in patients with intractable epilepsy have led to the hope that some of these deficits may be prevented by earlier definitive therapy [49,54,55]. Rasmussen has shown that the results of temporal lobectomy carried out in children are similar to those obtained in adults [49]. Surgical therapy in children is discussed more fully in Chapter 5.

Evaluation of likelihood of spontaneous cessation of attacks

The main problem in the selection of surgical candidates in childhood is to identify those patients who are likely to remit spontaneously. There are no absolute criteria which enable recognition of this group of children [54–58]. A stable habitual seizure pattern which shows no sign of improving over the years represents a major indication. Such a pattern is often quite unresponsive to medication. Complex partial seizures which develop after prolonged seizures associated with fever and are related to Ammon's horn sclerosis represent a good example of this type. Having started in childhood, the persistence of such a pattern by the midteens (15–16 years) suggests that the likelihood of lasting remission is very small, but convincing statistical data are unavailable.

Optimal imaging studies are important in childhood since the seizures associated with small, not readily identifiable, foreign tissue lesions are unlikely to remit.

Prevention of behavioral complications and the deteriorating child

The progressive deterioration of behaviour and of cognitive function in some children also represent indications for early consideration of surgical intervention. Development of pediatric neurology leading to better prognostic acumen has led to a reluctance to accepting as inevitable the deterioration which may accompany seizures related to demonstrable lesions. It is often the pediatric neurologist, aware of the poor prognosis, who urges consideration of a surgical approach which might arrest or hopefully reverse such a process. As in older patients, one may anticipate control in some but only palliation in others.

Rehabilitation following surgery

The potential for rehabilitation is generally considered early in the process of assessment. Many patients are quite capable of adjusting to their new seizure-free or improved status, whereas others require guidance or help from family or professionals. A postoperative convalescence of 2 or 3 months is advisable and should be taken into account in the early stages of planning. Plans for continued postoperative medical treatment should be discussed during the initial session of interpretation in order to dispel any misconceptions. Continued antiepileptic treatment is advised for at least 2 or 3 years with carbamazepine or phenytoin monotherapy if at all possible. Gradual reduction to a level with few side effects is the aim after the first postoperative year. After another year or two, the treatment options are discussed further with patient and family and, hopefully, decisions on cessation or continuation of medication as well as dosage and levels are made jointly. Despite the manifest motivation of this group of people for good seizure control, attitudes vary widely and decisions are often made without medical advice.

Patterns of outcome

The possible patterns of outcome are also discussed early with patients and family since this may play a part in their decision to proceed with more complete evaluation. Outcome varies with many factors including localization. In temporal lobe epilepsy there may be freedom from attacks, persistence of auras which progressively diminish, partial seizures arising from residual frontal, suprasylvian or posterior temporal areas, or occasional major seizures different from the preoperative habitual patterns. Sometimes seizures similar to the original attacks return after a period of freedom.

Lingering prejudice in the neurologic community

Inversely correlated with experience: can one operate on the left hemisphere? Trading one cicatrix for another?

Despite the recent upsurge of interest in surgical treatment of epilepsy, considerable prejudice against such an approach remains among some members of the neurologic community. This is usually inversely correlated with experience and knowledge in this area. The following excerpt from a recent medical report illustrates this type of prejudice very well: " . . . surgery for the relief of seizures is not the best way to go and particularly in complex partial seizure disorder. If they did remove his left temporal lobe he might not be able to understand anything anybody said and may also have difficulty with regard to some function that he already has and could potentially have some paresis although the motor strip *per se* is not involved. The other problem with surgery for seizures is the fact that often within five years the seizures will come back along the suture line of where the surgery was done" [anonymous neurologist]. This retarded patient was subsequently referred for investigation, studied, underwent an operation, and has been seizure-free since, to the enormous relief of the family. It is of course possible to operate on the left, or dominant hemisphere, provided sufficient information about language localization is available, and speech areas are respected. Results of left temporal lobectomy [48,50], for instance, are similar to those obtained after right-sided removal. A clean postsurgical cicatrix seems preferable to a posttraumatic or posthemorrhagic lesion. It was not really possible until now to assess the tendency to develop gliotic reactions following seizure surgery, nor the putative effect of such a process in areas surrounding the re-magnetic resonance imaging (MRI) studies promise to throw much light on this problem and its possible significance in the surgical treatment of epilepsy.

Some special problems

Tuberous sclerosis

It is likely that the deterioration of intelligence and poor prognosis in tuberous sclerosis are related more to the epileptic process than to the cortical lesions or the periventricular calcified areas. Patients with tuberous sclerosis who have a stable pattern of partial seizures may prove to have a localized area of epileptogenic discharge which may be accessible to surgical treatment [59]. MRI may help clarify the localization of epileptogenic areas since abnormal cortical architecture can now be visualized in this way.

"Forme fruste of tuberous sclerosis"

Architectonic abnormalities in the cortex sometimes protruding into the underlying white matter may be seen by CT scan in the forme fruste of tuberous sclerosis described by Perot *et al.* [59]. As displayed by MRI, the lesions are considerably more widespread. The pathologic changes resemble those of tuberous sclerosis with giant cells. There are no characteristic periventricular calcifications, skin and other organs are not involved, and there is no positive family history. The relationship of this disorder to classical tuberous sclerosis remains quite uncertain [60].

Sturge–Weber syndrome

Patients with Sturge–Weber syndrome whose seizures are severe enough may also benefit from surgical therapy [61]. The extent of the pial angiomatosis is impossible to demonstrate with current imaging techniques. While the patients are receiving medication, the EEGs are often unrevealing. Reduction of medication enables the epileptogenic discharges to emerge and an electroclinical correlation to be established. Treatment strategies vary from removal of the epileptogenic area [61] to callosal section, removal of the calcified areas and hemispherectomy in infancy [62]. The latter procedure does not always appear justified in view of the great variation in the severity of epilepsy associated with Sturge–Weber syndrome; certainly there are some infants who have severe seizures and who subsequently are left severely retarded and these should have the benefit of aggressive medical treatment at the onset before surgery during infancy is considered.

Focal cortical dysplasia

Focal cortical dysplasia was described by Taylor *et al.* [63], and small dysplastic epileptogenic lesions have been encountered recently by Silfvenius *et al.* and Sourander *et al.* [64,65]. Cortical dysplasia is also found surrounding areas of focal macrogyria and the epileptogenic abnormality is usually peripheral to the area of maximal architectonic abnormality which can be visualized by CT or MRI scanning [60]. In such patients as well as in those with the forme fruste of tuberous sclerosis surgical treatment usually leads to improvement but not to complete suppression of the epileptogenic abnormality, probably because of the widespread nature of the lesions.

Chronic encephalitis of Rasmussen type

Chronic encephalitis, of the type described by Rasmussen and McCann [66], presents in children with intractable seizures and epilepsia partialis continua. It progresses to cause severe neurologic disability. A viral etiology has long been suspected, but has still not been proven. The possibility of an autoimmune disorder must also be considered. In patients whose seizures are life-threatening because of excessive secretions or other causes, removal of epileptogenic tissue may be of benefit [1]; whether the precentral gyrus can be removed depends on the degree of hemiparesis. Where there is no useful fine finger movement, a functional hemispherectomy can be carried out [24,25] without further functional loss and with good seizure control.

Prospect

Surgical treatment is clearly not the ideal answer to the problem posed by severe epilepsy. Better drugs, prevention, and eventually manipulation of the genetic component of the epilepsy, when that will be understood, may render surgical therapy obsolete. In the meantime, patients with uncontrollable epilepsy should have access to appropriate investigation and the benefit of surgical therapy which in many instances may lift the cloud under which they live.

Evaluation of patients for epilepsy surgery at the West Haven VA/Yale–New Haven Epilepsy Unit

Peter D. Williamson

Introduction

The past decade has witnessed a progressive expansion in the number of epilepsy programs that offer modern surgical treatment for patients whose seizures cannot be controlled with medications. Despite the increasing numbers of programs, there is no standard or agreed-upon methodology used in the presurgical evaluation of these patients. To some extent, each program develops its own personality or style dependent upon individual experiences and philosophies and available facilities and technologies. Programs will, therefore, use different selection criteria, investigative techniques and surgical approaches. While one would hope that a more unified approach will evolve in the future, our current state of understanding promotes a certain degree of diversity. This is healthy, as through diversity new techniques are developed and different experiences are accumulated for eventual comparison among the different epilepsy surgery programs. Almost certainly no one technique or methodology will emerge as universally superior, but rather different specific approaches will apply depending on individual circumstances. The following discussion describes our approach at the West Haven VA/Yale –New Haven Epilepsy Surgery Program.

Presurgical evaluation

The presurgical evaluation of patients for possible surgical intervention is a team approach utilizing the specific skills and abilities of the different personnel involved in the program. The goal of the evaluation is to determine, as well as possible, the type of surgery most appropriate for each patient or, conversely, if surgery is contraindicated. The evaluation proceeds through an orderly series of stages or phases using progressively more invasive procedures. Throughout the process and at certain points, decisions are required. Some decisions can be made "on-line" by the physician primarily responsible for the patient's care while others are best addressed using the entire team. The different phases of evaluation will be described first and then the decision-making processes will be examined.

Phase I

History

Phase I is a thorough, comprehensive, noninvasive evaluation of each patient being considered for surgery. An accurate, detailed history is an essential first part of this phase. All sources are utilized including the patient, family, close friends, and referring physicians. The history is augmented throughout all phases of evaluation as pertinent information is uncovered. The frequency, duration, and clinical characteristics of the seizures are carefully defined. Information concerning subjective experiences during seizures can only be described by the patient and these symptoms are noted and characterized. Auras or warnings and other symptoms may have occurred previously but are no longer present. These remote symptoms may have important localizing significance and their occurrence is actively sought. Circumstances of birth and early development, the occurrence of febrile seizures, central nervous system infections, or head trauma are relevant considerations in the history of patients with epilepsy as are family history of seizures or other diseases, school and work performance, and psychosocial adaptation. The chronology of the patient's epilepsy is documented from age of onset and first seizure type to the current condition. Rarely do seizures remain static from childhood through adolescence and into adulthood. The evolution of seizures, the response to different medications, and precipitating events are additional considerations that are defined. Thorough medical, psychiatric, and psychosocial histories are obtained as they may have an important impact upon surgical decisions.

Whenever potentially significant information is uncovered, it must be characterized in detail. For example, the occurrence of a febrile seizure needs to be defined. A single, brief seizure during a febrile episode probably has little significance whereas repeated or prolonged febrile seizures or the occurrence of transient neurologic deficits following febrile seizures can be of definite importance. The same is true of a history of head trauma, central nervous system infections, early seizure signs and symptoms, and any and all of the potentially pertinent historical information. While it may be argued that such thorough and detailed historical documentation is in keeping with good medical practice, this is not always realized. However, when evaluating patients for possible epilepsy surgery, there are numerous variables that must be considered, any one of which can alter decisions. A thorough history will yield vital information concerning these variables.

Examination

A careful, complete, general physical examination is performed in order to detect any unsuspected medical conditions. A thorough neurologic examination is designed to define obvious abnormalities and to detect subtle findings. All patients undergo formal visual field testing.

Closed-circuit television and simultaneous electroencephalographic monitoring

The value of intensive video-EEG monitoring has been well established [67,68] and we consider such monitoring to be a crucial part of the evaluation. EEG monitoring consists of 16-channel recording using standard 10–20 bipolar parasagittal and temporal montages. Different or special montages are selected as indicated. EEG monitoring is continuous for 24 hours for as many days as necessary to record three or more habitual seizures. The EEG is recorded on standard paper chart recorders or multiplexed and stored on magnetic videotape. Audio/video monitoring is done using monochromatic, low-light, video cameras and is recorded on videotape using standard split-screen technology to include both the patient and the EEG [69]. During monitoring, waking and sleeping interictal records are repeatedly reviewed to detect and localize paroxysmal abnormalities. Medication withdrawal is commonly used to precipitate seizures. When patients are on multiple anticonvulsant drugs one medication at a time is withdrawn. For reasons of expediency, the drug with the shortest half-life is usually selected first. When patients are on monotherapy the drug is withdrawn by incremental amounts. Anticonvulsant drug withdrawal is rarely associated with convulsive status epilepticus, however, it does occasionally result in the development of secondarily generalized convulsive seizures even in patients who have never or rarely experienced this type of seizure. Patients and their families are therefore always forewarned of this possibility. When seizures occur during monitoring, every attempt is made to examine the patient early in the seizure, during the seizure, and throughout the postictal period. The nurses, who have been specially trained to perform these examinations, provide test phrases and determine level of contact during seizures, check autonomic function such as pupil size and reactivity, observe and report any findings not always apparent on videotape such as eye deviation or minor focal clonic activity and test for focal neurologic signs during the postictal period such as visual field cuts, language deficits and hemipareses [70]. The goals of video-EEG monitoring are (1) to document seizures; (2) to establish seizure type or types; (3) to define interictal and ictal scalp EEG patterns; and (4) to determine ease of recording seizures.

Neuroimaging

The introduction of CT in the mid-1970s and the development of MRI a decade later have had major importance in the presurgical evaluation of patients with medically intractable epilepsy. Unsuspected, potentially epileptogenic lesions are detected increasingly frequently [71–74]. The significance of these lesions cannot be disputed as their resection is associated with a high percentage of seizure relief [75–77]. Furthermore, since over half these lesions prove to be neoplastic [78], their detection imparts a certain degree of urgency to the evaluation. All patients, therefore, have CT scans and MRIs prior to or as part of the Phase I evaluation.

Neuropsychologic testing

Extensive neuropsychologic testing is a standard part of the Phase I presurgical evaluations. This includes examination of upper extremity strength and dexterity, sensory perceptual examinations in three major modalities (auditory, visual, tactile), speech and language testing, quantification of both immediate and delayed verbal and nonverbal memory, evaluation of intellectual function (WAIS-R) and assessment of personality structure (MMPI). The aims of these tests are not only to detect potentially lateralizing and/or localizing deficits [79] but also to define strengths and weaknesses that might relate to the ability to tolerate the presurgical evaluation and the results of surgery. The presurgical neuropsychological test results also provide a valuable baseline for comparison with postoperative testing.

Psychiatric evaluation

All patients undergo formal psychiatric evaluation. This is done not only to define or look for psychopathology but also as an additional estimate of the patient's ability to tolerate the presurgical evaluation, particularly if intracranial electrodes are required. The psychiatric examination is also used to predict the patient's reaction to or ability to cope with the results of surgery and to decide whether or not active intervention and counseling might be anticipated following surgery.

Phase II

All patients who complete the Phase I evaluation and who are still considered surgical candidates undergo bilateral carotid angiography and bilateral carotid Amytal testing. The Amytal testing is done to determine hemispheric language dominance and lateralized memory function. A bolus injection of 130 mg of Sodium Amytal in 10 cm^3 of solution is used for each injection. Injections are separated by at least 30 minutes. Memory function is tested by presenting six test objects (two pictures, one colored geometric shape, two words, one simple mathematical problem). The start of test object presentation is determined by the development of contralateral hemiplegia and/or muteness. Object presentation is performed during the first 2–2½ min after injection with the position of presentation recognizing the hemianopic visual field. Ten minutes after injection, the patients are tested for recall. Two or more correct responses on spontaneous recall or multiple-choice recognition is considered a memory pass. Forced guessing is not included in the pass/fail equation.

Phase III

If it is decided that intracranial monitoring is required the patient enters the third phase of evaluation. Placement and numbers of depth and/or subdural electrodes are dictated by the results of the previous evaluations in each patient. As in Phase I, monitoring is continuous until three or more seizures have been captured. EEG recording is done using continuous 16-channel paper write-out or multiplexed 16-channel reformatted videotape recording. In addition, EEG is recorded digitally in parallel using a 64-channel computerized system [80]. Video recording is performed using techniques identical to that in

Phase I. Functional mapping using subdural strip and grid electrodes is performed when indicated [81,82]. Electrical stimulation for functional mapping is done using adjacent electrode pairs and a constant current stimulator. Stimulation parameters are 50 Hz biphasic pulses with 0.5 msec duration applied for 5 seconds. Current strength is begun at 1 mA and increased by 0.5 to 1 mA increments to a maximum of 10 mA. Current is increased until signs or symptoms are elicited or until an after-discharge or seizure occurs.

Event-related potentials are recorded from depth and subdural electrodes. Somatosensory evoked potentials are used to augment cerebral localization when subdural electrodes are placed over the central convexity. Preliminary data from studies of event-related potentials from depth electrodes suggest they might have clinical relevance in terms of localization and lateralization [83–85].

Phase IV surgery

Upon completion of Phases I and II, and when indicated Phase III, patients who are considered appropriate candidates for surgery are offered operative procedures. Surgical options vary, depending upon the findings from the preoperative evaluation. They include cortical resections aimed at eliminating or at least greatly reducing seizures and palliative procedures such as section of the corpus callosum. Some of the indications for different surgical options are discussed below and are examined in detail elsewhere in this volume.

Follow-up

All patients who have undergone epilepsy surgery have periodic outpatient evaluations. These routinely occur at 2 weeks, 3 months, 6 months, and 1 year postsurgery, and yearly thereafter. Routine postoperative follow-up assumes that the patients have had an excellent result following surgery. If surgical results have been unsatisfactory and disabling seizures persist the patients undergo extensive inpatient evaluations, dependent upon individual circumstances. When the findings suggest that persistent seizures are due to residual epileptogenic tissue in the region of the previous operation or due to epileptogenic tissue in another, but still surgically accessible area these patients may undergo a repeat of all indicated phases of evaluation aimed towards further surgery. In practice, there are numerous options that have to be considered in patients in whom surgical intervention has failed. We consider it imperative that these patients not be abandoned. Of equal importance is that additional surgery not be attempted unless there is a reasonable chance of success.

Additional patients requiring periodic evaluation are those in whom extensive presurgical studies have failed to localize the region of seizure origin and in whom disconnection procedures were deemed inappropriate. Hopefully, improved knowledge of different seizure types combined with advances in technology will eventually allow us a better understanding of these patients and a better management of their epilepsy. The introduction of MRI has already shown this to be true.

Decisions during patient evaluation

Throughout the course of the presurgical evaluation there are a number of decisions that must be made. Some are straightforward while others are difficult, and often specific to a particular patient. While an examination of all the possible combinations of variables that might influence the decision-making process is simply not possible, there are general considerations that can be examined. During the initial evaluation there are several issues that must be addressed.

Does the patient have epilepsy? In most patients referred for epilepsy surgery, the diagnosis of epilepsy will have been established. Occasionally, some doubt will exist. When this occurs the usual concern is the possibility that some or all of the patient's attacks are pseudoseizures. Considering the wide variety of seizure manifestations, only exceptionally will it be possible to resolve this issue during an initial interview. It is very unlikely, however, that a patient with pseudoseizures will escape detection during the initial phase of evaluation.

Does the epilepsy significantly interfere with the patient's life? While this important question must be answered for each patient being considered for surgery, there is no standard formula for answering it. Perceptions of the patient, the family, and the physician concerning the impact of seizures upon lifestyle can differ widely. Recurrent convulsive status epilepticus or frequent tonic seizures with falling can result in permanent neurologic damage or even death. In this case, there is certainly no argument. Conversely, a patient who has one or two mild partial seizures per month represents a situation that requires examination of many different variables to determine degree of disability. For example, this seizure frequency–severity combination would be incompatible with a career as an airline pilot, whereas it would hardly represent a handicap for a socially withdrawn, mildly retarded individual. Expectations and goals of the patient and family need to be carefully assessed and thoroughly discussed. The patient's motivation, willingness and ability to undergo the extensive evaluation process must be taken into consideration. Specific answers to the many questions concerning the overall incapacity imposed by seizures can often only be estimated during the initial interview but the issues usually become much clearer during the Phase I evaluation. Some of the specific issues will be discussed below when considering contraindications to surgery.

Early in the evaluation, after discussing the risks, goals, and options, the patient and/or the family are asked exactly what would be the effect of suddenly stopping seizures. Sometimes the results are surprising. A chronically unemployed middle-aged male patient with relatively mild partial seizures, after discussing the risks involved and the extensive presurgical evaluation required, was asked the question. He answered, quite sincerely, that elimination of seizures would allow him to learn how to scuba dive. When further questioning documented that this was indeed his compelling reason for seeking epilepsy surgery, he was dropped from the program. This is probably the most extreme inappropriate response we have encountered. A frequent response, particularly from teenagers, is that they would be able to drive. While this might be considered a trivial response, driving is an important function in our mobile society and, with our younger patients, there are strong peer-pressure implications. More mature responses include independence, employability, and improved social opportunities. A severely socially withdrawn, overly protected, and naive patient might anticipate that their life would suddenly blossom following successful epilepsy surgery. While improved lifestyle is one of the goals, unrealistic expectations must be discouraged. Parents of children with severe epilepsy with associated recurrent convulsive status epilepticus and frequent injury-producing falls hardly need be queried regarding the beneficial effects of seizure elimination. They will grasp at any straws. Rarely will surgery prove curative in these patients so, goals must be clearly defined.

Is there a reasonable chance the seizures originate in a surgically accessible region of the brain? While the answer to this question is one of the obvious goals of the entire presurgical evaluation, early predictions based on seizure descriptions and referral data are usually possible. If, for example, seizures are described as beginning with an unpleasant abdominal sensation, followed by loss of contact and aimless, semipurposeless activity preceding several minutes of confusion and the referral information contains descriptions of repeated EEGs demonstrating consistent anterior temporal sharp waves on one side, a reasonable assumption would be seizure origin in the medial temporal region. If similar seizures were described as beginning with sudden loss of vision or flashing colored lights a different assumption would be made [86] Conversely, if seizures are described as sudden stiffening of the body often resulting in falls, brief staring spells and recurrent convulsive episodes and prior EEGs demonstrate diffuse slow spike-wave complexes, the chance of finding a resectable focus would be remote. These initial findings affect the content of discussions with the patient and family and provide direction for subsequent evaluation. Results of the subsequent evaluation can, however, alter early assumptions.

Is the patient medically intractable? Defining medical intractability is not simple and will vary to some extent for each patient. In general, we consider patients medically intractable when reasonable trials of all major anticonvulsant drugs alone and in combination have failed to control incapacitating seizures. What are reasonable trials? Currently therapeutic serum anticonvulsant levels should be documented but a history of persistent seizures despite increasing a drug to clinical toxicity is considered adequate. Sufficient trial duration depends on seizure frequency. When seizures are occurring daily despite therapeutic drug levels, a month is enough time. Less frequent seizures will usually require longer. How many drugs should be tried and in what combinations has never been precisely defined. The current trend is towards monotherapy first, with a second drug added later, as necessary.

Some patients will develop allergic responses to some or even most anticonvulsant drugs and these usually cannot be used. Other patients cannot tolerate even modest doses of medications because of undesirable side effects. On the other hand, some patients are reluctant to take medications for various psychosocial reasons despite achieving complete seizure control when serum levels are in the therapeutic range. Poor compliance requires education, not presurgical evaluation. Seizure control at the expense of chronic disabling toxicity is not acceptable, particularly in patients who stand a good chance to benefit from surgery. Indeed, practitioners who refuse to consider the possibility of surgery while maintaining their patients on multiple drugs at toxic levels, despite poor seizure control, with the expectation that a new miracle drug is just over the horizon are often doing their patients a disservice.

In conclusion, medical intractability is determined combining experience with common sense. If there is any doubt that medical therapy has been sufficient, additional attempts at medical management are mandatory. The long waiting periods for evaluation in our program provide ample time for any medication adjustment. Occasionally this results in satisfactory seizure control. Unfortunately, this control is usually transient.

Are there contraindications to surgery? There are few absolute contraindications to surgery. Some are obvious such as the unlikely possibility that a patient referred for surgery is found to have primary generalized epilepsy. Patients with progressive incurable medical or neurologic diseases would be inappropriate surgical candidates. Active psychoses or severely disturbed behaviors are generally considered absolute contraindications since these patients would be incapable of cooperating during the extensive presurgical evaluation. A history of psychosis or unstable psychologic function are relative contraindications that need to be assessed individually.

Degree of mental retardation is an issue that is frequently raised in discussions of surgical candidacy. This issue encompasses social and ethical questions for which there are no standard answers. If mental retardation is equated with poor results following surgery, then surgery should be contraindicated in these patients. This seems to be the case in patients who have had corpus callosum section with low IQs [87]. Since our early experience with callosal section agrees with this observation we would not normally consider this procedure in patients with IQs of <50. Evaluation for resective surgery usually requires a certain amount of patient cooperation, particularly if intracranial electrodes are needed. If mental incapacity precludes cooperation, adequate evaluation may not be possible. While we use an IQ of 70 as a lower limit for resective surgery we recognize exceptions. For example, a patient with infantile hemiplegia, mental retardation, disruptive behavior, and severe epilepsy may experience dramatic improvement in cognitive and behavioral function as well as seizure control following functional hemispherectomy. Nor could it be justified to exclude surgery in a retarded patient in whom a probable causative mass lesion had been detected.

Age is another factor when considering patients for epilepsy surgery. Is there an upper age limit? Patients 50 years of age or older with lifelong histories of epilepsy are not likely to benefit much, even with successful epilepsy surgery. While we use the upper limit of 50 years of age as a relative contraindication for surgery, we again recognize exceptions. We used to consider 10 years of age as a lower limit for surgical evaluation but we no longer recognize lower age limits. When medically refractory seizures are documented in younger children, we now evaluate them for surgery. However, the criteria used to identify such children have not been firmly established. Patients with the various benign childhood epilepsy syndromes must be rigorously excluded. This is usually not a problem as such children have identifiable clinical seizure and EEG characteristics and rarely fail antiepileptic drug therapy. If, however, there is any doubt, surgical consideration is delayed.

Thus, while there are only a few absolute contraindications for epilepsy surgery, we recognize a number of relative contraindications. The degree that these factors will affect decisions concerning surgery will depend upon all of the circumstances of each patient's particular situation. Our aim is to be flexible and to avoid overly strict exclusion criteria. Demands upon limited resources and the time and expense involved in presurgical evaluation impose the possibility of preselection, favoring the younger, best candidates. Admittedly, these patients would benefit most from epilepsy surgery, the program statistics would be excellent, and the medical economists would be satisfied. We avoid exclusion criteria based on psychologic or economic issues and rely on accepted medical principles. Failure to do so would deprive many patients of procedures that may be of enormous benefit to them or their families. Successful epilepsy surgery does not equate with the patient obtaining a college degree or becoming a community leader. Furthermore, concentrating only on the most ideal surgical candidates would narrow our perspectives of epilepsy. The difficult challenging cases are the ones that teach us the most and broaden our understanding of epilepsy [88,89].

Epilepsy surgery conference

Upon the completion of Phase I each patient is formally presented at a weekly epilepsy surgery conference. Pertinent historical data, seizure descriptions, referral information, and physical findings are reviewed. Results of neuropsychologic testing and EEG monitoring are evaluated for lateralizing/localizing features and congruency. The psychiatric assessment, neuropsychologic testing and opinions of those who have interreacted with the patient and family are discussed in terms of general intelligence and ability to cooperate with and tolerate eventual procedures and evaluations. All neuroimaging studies are reviewed and compared to other findings. Videotaped seizures are examined for possible localizing or lateralizing clinical seizure characteristics.

Upon completion of the data review, discussions are held to determine if the patient is an appropriate candidate for surgery. If the decision is in favor, the second phase of the evaluation is scheduled. If there are controversies or inconsistencies, it may be necessary to repeat or expand certain aspects of the Phase I evaluation. If there are clear contraindications to surgery, the evaluation will be terminated.

After the second phase of evaluation has been completed, the patient is again discussed. We recognize that the intracarotid Amytal test is far from ideal, particularly with regard to memory function, but at present there are no accepted alternatives. We use the results of this procedure to direct subsequent evaluation. For example, if the results of the Phase I evaluation had suggested right temporal seizure origin but Amytal testing failed to demonstrate left memory, then our approach would have to be modified. Options in this situation would include repeating the Amytal test using incremental doses of Amytal, recommending bilateral intracranial electrode placements in a patient in whom intracranial recording might have been avoided or doing more extensive intracranial electrode placements than had previously been anticipated. The option selected would depend on previously accumulated data. Finding bilateral intact memory in a patient who had previously been thought to have seizures originating in either temporal lobe would also influence our decisions concerning the need for intracranial recording and the placement strategies concerning depth and subdural electrodes. Complete and repeated bilateral memory failure would cause us to pause before considering further presurgical evaluation in a patient with suspected temporal lobe seizure origin. Determination of side of language dominance is of obvious importance when considering the side and site of proposed surgery. The implications of detecting mixed cerebral dominance in a patient being considered for callosal section are discussed elsewhere in this volume.

After the results of the Phase II evaluation have been assessed and compared to the findings from Phase I, final decisions are made concerning the need for intracranial electrodes. Specific details of electrode type and placement strategies are described in Chapter 3. Some general considerations concerning intracranial electrodes are discussed below.

When intracranial recording is performed, the results from each patient are again discussed in the weekly epilepsy surgery conference. After reviewing all of the pertinent intracranial electroencephalographic data and comparing it with all of the other previously accumulated data, decisions are made concerning localization of seizure onset. If, at the end of this review, lateralization and localization cannot be achieved, several options are possible. If the patient has unlateralized, but predominantly frontally localized seizure activity, consideration is given to an anterior two-thirds corpus callosum section [90]. If the data strongly suggest lateralized but unlocalized seizure onset, the possibility of a second intracranial electrode exploration at another date is discussed. Similarly, if the seizures are unlocalized or unlateralized, but the clinical seizure characteristics strongly suggests a single region of seizure onset, consideration is also given to a second exploration. If there is no suggestion of possible localized onset to one region of the brain and if the seizure characteristics, both electrical and clinical, suggest multifocal onset in a pattern that would probably not benefit from callosal section then the patient is considered a localization failure and additional studies are not justified. Complete failure to localize after such extensive investigations represents one of the most frustrating experiences encountered, both for the patient and ourselves. As discussed previously, we continue to follow or at least keep track of these patients in the hopes that some future medical, surgical, or diagnostic development might prove beneficial.

Intracranial electrodes

The decision whether or not to use intracranial electrodes remains a controversial issue. Some programs use them scarcely at all and rely almost entirely on the findings from noninvasive evaluations, while others use intracranial recording on almost all patients. Proponents of intracranial recording state that this technique will allow patients to have surgery who would have otherwise been denied it, and that it will prevent surgery or indicate a different type of surgery in patients who otherwise would have undergone inappropriate operations. Those opposed to the extensive use of intracranial recording feel that most good surgical candidates can be selected on the basis of noninvasive studies and that depth electrode recordings are performed mainly on patients who are not very good surgical candidates. Depth electrode evaluations are also opposed because of the risk and tremendous time and expense involved. There must be some good middle ground. Contrary to publicized opinion, our program does not recommend depth electrode implantations for all patients being considered for epilepsy surgery. While admittedly, early in our program, almost all patients underwent depth electrode placements, significant advances in technology, namely neuroimaging, and experience gained over the past 19 years have caused us to change our strategies. While we still maintain a low threshold for intracranial electrode placement, we do recognize exceptions.

Surgical candidates not requiring depth electrodes

Mass lesions Small, well circumscribed, mass lesions are commonly detected using modern neuroimaging techniques. When such lesions are found in the course of evaluating patients with epilepsy and when the other findings are in general agreement with the location of the lesion, these patients go to surgery without intracranial monitoring. This assumes the lesion is not located in or near a critical area.

Large unilateral destructive lesions Patients with hemiplegia acquired early in life and disabling seizures present some special considerations. If the upper extremity is truly plegic with little or no useful hand and finger movement, these patients can proceed directly to surgery for a functional hemispherectomy. When the paresis is not complete and there is significant residual function in the distal upper extremity, hemispherectomy should be avoided. If, in this situation, the atrophic lesion is large or multifocal, a partial or complete callosal section may be recommended. This often produces surprisingly good results [90,91]. Some hemiparetic patients by virtue of lesion size or location or because of clinical seizure characteristics can benefit from localized excisions. However, these patients often require intracranial monitoring for a better definition of region of seizure origin.

Corpus callosotomy As noted above, some patients with incomplete infantile hemiplegia syndromes will benefit from callosal section. Corpus callosotomy will be recommended in other patients after intracranial monitoring has failed to demonstrate seizure localization. Some patients will have clearly unlocalized multifocal or diffuse epilepsy demonstrated during the initial phases of evaluation. We consider these patients for callosal section at the end of phase II. A more detailed discussion of the selection criteria used for callosal section is given in Chapter 4.

Localized resection without mass lesions In the past, we implanted depth electrodes in all those patients who did not have clear-cut lesions as the probable cause of their seizures. Years of experience and the introduction of new technology have changed our philosophy concerning patients with probable temporal lobe seizure origin. When history, clinical seizure characteristics, scalp EEG findings, and neuropsychologic studies are all clearly in agreement, these patients are considered for surgery without intracranial monitoring. If, in addition, the MRI demonstrates signal abnormalities in the correct mesial temporal region [92], intracranial electrodes are definitely not indicated. We consider this finding so important that its absence, i.e. perfectly normal appearing mesial temporal structures on MRI, will cause us to pause before recommending surgery without intracranial monitoring. When findings from any of the investigations are not congruent with a lateralized medial temporal onset, then we will recommend that the patient does not proceed directly to surgery. For example, a history of elementary visual symptoms preceding seizures many years previously, clearly more than one type of seizure, seizures not characteristic of temporal lobe origin, or neuropsychologic findings strongly suggesting abnormalities on the side opposite EEG localization would cause us to recommend intracranial monitoring.

Reasons for intracranial monitoring

Patients with temporal lobe-type seizures Reasons for implanting electrodes in patients with complex partial seizures of presumed temporal lobe origin can be adduced from the preceding discussion on why we do not implant some of these patients. While, admittedly, as previously mentioned, our threshold for recommending intracranial monitoring is low, there is a reason for this. We have found that when findings are divergent in any way, the potential for unexpected findings from intracranial monitoring is high.

Patients with suspected extratemporal seizure origin In the absence of an unequivocal circumscribed lesion as the probable cause of seizures, patients with suspected extratemporal seizure origin have intracranial electrode placements. The only exception from our program was a young patient with chronic encephalitis of the Rasmussen type who underwent a local cortical resection for epilepsy partialis continua. Indeed, even with the increased awareness of extratemporal epilepsy, and the use of intracranial monitoring to study these patients, accurate localization often proves elusive. These patients constitute a challenge for the next decade.

Patients with lesions The need to study some patients with large atrophic lesions was previously mentioned. Basically this occurs when the patient has considerable residual function of the involved side and the goal is to perform a limited resection. Intracranial electrodes are indicated for two reasons when well circumscribed mass lesions are detected: (1) if the lesion lies in or near a critical area, a grid of subdural electrodes is placed over the lesion and the critical area with additional electrodes placed as indicated, allowing both detailed extraoperative functional mapping of the area of concern and the detection of the region of seizure origin in relationship to the lesion; and (2) when the data obtained during Phase I and II of the evaluation are not congruous or extremely confusing. In this situation, the lesion may not be the cause of the seizures or the lesion may be precipitating the seizures by unexpected means. For example, a deep-seated right frontal lesion might be an incidental finding in a patient with left medial temporal epilepsy or a parietal lesion might be responsible for producing seizures that have the appearance of bilateral independent temporal lobe epilepsy.

Justification for intracranial electrodes

Risk is often mentioned as mitigating against the use of intracranial electrodes. While risks exist and cannot be eliminated, they must be taken into perspective. Hemorrhage is the most significant risk associated with depth electrodes. We have had intracerebral hemorrhages develop in three patients within the first 12 hours of electrode placement. In one, hemorrhage resulted in permanent disabling neurologic deficits, while in the other two, neurologic impairment was transient, followed by complete recovery. Hemorrhage with serious consequences is therefore a risk, but a small one. Infection is another potential complication of intracranial electrode monitoring. While we have documented infection in approximately 15 patients, it has always been due to an opportunistic organism; has always occurred at the time of electrode removal; and has always responded rapidly to antibiotics. We have had no intracerebral abscess although one patient may have had mild cerebritis. Complications from subdural electrodes also occur. Hemorrhage is probably less likely than with depth electrodes and we have not detected hemorrhage in any of our patients. The occurrence of a subdural hemorrhage at another medical center has been reported but this was associated with an early, fairly rigid, subdural grid electrode. Infection has also been reported and it has occurred in one of our patients. As with the other infections, it responded promptly to antibiotics. Another patient developed cerebral edema following a rather extensive bilateral subdural electrode placement necessitating premature electrode removal. Thus, with one exception, complications have not been a factor in terms of producing permanent residual neurologic deficits in our program.

Time and expense are often cited as undesirable features of intracranial recording. We will certainly attest to the considerable time and energy that must be devoted to these patients. The overall expense, however, is usually less than that of coronary bypass surgery. Considering the relative, and in many cases, the absolute young age of these patients and the high success rate of epilepsy surgery, one can hardly argue that it is not justified on the basis of expense.

Conclusion

The West Haven VA/Yale–New Haven Epilepsy Surgery Program began in 1971 and evolved over the next 19 years. We started with three interested physicians, a few nurses, and one EEG technician. Currently, over 40 people are directly involved with the program, providing patient care and conducting clinical and basic research. Initially, only a few patients were evaluated for surgery each year while now we do six to eight Phase I evaluations and three to four Phase III evaluations per month. Although the basic scheme of the evaluation process has remained the same, methodology, goals, and approaches have changed to reflect new technology and accumulated experience.

Epilepsy surgery programs provide a unique opportunity for research [93]. Indeed, prolific research activity is an integral part of most well established epilepsy surgery programs as witnessed in the proceedings of national and international epilepsy conferences during the past few years. Clinical and research efforts from the numerous programs unquestionably enhance our knowledge of epilepsy but these efforts also provide fuel for controversy. Prefacing the publication from the 1986 Palm Desert Epilepsy Surgery Symposium, Dr Jerome Engel concluded "... that efforts must be directed toward defining the specific indications for particular diagnostic tests and surgical procedures rather than attempting to prove general superiority of one over another." [94]. We thoroughly agree.

References

1 McNaughton FL, Rasmussen T. Criteria for Selection of Patients for Neurosurgical Treatment. *Advances in Neurology* No. 8. Raven Press, New York, 1975, pp 37–48.

2 Jackson JH. On the anatomical, physiological, and pathological investigation of epilepsies. *West Riding Lunatic Asylum Medical Reports.* 1873; **3**: 315. Reprinted in J Taylor (ed) *Selected Writings of John Hughlings Jackson.* Hodder and Stoughton, London, 1931, pp 90–111.

3 Horsley, Sir V. Brain Surgery *Br Med J* 1986; **2**: 670–675.

4 Penfield W, Jasper H, *Epilepsy and the Functional Anatomy of the Human Brain.* Little, Brown, Boston, 1954.

5 McNaughton FL. Observations on diagnosis and treatment. In Penfield W, Jasper H (eds) *Epilepsy and the Functional Anatomy of the Human Brain.* Little, Brown, Boston, 1954, pp 540–568.

6 Falconer MA, Taylor DC. Temporal lobe epilepsy: clinical features, pathology, diagnosis and treatment. In Price JH (ed) *Modern Trends in Psychological Medicine.* Butterworth, London, 1970, pp 346–373.

7 Walker E. Surgery for epilepsy. In Vinken, Bruyn (eds) *Handbook of Clinical Neurology,* Vol. 15, 1974, p 739.

8 Green JR. Surgical treatment of epilepsy during childhood and adolescence. *Surg Neurol* 1977; **8**: 71–80.

9 Jensen I. Temporal lobe epilepsy: on whom to operate and when. In Penry JK (ed) *VIIIth Epilepsy International Symposium.* Raven Press, New York, 1977, pp 325–331.

10 Glaser GH. Treatment of intractable temporal lobe–limbic epilepsy (complex partial seizures) by temporal lobectomy. *Ann Neurol* 1980; **8**: 455–459.

11 Delgado-Escueta AV, Treiman DM, Walsh GO. The treatable epilepsies. Part I. *New Eng J Med* 1983; **308**: 1508–1514.

12 Delgado-Escueta AV, Treiman DM, Walsh GO. The treatable epilepsies. Part II. *New Eng J Med*

1983; **308**: 1576–1584.

13 Delgado-Escueta AV, Walsh GO. The selection process for surgery of intractable complex partial seizures: surface EEG and depth electrography. *ARNMD US* 1983; **61**: 295–326.

14 Ward AA, Jr. Perspectives for surgical therapy of epilepsy. *ARNMD US* 1983; **61**: 371–390.

15 Elwes RDC, Johnson AL, Shorvon SD, Reynolds EH. (1984): The prognoses for seizure control in newly diagnosed epilepsy. *New Eng J Med* 1984; **311**: 944–947.

16 Sammaritano M, de Lotbiniere A, Andermann F, Olivier A, Gloor P, Quesney LF. False lateralization by surface EEG of seizure onset in patients with temporal lobe epilepsy and gross focal cerebral lesions. *Epilepsia* 1984; **25**: 664–665.

17 Morrell F. Secondary epileptogenesis in man. *Arch Neurol* 1985; **42**: 318–335.

18 Oliver A, Gloor P, Andermann F, Ives J. Occipitotemporal epilepsy studied with stereotaxically implanted depth electrodes and successfully treated by temporal resection. *Ann Neurol* 1982; **11**: 428–432.

19 Engel J, Jr, Crandall PH. Falsely localizing ictal onsets during depth EEG telemetry during anticonvulsant withdrawal. *Epilepsia* 1983; **24**: 344–355.

20 Ochs R, Gloor P, Quesney LF, Ives J, Olivier A. Does head-turning during a seizure have lateralizing or localizing significance? *Neurology* 1984; **34**: 884–890.

21 Wyllie E, Lüders H, Morris HH, Lesser R, Dinner DS. The lateralizing significance of versive head and eye movements during epileptic seizures. *Program American Epilepsy Society Annual Meeting, New York* Am. Epilepsy Soc, 1985, p 50. Abstract.

22 Remillard GM, Andermann F, Rhisausi A, Robbins N. Facial asymmetry in patients with temporal lobe epilepsy. A clinical sign useful in the lateralization of temporal epileptogenic foci. *Neurology* 1977; **27**: 109–114.

23 Remillard GM, Ethier R, Andermann F. Temporal lobe epilepsy and perinatal occlusion of the posterior cerebral artery. *Neurology* 1974; **23**: 1001–1009.

24 Rasmussen T. Hemispherectomy for seizures revisited. (The 1982 Penfield lecture.) *Can J Neurol Sci* 1983; **10**: 71–78.

25 Tinuper P, Andermann F, Villemure J-G, Rasmussen TB, Quesney LF, Avoli M. Current status of hemispherectomy for seizures. XVIth *Epilepsy International Symposium*, Hamburg, 1985. Abstract.

26 Penfield WP, Ward A. Calcifying epileptogenic lesions; hemangioma calcificans. Report of a case. *Arch Neurol Psychol* 1948; **60**: 20–36.

27 Falconer MA, Serafetinides FA, Corsellis JAN. Etiology and pathogenesis of temporal lobe epilepsy. *Arch Neurol* 1964; **10**: 233–248.

28 Sammaritano M, Andermann F, Melanson D, Guberman A, Tinuper P, Gastaut H. The syndrome of epilepsy and bilateral occipital cortical calcification. In: *1985 Program American Epilepsy Society Annual Meeting, New York.* Am. Epilepsy Soc., 1985.

29 Wyler AR, Bolender NF. Preoperative CT diagnosis of mesial temporal sclerosis for surgical treatment of epilepsy. *Ann Neurol* 1983; **13**: 59–64.

30 Kuzniecky R, De La Sayette V, Ethier R, Melanson D, Robitaille Y, Andermann F, Berkovic S, Olivier A, Feindel W. Magnetic resonance imaging in temporal lobe epilepsy: pathological correlations. *Ann Neurol* 1987; **22**: 341–347.

31 Berkovic S, Andermann F, Ethier R, Melanson D, Robitaille Y, Kuzniecky R, Peters T, Olivier A, Feindel W Hippocampal sclerosis in temporal lobe epilepsy demonstrated by magnetic resonance imaging. *Ann Neurol.* In press.

32 Marciani MG, Gotman J, Andermann F, Olivier A. Patterns of seizure activation after withdrawal of antiepileptic medication. *Neurology* 1985; **35**: 1537–1543.

33 Engel J, Jr, Crandall P, Rausch R. The partial epilepsies. In Rosenberg RN, Grossman RG, Schochet S, Heinz ER, Willis D (eds) *The Clinical Neurosciences*, Vol. 2, Churchill Livingstone, Edinburgh, 1983, pp 39–80.

34 Sadler RM, Blume WT. Co-occurrence of temporal epileptiform potentials and generalized spike wave discharges. *Epilepsia* 1984; **25**: 654.

35 Ludwig B, Ajmone Marsan C, Van Buren J. Cerebral seizures of probable orbitofrontal origin. *Epilepsia* 1975; **16**: 141–158.

36 Williamson PD, Spencer SS, Spencer DD, Mattson RH. (1981): Complex partial seizures with occipital lobe epilepsy. *Epilepsia* 1981; **22**: 247–248.

37 Taylor L. Psychological assessment of neurosurgical patients. In Rasmussen TB, Marino R (eds) *Functional Neurosurgery*. Raven Press, New York, 1979, pp 165–180.

38 Milner B. Hemispheric specialization: scope and limits. In Schmidt FO, Worden FG (eds) *The Neurosciences: Third Study Program*. MIT Press, Boston, 1974.

39 Engel J, Jr, Kuhl DE, Phelps ME, Crandall PH. (1982): Comparative localization of epileptic foci in partial epilepsy by PET and EEG. *Ann Neurol* 1982; **12**: 529–537.

40 Engel J, Jr, Kuhl DE, Phelps ME. Functional imaging of the epileptic brain with positron emission tomography. In: Rose FC (ed) *Research Progress in Epilepsy*. Pitman, London, 1983, pp 301–314.

41 Yamamoto YL, Ochs RF, Gloor P, Ammann W, Meyer E, Evans AC, Cooke B, Sako K, Gotman J, Feindel W, Diksic M, Thompson CJ, Robitaille Y. Patterns of rCBF and focal energy metabolic changes in relation to EEG abnormality in the interictal phase of partial epilepsy. In Baldy Moulinier M, Ingvar DH, Meldrum BS (eds) *Current Problems in Epilepsy: Cerebral Blood Flow, Metabolism and Epilepsy*. John Libbey, London, 1983, pp 51–62.

42 Gotman, J. Measurement of small time differences between EEG channels: method and application to epileptic seizure propagation. *EEG Clin Neurophys* 1983; **54**: 501–514.

43 Savard G, Andermann F, Remillard GM, Olivier A. Post-ictal psychosis following partial complex seizures is analogous to Todd's paralysis. *XVIth Epilepsy International Symposium*, Hamburg, 1985. Abstract.

44 Savard G, Andermann F, Olivier A. The disinhibition syndrome: a behavioural disorder in patients with severe bitemporal epilepsy. *XVIth Epilepsy International Symposium*, Hamburg. 1985. Abstract.

45 Jensen I, Larsen JK. Mental aspects of temporal lobe epilepsy. Follow-up of 74 patients after resection of a temporal lobe. *J Neurol Neurosurg Psychiat*. 1979; **42**: 256–265.

46 Taylor DC, Falconer MA. Clinical, socio-economic and psychological changes after temporal lobectomy for epilepsy. *Br J Psychiatry* 1968; **114**: 1247–1261.

47 Taylor DC. Mental state and temporal lobe epilepsy. *Epilepsia* 1972; **13**: 727–765.

48 Rasmussen TB. Surgical aspects of temporal lobe epilepsy. Results and problems. *Acta Neurochir Wien* (Suppl) 1980; **30**: 113–116.

49 Rasmussen T. (1983): Cortical resection in children with focal epilepsy. In Parsonage M, Grant R, Craig AG, and Ward A (eds) *Advances in Epileptology. XIVth Epilepsy International Symposium*. Raven Press, New York, 1983, pp 249–254.

50 Rasmussen TB. Surgical treatment of complex partial seizures. Results, lessons, and problems. *Epilepsia* 1983; **24** (Suppl 1): 65–76.

51 Rausch R, Crandall PH. Psychological status related to surgical control of temporal lobe seizures. *Epilepsia* 1982; **23**: 191–202.

52 Wieser HG, Yasargil MG. Selective amygdalohippocampectomy as a surgical treatment of mesiobasal limbic epilepsy. *Surg Neurol* 1982; **17**: 445–457.

53 Wieser HG. Selective amygdalohippocampectomy: Indications, investigative techniques and results. In Symon L *et al.* (eds) *Adv Technol Neurosurg* Vol. 13, Springer, Vienna, 1986.

54 Andermann F. Selection and investigation of candidates for surgical treatment of temporal lobe epilepsy in childhood and adolescence. In Blaw M, Rapin L, Kinsbourne M (eds) *Topics in Child Neurology*. Spectrum, Englewood Cliffs, NJ, 1977, pp 167–171.

55 Falconer MA. Place of surgery for temporal lobe epilepsy during childhood. *Br Med J* 1972; **2**: 631–636.

56 Lindsay J, Ounsted C, Richards P. The long-term outcome in children with temporal lobe seizures. I. Social outcome and childhood factors. *Dev Med Child Neurol* 1979; **21**: 285–298.

57 Lindsay J, Ounsted C, Richards P. The long-term outcome in children with temporal lobe seizures. II. Marriage, parenthood, and sexual indifference. *Dev Med Child Neurol* 1979; **21**: 433–440.

58 Lindsay J, Ounsted C, Richards P. The long-term outcome in children with temporal lobe seizures. III. Psychiatric aspects in childhood and adult life. *Dev Med Child Neurol* 1979; **21**: 630–636.

59 Perot P, Weir B, Rasmussen T. Tuberous sclerosis: surgical therapy for seizures. *Arch Neurol* 1966; **15**: 498–506.

60 Andermann F, Olivier A, Melanson D, and Robitaille Y. Focal cortical dysplasia, macrogyria, and epilepsy: a study of 15 patients. *XVIth Epilepsy International Symposium*, Hamburg, 1985. Abstract.

61 Rasmussen T, Mathieson G, Leblanc F. Surgical therapy of typical and a forme fruste variety

of the Sturge–Weber syndrome. *Arch Suisses Neurol Neurochir Psychiat* 1972; **111**: 393–409.
62 Hoffman HJ, Hendrick EB, Dennis M, Armstrong D. Hemispherectomy for Sturge–Weber syndrome. *Child's Brain* 1979; **5**: 233–248.
63 Taylor DC, Falconer MA, Bruton CJ, Corsellis NA. Focal dysplasia of cerebral cortex in epilepsy. *J Neurol Neurosurg Psychiat* 1971; **34**: 369–387.
64 Silfvenius H, Blom S, Zetterlund B, Sourander P, Nordborg C. Mild cortical dysplasia in patients with intractable seizure: early surgical results. *XVIth Epilepsy International Symposium*, Hamburg, 1985. Abstract.
65 Sourander P, Nordborg C, Silfvenius H, Blom S, Zetterlund B. Mild cortical dysplasia with intractable seizures: histological studies on 10 cases. *XVIth Epilepsy International Symposium*, Hamburg, 1985. Abstract.
66 Rasmussen TB, McCann W. Clinical studies of patients with focal epilepsy due to "chronic encephalitis". *Trans Am Neurol Assoc* 1968; **93**: 89–94.
67 Mattson RH. Value of intensive monitoring. In Wada JA, Penry JK (eds) *Advances in epileptology. Xth Epilepsy International Symposium*. Raven Press, New York, 1980, pp 43–51.
68 Gumnit RJ (ed). *Advances in Neurology: Intensive Neurodiagnostic Monitoring*. Raven Press, New York, 1980, 309 pp.
69 Porter RJ. Methodology of continuous monitoring with videotape recording and electroencephalography. In: Wada JA, Penry JK (eds) *Advances in Epileptology. Xth Epilepsy International Symposium*. Raven Press, New York, 1980, pp 35–42.
70 Fay ML, Mattson RH. Clinical testing during intensive monitoring of ictal events. In: Wada JA, Penry JK (eds). *Advances in Epileptology. Xth Epilepsy International Symposium*. Raven Press, New York, 1980, pp 65–68.
71 Bracchi M, Battaglia G. Neuroradiology in epilepsy. In: Broggi G (ed) *The Rational Basis of the Surgical Treatment of Epilepsies*. John Libbey, London, New York, 1988, pp 103–106.
72 Rich KM, Goldring S, Gado M. Computed tomography in chronic seizure disorder caused by glioma. *Arch Neurol* 1985; **42**: 26–27.
73 Sperling MR, Sutherling WW, Nuwer MR. New techniques for evaluating patients for epilepsy surgery. In: Engel J (ed) *Surgical Treatment of the Epilepsies*. Raven Press, New York, 1987, pp 235–257.
74 Theodore WH, Dorwart R, Holmes M, Porter RJ, DiChiro G. Neuroimaging in refractory partial seizures: comparison of PET, CT and MRI. *Neurology* 1986; **36**: 750–759.
75 Boon PA, Williamson PD, Fried I, Spencer DD, Novelly RA. Intracranial intraaxial space-occupying lesions in patients with intractable partial seizures. *Epilepsia* 1988; **29**: 672–673.
76 Daumas-Duport C, Monsaingeon V, Vedrenne C, Munari C, Bancaud J, Chodkiewicz JP. Complex neuroepithelial tumors in epilepsy surgery. A series of 20 cases. In Broggi G (ed) *The Rational Basis of the Surgical Treatment of Epilepsies*. John Libbey, London 1988, pp 149–167.
77 Spencer DD, Spencer SS, Mattson RH, Williamson PD. Intracerebral masses in patients with intractable partial epilepsy. *Neurology* 1984; **34**: 432–436.
78 Gumnit RJ. Postscript: Who should be referred for surgery?. In Engel J (ed) *Surgical Treatment of the Epilepsies*. Raven Press, New York, 1987, pp 71–74.
79 Rausch R. Psychological evaluation. In Engel J (ed) *Surgical Treatment of the Epilepsies*. Raven Press, New York, 1987, pp 181–195.
80 Darcey TM, Williamson PD. Computer system for automated seizure detection, recording, and reformatting. In Wolf P, Dam M, Janz D, Dreifuss FE (eds) *Advances in Epileptology* Vol 16. Raven Press, New York, 1987, pp 269–272.
81 Lesser RP, Luders H, Klem G, Dinner DS, Morris HH, Hahn JF, Wyllie E. Extraoperative cortical functional localization in patients with epilepsy. In Whitaker HA (ed) *Studies in Neuropsychology*. Erlbaum Assoc, Hillsdale NJ, 1985.
82 Luders H, Lesser RP, Dinner DS, Morris HH, Hahn JF, Friedman L, Skipper G, Wyllie E, Friedman D. Commentary: chronic intracranial recording and stimulation with subdural electrodes. In Engel J, Jr (ed) *Surgical Treatment of the Epilepsies*. Raven Press, New York, 1987, pp 297–321.
83 McCarthy GM, Darcey TM, Wood CC, Williamson PD, Spencer DD. Asymmetries in scalp and intracranial endogenous ERPs in patients with complex partial epilepsy. In Engel J, Ojemann GA, Luders HO, Williamson PD (eds) *Fundamental Mechanisms of Human Brain Function*. Raven Press, New York, 1987, pp 51–59.
84 McCarthy GM, Wood CC, Williamson PD,

Spencer DD. Task-dependent field potentials in human hippocampal formation. *J Neuroscience*, submitted.
85 Meador KJ, Loring DW, King DW, Gallagher BB, Gould MJ, Flanigan HF, Smith JR. Limbic evoked potentials predict site of epileptic focus. *Neurology* 1987; **37**: 494–497.
86 Williamson PD, Spencer SS. Clinical and EEG features of complex partial seizures of extratemporal origin. *Epilepsia* 1986; **27** (Suppl 2): S46–S63.
87 Wilson DH, Reeves AG, Gazzaniga MS. "Central" commissurotomy for intractable generalized epilepsy: series two. *Neurology* 1980; **32**: 687–697.
88 Williamson PD. The symptomatic localization-related epilepsies — problems with subclassification. *Yale J Biol* 1987; **60**(2): 60–77.
89 Williamson PD. Frontal lobe seizures: problems with diagnosis and classification. In Delgado-Escueta AV (ed) *Frontal Lobe Seizures and Epilepsies*. Raven Press, New York. In Press.
90 Williamson PD. Corpus callosum section for intractable epilepsy. In Reeves AG (ed) *Epilepsy and the Corpus Callosum*. Plenum Press, New York, 1985, pp 243–257.
91 Goodman RN, Williamson PD, Reeves AG, Spencer SS, Spencer DD, Mattson RH, Roberts DW. Interhemispheric commissurotomy for congenital hemiplegics with intractable epilepsy. *Neurology* 1985; **35**: 1351–1354.
92 McLachlan RS, Black S, Nicholson RL, Blume T. Nuclear magnetic resonance, a new approach to the investigation of refractory temporal lobe epilepsy. *Epilepsia* 1985; **26**: 555–562.
93 Engel J, Ojemann GA, Luders HO, Williamson PD (eds) *Fundamental Mechanisms of Human Brain Function*. Raven Press, New York, 1987, 288 pp.
94 Engel J (ed) Preface. In *Surgical Treatment of the Epilepsies*. Raven Press, New York, 1987, pp v–vi.

Comment

Susan S. Spencer

This chapter addresses patient selection criteria for resective procedures. Dr Andermann gives an excellent overview which discusses all the issues surrounding, preceding and following upon consideration, evaluation and performance of resective procedures for uncontrolled epilepsy. His literature review and his guiding comments reflect decades of experience and constitute pearls of wisdom which even seasoned epilepsy surgeons and neurologists would do well to heed. Entwined in this discussion of issues is a description of the methods by which surgical candidates for resection are evaluated at the MNI. Dr Williamson describes, with a more restricted approach, details of testing at another center.

Both authors provide a contrast between the two centers that are perhaps the most divergent with respect to patient evaluation, yet what emerges is the number of similarities in philosophy. Initial patient selection and its dependence upon seizure characteristics, lifestyle, IQ, age, diagnosis, etiology, and examination is approached in much the same way. Neither author can give a set of rules as to the candidates to select, but both provide insights into the issues to be considered. Neuropsychologic examination, CT, and MRI are important localizing studies at each center.

The divergence occurs with respect to electrographic criteria considered imperative in presurgical evaluation and determination of resective candidates. While the MNI may utilize repeated scalp EEGs incorporating sphenoidal electrodes but not intensive monitoring in rare situations, Yale demands intensive monitoring of seizures and may not use sphenoidal electrodes, yet intensive monitoring for seizure onset is also done at MNI in most instances. Both centers indicate situations in which intracranial monitoring is considered essential, but the threshold is clearly lower at Yale than in Montreal. Either subdural or depth EEG may be employed at either of these centers.

Other epilepsy surgery centers fall somewhere between these two extremes. They may always require intensive monitoring of seizure onset with scalp electrodes more often than MNI, but use intracranial electrodes less often than Yale. Not all centers use depth or subdural electrodes but may prefer or restrict intracranial study to one or the other. These issues are discussed in more detail in Chapter 3. All agree, however, that convergence of localizing information from multiple diagnostic studies enables surgery without intracranial monitoring in some patients.

Neither author addresses patient-outcome directly. Multiple reports indicate 60–90% excellent results after resective procedures for uncontrolled epilepsy. Excellent results are defined as no seizures or only auras with at least 2 year follow-up. Although it might be anticipated that results would depend on the exact criteria for patient selection and on the surgical approach used, so far reported results are much the same regardless of these variables. More recent reports indicate improved response-rate suggesting more expertise as experience is gained in patient selection. Less rigid criteria for patient selection diminish the excellent response rate at some institutions. The recent advent of revised surgical approaches may provide some more variability, but additional reports and longer follow-up are needed. Similarly, combinations of intracranial recording methods may eventually be shown to enable more precise patient selection for cure.

As Dr Andermann points out, strict patient selection criteria may also deprive some patients from an improvement, if not cure, of their uncontrolled seizure disorder. Further definition of the goals and mechanisms of follow-up procedures are essential. In the future, technologic and conceptual advances in localization by electrical, clinical and imaging studies as well as advances in diagnosis hold the promise of streamlined evaluation, decreased risk, decreased cost, and increased efficacy. We agree that prevention and genetic approaches may become important in the future, but we suspect that uncontrolled epilepsy of a focal, potentially resectable, nature is here to stay.

chapter 3

Intracranial Recording

Susan S. Spencer

Indications

Chapter 2 illustrates the manner in which the evaluation methods for epilepsy surgery at various centers employ similar techniques with uniform standards of interpretation, which are then combined to determine the need for further evaluation and suitability of the patient for surgery. Centers may, however, differ with respect to the exact criteria for final decisions in these two regards. These differences often evolve from the experience and facilities at a given institution. Nevertheless, uniform agreement exists that multiple methods of localization should be concordant with EEG localization to a specific cerebral area for the decision to proceed to a resective surgical procedure. If precise localization is elusive because scalp EEG does not localize sufficiently or because other localizing studies disagree, but seizures are stereotyped and a single localization of origin is suspected, further evaluation is necessary to consider surgery. This usually involves intracranial recording of EEG activity [1–3].

Implantation of intracranial electrodes always follows extensive prior evaluation from which the sites for electrode placement are derived. (It is generally assumed that, in situations where no localizing criteria provide any guidance, intracranial investigation will also be fruitless. Although occasional study is performed in such patients, the benefit : risk ratio must be carefully assessed.) The prior evaluation is described in detail in Chapter 2.

Intracranial EEG may be studied by depth (intracerebral) or subdural or epidural electrode implantation for chronic or acute recording. Although interictal localization of spikes is often more valuable than ictal localization from scalp EEG, the ictal recording is preferred for intracranial EEG localization. Since acute recording usually cannot encompass ictal events, chronic recording is preferred and will be exclusively addressed in this chapter.

Some authors list specific criteria for one or another intracranial recording method [2]. In my view, with the presently available published information, such distinctions are often arbitrary. In this chapter, I will describe the electrodes used for depth, subdural, and epidural recording, the implantation techniques, risks, technical aspects of recording, interpretation, and results. Especially with respect to results, every attempt will be made to contrast these intracranial recording methods to obtain a set of recommendations with as much specificity as present literature permits.

Electrodes

Depth electrodes

Construction Electrodes for implantation within the brain may be constructed of platinum, stainless steel, platinum–iridium alloys, or gold, but silver is toxic to the brain and should not be employed [4,5]. These electrodes are often constructed in the laboratory associated with an individual program to meet certain specifications, but several varieties are commercially available. Diameters vary from 0.5 mm to 3.0 mm. The shaft of these electrodes must be very smooth and the tip blunt, to prevent tissue and vascular trauma during insertion. Depth electrodes may provide bipolar recording from two nearby contacts at the tip of the electrode, usually on two separate wires, or multiple recording sites at predetermined distances along the entire length or part of the length of the electrode [2]. Multicontact electrodes are created by removing insulation at specific contact points on each of the multiple wires used to create a composite electrode (6–18, usually) or by wrapping stainless steel "collars" at specific distances along a polyurethane catheter, which connect to an equivalent number of stainless steel wires running along the inside of the catheter. Since these contacts are small, they record from a limited area. As such, they are capable of precise localization, but can "miss" seizure onsets that occur at only small distances from the contacts.

Depending on the metals and insulation used and their thicknesses, but mostly on the method of construction, depth electrodes may be flexible or rigid. Flexible electrodes are inserted by means of an introducer, which has traditionally been located alongside the electrode itself. Prior teaching held that placement of rigid electrodes was somewhat more accurate because the tip of the flexible electrode might be pulled back slightly from its target area with removal of the introducer, a process not required with rigid electrode placement. Recent modifications in electrode construction, however, have focused on this difficulty with flexible electrodes by placing the introducer along the central hollow shaft of the polyurethane catheter, around which the electrode contacts are located.

Implantation Depth electrodes are usually placed bilaterally in preselected sites dictated by the earlier patient evaluation. Most commonly, temporal lobe structures are studied in patients with bitemporal scalp EEG abnormalities. In these situations, because the hippocampus has been implicated as the site of pathology in most patients with temporal lobe epilepsy [6] depth electrodes are inserted into the hippocampal and amygdalar areas through lateral or posterior approaches. When the lateral approach is used, six to eight recording sites along the electrode allow simultaneous recording of lateral temporal (neocortical) and medial temporal (hippocampal) activity along the same anterior–posterior plane, and multiple such electrodes will be placed to sample along the anterior–posterior dimension of the temporal lobe.

The posterior approach allows from eight to 18 medial recording sites, giving a more complete study of the anterior–posterior hippocampal electrical activity, but prevents simultaneous sampling of temporal neocortical structures with the same electrode.

Areas of frontal, parietal, and occipital lobes are similarly selected for study, based on previous localizing information. Structures within these lobes (akin to the hippocampus in temporal lobe epilepsy) are not specifically targeted, since the pathophysiologic substrate of extratemporal epilepsy has yet to be defined. Rather, imaging abnormalities or clinical characteristics of seizures often guide the sites of extratemporal electrode placement.

Implantation of depth electrodes is done under local or general anesthesia through twist drill holes or burr holes. When general anesthesia is employed, patients are awakened for actual electrode placement after coordinates and bone manipulation are complete, in order to allow early detection of major vascular complications. Stereotactic techniques employ the Todd Well's frame, the Lexell frame, computed tomography (CT) or magnetic resonance imaging (MRI). Electrodes are secured to the scalp or bone, or to an acrylic block fashioned for these purposes, and then connected to cables which are fixed to the scalp.

Subdural and epidural electrodes

Construction Subdural and epidural electrodes are also commercially available. Most common are strips (4–16 contacts) or grids (8 × 8 matrix) or round stainless steel contacts, each 5 mm–10 mm in diameter, embedded in silastic sheets [4]. Usually, contact points are separated by 10 mm. The electrode array can be cut and fashioned to cover the appropriate area. Less frequently, catheter-like subdural electrodes have been employed, consisting of multiple stainless steel contacts banded along the outside of a polyurethane catheter [2]. Since the contacts are slightly larger in subdural electrodes, compared to depth electrodes, they record from a slightly greater volume of brain.

Implantation Contrary to depth electrode techniques, subdural and epidural electrode arrays are often placed unilaterally, implying that localization has been narrowed down to one hemisphere and usually part of one hemisphere. Lately, bilateral (usually temporal) placement has been used [7]. Because hippocampal onset is associated with most cases of drug-resistant temporal lobe epilepsy, more medial temporal lobe placement of subdural grids has also been advocated [7]. Subdural and epidural electrodes are placed under general anesthesia through craniectomized burr holes (for strips) or a craniotomy (for grids). The silastic is secured to the dura and the wire cable from the grid or strip is secured to the scalp, to which it may exit through a separate stab incision. The bone may be replaced immediately or after grid removal.

Combined placement

When depth electrodes are used, particularly in temporal lobe study, and are placed with posterior approaches, simultaneous subdural electrodes may also be implanted to allow study of the temporal neocortex [8,9]. Lateral placement of depth electrodes allows simultaneous sampling of a limited number of locations in the temporal neocortex. Combinations of depth and subdural electrodes have been described to achieve what is thought to be the best study of areas suspected of seizure onset. These combined studies follow the same general placement protocols and have no greater risks than the individual studies combined, but obviously lengthen the time required for implantation.

Risks

Depth electrodes

Sixteen major complications of depth electrodes have been reported in the world literature, which includes 1 141 individuals undergoing such study [10]. This gives an incidence rate of 1.5% of major complications. More than 60% were intracranial hemorrhages, some followed by persistent neurologic deficit, and two patients died. Accepted practice dictates avoiding drugs which may affect platelet function, such as aspirin or valproic acid, for at least 2 weeks prior to implantation of depth electrodes or until the bleeding time is normal. Infectious complications are not as common after depth electrode implantation (three of 16 major complications reported), but Jakob–Creutzfeldt disease may be transmitted by intracerebral electrodes, which should therefore be suitably sterilized or preferably regarded as disposable. Minimal headache or other symptoms accompany depth electrode procedures acutely in the absence of other major complications, and patients are usually asymptomatic within 24 hours of implantation.

Subdural and epidural electrodes

Of 247 subdural and epidural studies reported in the world literature, five patients had major complications, which gives an incidence rate of 2% [10]. No hemorrhages, persistent deficits, or deaths have been reported after these studies. Cerebral edema appears to complicate the placement of large grids, an observation causing us to replace the bone flap only after the study is complete. Most major complications after subdural electrode implantation are caused by infections. Despite the lack of reported hemorrhage or slow virus transmission, precautions as for depth electrode implantation are recommended. Subacute headache, nausea, vomiting, and anorexia are common after subdural grid implantation and last for approximately 48 hours.

Technical aspects of recording

Montage selection

Intracranial electrodes should be employed in accordance with guidelines for patients with indwelling devices (Underwriters Laboratory-type A patient). Electrode impedances can be safely checked, after insertion, with currents in the range of 10 nA. Integrity of cables should be verified prior to insertion [2,3].

Depending on the number of contacts and the recording system available, it may not be possible to record continuously from all available contacts. All contacts are initially screened using referential and bipolar derivations, and those with maximal interictal activity, plus some sampling of each implanted electrode, are incorporated into an initial montage for continuous monitoring. Both deep (intracranial) and surface (subdural, epidural or, in their absence, scalp) sampling should be included in all montages. Frequent rescreening of all sites on all intracranial devices and review of ictal recording shortly after each seizure occurs are necessary. The montage should be reconfigured, based on changing patterns of interictal activity and ictal records, to achieve maximal information. A minimum of 16 channels is necessary to perform intracranial recording, although 32 are preferred, and in many situations 64 are desirable.

After electrode insertion and montage selection, patients are continuously recorded on EEG and videotape until multiple (three minimum) spontaneous seizures occur. The habitual nature of these spells is verified by the patient's family and personnel on the unit, and by comparison with previous videotaped seizures during scalp recording. Prolonged recording may be needed since anesthesia, and perhaps subdural grids, appear to suppress spontaneous seizure occurrence. For this reason, we recommend early decrease of antiepileptic medications, with discontinuation if necessary. With these techniques, a typical recording session lasts 1–2 weeks.

EEG transmission, storage, and retrieval

Of the various methods for EEG transmission available for long-term monitoring, including standard cable, ambulatory cassette, cable telemetry, and radiotelemetry, only standard cable and cable telemetry are appropriate for intracranial recording [11]. The need for many EEG channels with simultaneous video recording dictates this necessity. Similarly, because of the need for direct access to the data, monitoring of the data online, and multiple channels, EEG recording and storage is best performed on analog or digital tape, video cassette, or digital disk, with synchronized time code to a behavioral videotape recorder, or with split-screen behavioral monitoring. Continuous paper printout can also be used, but this eliminates the possibility of replay, manipulation of data, and computerized quantitative analysis, which are increasingly considered important aspects of this evaluation.

Ideally, computerized seizure detection and constant EEG technician or nurse observation would provide maximal information, assuring identification of all clinical and EEG events which usually, but not always, occur simultaneously. Various combinations of observer and EEG review are in use, however, employing combinations of direct observation, computerized detection, patient signaling, and spot sampling of EEG for interictal activity and quantification.

With respect to the large number of technical options available, the American Electroencephalographic Society has developed minimal standards for long-term monitoring of patients undergoing presurgical evaluation [11]. These incorporate the above considerations and specify the need for standard or cable telemetry with at least 12 channels of EEG, recorded by continuous paper printout or, preferably, by tape or disk with computer-assisted detection, both with a synchronized time code to a continuous videotape which records behavior. These methods assure the ability to review behavioral and EEG characteristics of all seizures, as well as samples of interictal activity. To facilitate detection of subclinical ictal discharges, and to quantify interictal abnormalities recorded from intracranial or scalp EEG, computerized assistance is invaluable. Although review of continuous hard copy EEG is also adequate, with the development of epilepsy centers with multiple monitoring beds, such labor-intensive methods are often not feasible. Many centers have written their own software for these purposes and commercially available software or computerized seizure and spike detection systems linked to EEG monitoring equipment are available. Such programs, by necessity, detect up to 80% of nonictal paroxysmal bursts and probably do not detect all seizures, but provide a remarkable amount of data reduction, nonetheless.

Data reduction by computer is distinct

from data analysis programs, which aim to extract additional information from the EEG signals. These have been applied to the study of pathways of seizure spread or to the detection of the area of seizure origin in instances of rapid spread. Such applications are too specialized to be within the scope of this chapter, and most such software is not commercially available [12].

Equipment operation

Utilization of continuous hard-copy EEG monitoring methods requires constant attendance by trained technicians or nurses. For obvious reasons, most centers now prefer EEG systems which store information on tape or disk. Tape systems require only that an individual changes tapes at specified times, provided computerized seizure detection is available. Otherwise, independent observation of patient behavior still necessitates additional personnel around the clock. It is advantageous, regardless of the presence of computerized seizure detection systems, to have nurses in attendance to examine patients at the time of, and immediately following, seizures. Such examinations can document transient neurologic deficits which may aid in localization of the focus.

In most cases, filter settings for intracranial EEG are similar to those for scalp EEG (low linear frequency one, high linear frequency 70), although selective filtering may be employed to increase the yield of information. The amplitude of EEG signals from intracranial recording requires lowered sensitivity, usually in the range of 15 μV/mm for subdural and 20–30 μV/mm for depth electrode signals. Although it is generally preferable to record multiple channels with equal sensitivities, individual channel modification may be necessary depending on inter-electrode distances and combinations of depth, subdural, and scalp contacts in a particular recording montage.

Intracranial stimulation

Depth electrodes

Stimulation through depth electrodes has been employed as a method of seizure focus localization, with the rationale that electrical stimulation of areas which approximate the cerebral region of habitual onset will provoke habitual seizure activity. Unfortunately, the localization of seizures by electrical induction has proven to be less accurate than the recording of spontaneous ictal events [13]. This conclusion might have been predicted. Electrical stimulation may activate areas at a distance from the stimulus site. Therefore, electrical stimulation through depth electrodes, although useful as a confirmatory device for seizure focus localization, is not a primary method of localization.

Subdural electrodes

The above comments on localization of the seizure focus by stimulation through intracranial contacts apply also to subdural and epidural electrodes. Subdural and epidural electrode grids, however, provide an additional opportunity for stimulation to localize functional cerebral tissue [7]. The ability to localize spontaneous seizure onset and functional areas, using the same electrode grid, enables determination of the feasibility of resective surgery in certain situations and is therefore invaluable. The distribution and number of contacts available when depth electrodes are used usually prevent such functional localization. Cortical representation for motor, language, and perhaps memory function, has been shown to be somewhat variable, underlying the need for such individual localization prior to resective procedures near these areas [3]. Although localization of functional cerebral tissue has been done acutely in the operating room prior to resection of a previously identified epileptic focus, extraoperative localization utilizing subdural or epidural grids has the advantages of more leisurely protocols which facilitate accuracy. Such methods are applicable to mapping in the vicinity of structural lesions identified by imaging studies, as well as to cases where patients without structural lesions are being evaluated for epileptic foci close to language, motor, memory, or sensory areas.

Stimulation protocols generally include bipolar stimulation with biphasic 0.3 ms duration, 50 Hz pulses of 1–5 seconds duration, gradually increasing and rarely exceeding 15 mA. Maximum current used is determined by electrode size. Stimulation begins at 1–2 mA and increases until the maximal is reached, an after-discharge is induced, or positive or negative symptoms are elicited. Stimulation in primary afferent or efferent cortical areas produces positive effects (muscle twitching, visual phenomena, paresthesias), while stimulation of association areas produces negative effects (e.g. inability to speak). The area of brain stimulated is that between the two electrodes employed, as shown by Luders *et al.* [7].

Although concern over the harmful effects of stimulation is engendered by the increasing body of literature on kindling, no evidence exists for damage induced by stimulation of the type described above [7]. Stimulation protocols are time-consuming, requiring an expert team of physician, electroencephalographer, and psychologist, and constant attendance to the details of patient safety. For details of test protocols and results of stimulation, the reader is referred to the review article by Luders *et al.* [7].

Interpretation of intracranial EEG recordings

Background

Although basic background rhythms common to scalp EEG are represented in their expected anatomic distribution by intracranial EEG, the amplitudes, extent of distribution, and waveforms may differ to some degree. Scalp and bone attenuate cortical signals by up to 50 : 1 [14]. Experience is therefore necessary in the interpretation of the background activity to avoid ascribing undue significance to sharp activity of apparent high amplitude, which may represent only an amplified normal rhythm. This may be a problem with μ rhythm [7]. Asymmetry of background rhythms, however, is just as important a marker for abnormal cerebral electrophysiologic function as it is on the scalp EEG, and foci of slow activity are an accepted indication of abnormality. Just as in the interpretation of scalp EEG monitoring in uncontrolled epileptic patients, background abnormalities contribute to, but do not replace or equal, the localization obtained from the interictal and particularly the ictal epileptic events.

Interictal activity

With increasing use of computerized methods for quantification of interictal spikes, their localizing ability and relationship to other clinical and electrical data may become more clear. At present the controversy over the localizing accuracy of interictal spikes in scalp EEGs also applies to depth and subdural recordings. The present literature still provides no acceptable criteria for distinguishing primary from propagated interictal spikes [15].

The general definition of the interictal spike is applicable to depth and subdural recording (sharp wave distinct from background of <80 ms. duration) and morphology is perfunctorily similar. However, polarity, an important aspect of spike localization on the scalp EEG, loses its meaning in depth recording [12,15].

Interictal spikes in depth and subdural electrode recordings are mostly used to define the areas of depth or subdural electrode contacts for incorporation into montages which are limited to fewer channels than the number of electrode contacts. The interictal spikes recorded intracranially are given less weight for localization of the focus than the ictal events. This is because most intracranial recordings show an abundance of interictal spikes from multiple recording contacts and their association with multiple foci of spontaneous seizure onset is poor. In a Yale study of 47 patients who were investigated with depth and subdural electrodes simultaneously, interictal spikes were present in bilateral independent locations in 62% of patients with a single focus of seizure origin and in 93% of patients who were unlocalized or multifocal. Interictal spike frequency may change prior to or after seizures, but more data are needed to clarify this relationship and determine its usefulness in localization.

Ictal recordings

Seizure onset is more easily identified on intracranial recordings than scalp recordings, but the patterns of alteration of electrical activity resemble those seen much less frequently on the scalp EEG. Ictal discharge may be seen as a sudden change from background to electrode cremental activity, high frequency–low amplitude discharge, periodic spikes or spikes and slow waves, or rhythmic sharp discharge, with subsequent evolution into rhythmic slow, sharp, or spike activity at variable frequencies and amplitudes. Those experienced in interpretation of intracranial EEG believe that low amplitude high frequency discharge as the initial ictal event is the best indicator of the seizure focus, i.e., that its appearance suggests the recording electrode is in very close proximity to the seizure onset [12]. Nevertheless, other patterns of seizure onset, as described, can also provide localization sufficient to predict seizure cure after resection of the area so localized.

When abrupt seizure onset is identified in one to two electrode contacts, it is termed focal. A morphologically indistinguishable change in background detected simultaneously in several contacts (or often the entire sampling area of the hippocampus), has been termed regional seizure onset [2,3,12]. Despite the morphology, if the change is regional, it suggests to many interpreters a large epileptic zone or one removed from the lobe in question.

As the seizure spreads and is observed in other intracranial recording sites, involvement of areas distant from the initial region of seizure onset may show the same or different initial patterns and evolution. More often, subsequent involvement of the contralateral hippocampus is as clear as the initial seizure onset, with a morphologically similar sudden change in background. However, other areas are more gradually recruited with background slowing or rhythmic changes occurring over several seconds. Some areas of intracranial recording will show only slowing of background rhythms, often very early, without change to rhythmic or clearly identifiable paroxysmal patterns until secondary generalization has occurred. So far, no consistent observations have united these into identified groups of morphologic, temporal, or spatial characteristics associated with seizure onset in specific cerebral areas. However, the hope that this can be achieved has been expressed [10,12].

The interpretation of ictal EEG in intracranial records is dependent upon the simultaneous time-coded video recording of behavioral accompaniments without which it has no meaning [2]. In depth and subdural recordings, ictal EEG changes are expected to occur prior to clinical seizure onset; when they occur *following* clinical seizure onset, they imply seizure onset in an area other than that recorded by the implanted electrodes, with subsequent spread to the contacts in which they are first detected.

EEG events resembling ictal discharges occurring without simultaneous or subsequent clinical change are termed subclinical seizures. The meaning of their localization is not proven, but they are widely assumed to co-localize with the area of spontaneous clinical seizure onset.

Results

Patients whose presurgical evaluation requires implantation of intracranial electrodes are difficult localizing problems for whom, if surgery is to be considered, no other alternative exists. Taking into account the risks of intracranial implantation, it is appropriate to investigate not only the ability of these procedures to provide localization in this particular group of patients, but also their accuracy with respect to pathology, surgical outcome, and each other.

With respect to the yield of localization in otherwise unlocalized patients, both depth electrodes and subdural electrodes are reported by various groups, individually, to provide 60–80% successful localization [16–19]. Notably, although the groups overlap, subdurally-investigated patients are more often those with extratemporal, perhaps image-positive, prior evaluation while patients studied with depth electrodes more often include those localized to the temporal lobe who have had bitemporal, independent, interictal spikes on previous scalp EEG. It is impossible to completely eliminate this patient selection bias except by utilizing depth and subdural recordings in the same patients. This was done at Yale, as described above. In this study, 33 out of 47 previously unlocalized patients were localized by the combined study and all but four, including all temporal lobe seizure patients, exhibited initial seizure onset in the depth electrode [9].

Despite the nearly exclusive localization to extratemporal sites by subdural electrodes and to temporal sites by depth electrodes in this group, and a general bias towards using subdural electrodes for extratemporal localization at some centers, there is no evidence to indicate clearly that subdural electrodes are the preferred method of evaluation for extratemporal epilepsy. At Yale, 10 out of 109 patients studied with depth electrodes were localized to extratemporal sites, while 4 out of 47 depth-plus-subdural studies localized extratemporally. Half of the patients in the depth electrode, extratemporal-localized, group had positive imaging studies, while three out of four of those in the subdural, extratemporal-localized, group had positive imaging studies. The apparent superiority of subdural electrodes for extratemporal localization in this group was actually an artefact of the superiority of depth electrodes for temporal lobe localization. Extratemporal localization without imaging clues remains difficult by any method.

If the evidence suggests comparable yield from depth or subdural study in terms of localization, are depth or subdural electrodes comparable in accuracy? Accuracy can be judged by surgical outcome or pathology. The latter method indicates a considerably higher incidence of negative pathologic specimens in tissue resected on the basis of localization by subdural electrodes [10,20]. Pathologic confirmation of accuracy, however, requires appropriate pathologic analysis of the tissue resected and is therefore dependent on histopathologic methods in use and on the availability of intact tissue with which to pursue this goal. Because of our as yet incomplete understanding of the pathologic basis of epilepsy and because suction techniques for removal of medial temporal lobe structures at some centers prevent analysis of tissue, pathologic criteria are not always satisfactory.

Surgical outcome with respect to seizure control is the alternative scale against which to judge localizing accuracy of various intracranial recording techniques. (Improvement in seizures may reflect disconnection effects or variability of seizure frequency and is not a true standard either, but it is the only alternative.) Resection after depth-electrode investigation and localization reportedly produces 60–90% excellent results [1,19], while 60–70% of subdurally investigated and localized patients are reported to have good or excellent outcome after surgery [17,20,21].

Decreased success in seizure control of subdural identified foci might be ascribed to several factors. Most medically uncontrolled epileptic patients have temporal lobe epilepsy which is usually associated with hippocampal pathology [6]. Comparative studies have shown 5–15% of refractory temporal lobe seizures to arise in the temporal neocortex while the majority arise in the hippocampus, consistent with the pathologic findings [9]. Subdural electrodes, despite newer techniques for more medial insertion, do not directly sample the hippocampus, while depth electrodes do. Subclinical seizures, auras, and some clinical seizures arising in the hippocampus and seen on depth electrode recording were not detected by simultaneous temporal subdural recording [9,22]. The direct sampling of the hippocampus by depth electrodes also enables definition of the anterior–posterior extent of the seizure focus with its implications for modified surgical approaches, based on this information [1,18]. At least for temporal lobe epilepsy, the increased sensitivity and definition provided by depth electrodes enables increased patient selection; improved surgical success might well follow.

With respect to specificity, at least in temporal lobe epilepsy, in eight patients studied with bilateral temporal-lobe depth and subdural electrodes, seizure onset usually occurred in hippocampus and was first detected by depth electrodes. Eighty percent of seizures spread, eventually, to the temporal neocortex and if lateralized in the temporal neocortical recording, lateralization was consistently ipsilateral to the hippocampal onset [9]. Emphasizing the decreased sensitivity of the neocortical subdural electrode recording, these data also suggest the accuracy of temporal lobe lateralization with subdural electrodes. Another recent study, however, suggests possible false lateralization of temporal lobe epilepsy with subdural electrodes [22]. This issue has not been entirely resolved.

Other theoretical issues regarding accuracy should also be addressed. Extratemporal localization of seizures with initial or early spread to the temporal lobe might more often be mistaken for temporal lobe onset in subdural-electrode than in depth-electrode investigations. This speculation is based on the decreased sensitivity of subdural electrodes to hippocampal onset, and the fact that they reflect temporal lobe seizure onset later than the depth electrodes (and later in the clinical evolution of the event). In these terms, the combination of information from depth and subdural recordings sampling hippocampal and neocortical temporal lobe structures might help predict temporal or extratemporal onset. We studied 29 patients with temporal lobe seizure onset and simultaneous depth and subdural study. Surgical outcome and patterns of seizure onset were analyzed. Twenty-three had all of their seizures arising in one hippocampus recorded from the medially placed temporal lobe depth electrode; 16 out of 18 such patients who underwent operations had no further seizures after anteromedial temporal lobectomy of the identified temporal lobe. Six patients, however, had variable patterns of seizure onset, with initial changes in the depth electrode in some seizures and with initial changes in the subdural electrode or simultaneously in the depth and subdural electrode in some seizures, all in the same temporal lobe. None of the four patients in this group who underwent resection of that temporal lobe were cured. This kind of information may not be readily obtainable by just depth or subdural recording. Each needs to be interpreted in the light of other information and with respect to patterns of electroclinical correlation [9].

Summary

A review of the technicalities and results of intracranial electrode study for localization in uncontrolled epilepsy indicates a 1–2% risk of major complications after depth or subdural electrode insertion, but a higher risk of lasting deficit or death after depth electrodes; a 60–80% yield of localization by either technique in otherwise unlocalized patients; and a 60–90% success rate in patients who are selected for surgery after these techniques. Available data suggest increased sensitivity and specificity of depth-electrode recordings in temporal lobe epilepsy, but only one comparative report has used the techniques simultaneously to eliminate patient selection bias. In certain situations, combined recording may provide additional information of prognostic value. If cortical mapping for functional localization is needed, subdural grids are indicated. The goals of mapping and localization and the location of study must be balanced in the decision about the type of intracranial study to perform.

References

1 Spencer SS. Surgical options for uncontrolled epilepsy. In Theodore WH, Porter RJ (eds) *Epilepsy*. Neurological Clinics of North America, Vol. 4, No. 3. WB Saunders, Philadelphia, 1985, pp 313–330.

2 Engel J, Crandall PH. Intensive neurodiagnostic monitoring with intracranial electrodes. In Gumnit RJ (ed) *Intensive Neurodiagnostic Monitoring*. Advances in Neurology No. 46. Raven Press, New York, 1986, pp 85–106.

3 Ojemann GA, Engel J. Acute and chronic intracranial recording and stimulation. In Engel J, Jr (ed) *Surgical Treatment of the Epilepsies*. Raven Press, New York, 1987, pp 263–288.

4 Morris HH, Luders H. Electrodes. In Gotman J, Ives JR, Gloor P (eds) *Long Term Monitoring in Epilepsy*. Elsevier, Amsterdam, 1985, pp 3–26.

5 Cooper R, Crow JH. Toxic effects of intracerebral electrodes. *Med Biol Engineer* 1966; **4**: 575–581.

6 Babb TL, Brown WJ. Pathological findings in epilepsy. In Engel J, Jr (ed) *Surgical Treatment of the Epilepsies*. Raven Press, New York, 1987, pp 511–540.

7 Luders H, Lesser RP, Dinner DS, *et al.* Commentary: chronic intracranial recording and stimulation with subdural electrodes. In Engel J, Jr (ed). *Surgical Treatment of the Epilepsies*. Raven Press, New York, 1987, pp 297–321.

8 Spencer SS, Spencer DD, Williamson PD, Mattson RH. Simultaneous depth and subdural electrode investigation for localization of seizure onset. *Epilepsia* 1986; **27** (Suppl 2): 637.
9 Spencer SS, Williamson PD, Spencer DD, Mattson RH. Combined depth and subdural electrode investigation in uncontrolled epilepsy. *Neurology* 1990; **46**: 74–79.
10 Spencer SS. Controversies in epileptology: depth vs subdural electrodes. *J Epil* 1989: **2**: 123–127.
11 American Electroencephalographic Society. Guidelines for long-term neurodiagnostic monitoring in epilepsy. *J Clin Neurophysiol* 1985; **2**(4): 419–452.
12 Wieser H. Data Analysis. In Engel J, Jr (ed) *Surgical Treatment of the Epilepsies*. Raven Press, New York, 1987, pp 335–360.
13 Wieser HG, Bancaud, J, Talairach J, Bonis A, Szikla G. Comparative value of spontaneous and chemically and electrically induced seizures in establishing the lateralization of temporal lobe seizures. *Epilepsia* 1979; **20**: 47–59.
14 Abraham K, Ajmone-Marsan C. Patterns of cortical discharges and their relation to routine scalp electroencephalography. *EEG Clin Neurophysiol* 1958; **10**: 447–461.
15 Gloor P. Contributions of electroencephalography and electrocorticography to the neurosurgical treatment of the epilepsies. In Purpura DP, Penry JK, Walter RD (eds) *Neurosurgical Management of the Epilepsies*, Advances in Neurology No. 8. Raven Press, New York, 1975, pp 59–105.
16 Gloor P, Olivier A, Ives J. Prolonged seizure monitoring with stereotaxically implanted depth electrodes in patients with bilateral interictal temporal epileptic foci: how bilaterial is bitemporal epilepsy? In Wade JA, Penry JK (eds) *Advances in Epileptology, Xth Epilepsy International Symposium*. Raven Press, New York, 1980, pp 83–88.
17 Wyler AR, Ojemann GA, Lettich E, Ward A. Subdural strip electrodes for localizing epileptogenic foci. *J Neurosurg* 1984; **60**: 1195–1200.
18 Goldring S, Gregorie EM. Surgical management of epilepsy using epidural recording to localize the seizure focus. *J. Neurosurg* 1984; **60**: 457–466.
19 Spencer SS. Depth Electroencephalography in selection of refractory epilepsy for surgery. *Ann Neurology* 1981; **9**: 207–214.
20 Rosenbaum TJ, Laxer KD, Vessely M, Smith WB. Subdural electrodes for seizure focus localization. *Neurosurgery*. 1986; **19**: 73–81.
21 Goldring S. A method for surgical management of focal epilepsy, especially as it relates to children. *J Neurosurg* 1978; **49**: 344–356.
22 Sperling MR, O'Connor MJ. Depth electrodes are superior to subdural electrodes for recording temporal lobe seizures. *EEG Clin. Neurophysiol* 1988; **70**: 42p.

Comment

Allen R. Wyler

There is little doubt that both interictal or ictal scalp EEG have too high an error rate to be used for selecting candidates for epilepsy surgery because (1) they are insufficiently localizing in greater than 60% of cases; and (2) for those patients who have a localizing EEG, they are falsely localizing or lateralizing in approximately 30% of cases [1]. If additional data, such as neuropsychologic tests and neuroimaging information, are considered in conjunction with the EEG, the localization error rate can be lowered to approximately 10–15%. Further evidence demonstrates that interictal recordings have less localizing value than ictal scalp recordings [1]. Furthermore, there is little doubt that intracranial recordings are superior to scalp recordings for the reasons reviewed in this chapter. After taking all this into account, one is faced with the following dilemma: (1) scalp recordings are obviously safer than invasive recordings; (2) but scalp recordings will result in rejecting many patients who would be excellent surgical candidates; (3) and of those patients accepted for surgery based on scalp recordings, some will fail because the wrong lobe or hemisphere has been operated upon. One solution to this dilemma is to operate only upon patients with obvious structural lesions which correlate with clearly unilateral epileptiform scalp foci. That solution is unacceptable for the obvious reason that it denies surgery to the vast majority of patients who would benefit.

It is evident that invasive monitoring yields a clearer identification of who should, and who should not undergo resective surgery. It would, therefore, seem logical that patients who have undergone invasive monitoring should have better surgical outcomes than patients who have not undergone such monitoring. Evaluation of my own surgical experience has shown that 90% of my patients who underwent temporal lobectomy based on data from subdural strip electrode (SDSE) ictal monitoring have had excellent results. By comparison, patients who underwent temporal lobectomy after only scalp monitoring have had only a 60% success rate [1]. (These data are based on a retrospective study, and therefore are subject to criticism.) Another way of looking at the question is to evaluate surgical failures. At our center we routinely completely reevaluate patients who have failed epilepsy surgery done either by ourselves or others. We have found that approximately 15% of patients failed because the wrong lobe was operated upon, and none of those patients had undergone invasive monitoring (Wyler, unpublished data). In addition, if the wrong lobe has been resected, the patients will often become worse both cognitively and emotionally. Therefore, from our perspective it appears that the use of scalp electrode EEG is associated with a real (rather than hypothetical) morbidity. By comparison, our complication rate for intracranial monitoring with SDSEs is 1% (treatable infections). We have concluded that invasive recordings are well worth their risk, and now require ictal invasive monitoring on all patients with nonlesional complex seizures before proceeding with resective surgery. For patients with atonic, tonic, clonic, or tonic–clonic seizures (verified by video monitoring) and generalized ictal discharges we proceed with corpus callosotomy without invasive monitoring.

The next question is, what type of invasive recording method is best? This debate really concerns only depth electrodes and SDSE and does not include large grid arrays. Also the controversy does not include epidural electrodes because they cannot record from important cortical areas as inter-hemispheric fissure or basal temporal lobe. In my opinion, the only indication for epidural recordings is when either depth or subdural electrodes cannot be used, as for example, when the subdural space is obliterated from previous surgery. It should be remembered that large subdural grids are usually implanted unilaterally and therefore, the side of insertion has already been determined by scalp recordings. The primary indication for subdural grid arrays is to explore cortex adjacent to *known epileptogenic foci* with prolonged electrocorticography and "functional mapping" (through electrode stimulation). This technique can identify cortex associated with ictal onset and its functional relationship to surrounding areas. An example is the evaluation of cortical function surrounding a brain tumor suspected of being in or near "eloquent" cortex. This approach is preferred to the alternative method of acute corticography and stimulation during craniotomy performed with an awake patient because (1) the grid can be used on patients of various ages and psychiatric predispositions who are not candidates for local anesthesia; (2) acute recordings usually provide only interictal data which, even with direct cortical recordings, is inferior to ictal data; and (3) the grid allows more time for careful evaluation than is present in the operating room.

In contrast with grid electrode arrays (a method which assumes known lateralization of the focus) SDSE are commonly used to lateralize as well as localize an epileptogenic focus. As such, they are implanted in an "exploratory" montage, which is always bilateral. Because SDSE are inserted through a small burr hole, whereas grids are applied through a large craniotomy flap, the associated infection rates and general morbidity are considerably less for SDSE than they are for grid arrays. However, some authors have combined the morbidity of the two methods and have used that figure when comparing the morbidity of SDSE to that of depth electrodes. If the respective morbidity rates of subdural grids, subdural strips, and depth electrodes are separated and ranked, the grids have the highest frequency of problems, and the strips the lowest associated morbidity. In addition, the severity of complications associated with strips seems to be less than what has been known with depth electrodes. In our Memphis series of over 200 SDSE patients (an average of eight electrodes per patient) we have had one case of meningitis, and one scalp wound infection; a total morbidity rate of 1%.

There remains a great deal of controversy concerning the relative localizing value of exploratory depth and SDSE investigations. There is no question that the closer one places an electrode to the source of a signal, the more likely one is to record the signal. Thus, a SDSE placed under the temporal lobe will demonstrate more spikes originating from mesial temporal structures than will scalp or sphenoidal electrodes. Likewise, depth electrodes inserted into hippocampus will yield more spike activity from hippocampus than will a SDSE placed over parahippocampal gyrus. However, as Dr Spencer pointed out, most seizures do not begin with spike activity, and as with scalp recordings, interictal depth recordings of spikes alone are of little value in localizing epileptogenic foci. The essential question is: does one need to record exactly from hippocampus to select the correct temporal lobe for resection, or can recordings from parahippocampal gyrus be sufficient for excellent surgical selection? I, for one, am not sure this question has been suitably answered. Most studies which have compared results of depth and strip electrodes have several confounding variables associated with them including the placement of subdural strips only unilaterally in some cases. Moreover, judging the two techniques by surgical outcome between centers is fraught with uncontrolled variables such as individual center selection bias, nonstandardized surgical techniques, and removal of different temporal structures. At our center, virtually 100% of our temporal lobectomy cases selected by SDSE ictal monitoring have had positive pathology on microscopic examination of mesial temporal lobe tissue.

In my opinion there has been no

conclusive study to show superiority of depth electrodes to SDSE for selecting candidates for either temporal or extratemporal resections. Because depth electrodes can record directly from hippocampus whereas SDSE can, at best, record from parahippocampal gyrus it is *theoretically* attractive to assume depth electrodes are superior when evaluating patients with suspected temporal lobe foci. However, that bias also assumes that the entire epileptogenic focus is contained within hippocampus — an assumption not yet proven. The fact is, when evaluating patients with idiopathic (nonlesional) epilepsy, > 90% will harbor mesial temporal lobe foci. And although the most conspicuous histopathology is contained within the hippocampus, it is still not known if such changes are entirely cause or effect. Moreover, not all patients who undergo selective mesial amygdalohippocampectomy are rendered seizure-free. The point is, we are uncertain of the exact structures involved in the initiation of seizures for all patients with idiopathic temporal lobe epilepsy, and until we are, we cannot be sure of exactly where one should record within the temporal lobe to generate the best possible outcome from surgery. However, what we do know is that invasive ictal monitoring provides superior localization to scalp recordings and remains the singularly most accurate method for correctly choosing patients to undergo surgery.

Reference

1 Wyler AR, Richey ET, Hermann BP. Comparison of scalp to subdural recordings for localizing epileptogenic foci. *J Epil* 1989; **2**: 91–96.

chapter 4

Selection of Patients for Corpus Callosum Section

Sherrill J. Purves

Division of the corpus callosum (CC) has attracted renewed interest recently as a surgical method of treatment for medically intractable seizures in patients who are not eligible for focal cortical resections. In his 1985 review of the subject, Williamson [1] found reports of only 65 callosotomy patients. By 1988 detailed assessments of 185 cases from 11 centers were available with indications from several centers of additional experience but with the later cases not described in adequate detail for analysis [6,15–18]. This literature is summarized in Table 4.1 and forms the basis for this critical analysis.

If successful outcome after callosotomy is defined as an 80% or more reduction in seizure frequency, then 53% of the patients described in Table 4.1 with generalized tonic–clonic seizures (GTCS) or drop attacks had successful results. If a 50% or more reduction of seizure frequency is accepted as a good result then 82% of these patients have benefited. Many centers have also reported a marked modification in the severity of seizure patterns in most patients but this parameter is much more difficult to quantify. In the papers that reported akinetic or drop attack seizures separately 67% (28/42) of patients show a significant improvement. Success rates from different centers vary widely with 50–100% improved from GTCS pattern, and 22–79% of patients with atonic–tonic or akinetic drop attacks improved. Such variability may depend upon selection of patients, operative approach, extent of section and period of follow-up. A discussion of these factors in the selection of patients for a good outcome is presented below.

Historical perspective

The first report of surgical division of commissural pathways to prevent a spread of epileptic seizures was made by Van Wagenen and Herren in 1940 [19]. The number of patients in this original series may have been as many as 26, according to Williamson [1]. Follow-up data was limited. In the early

TABLE 4.1 Results of partial or complete microsurgical CC section reported in the literature after 1977. Seizure reduction refers to GTC and atonic–tonic or akinetic seizures unless otherwise indicated

Author(s)	Number of cases fully reviewed	Anterior or partial section	Complete section (1- or 2-stage)	Number of patients with >80% seizure reduction	Number of patients with 50–80% seizure reduction	Comments
Wilson *et al.* [2,3] (Dartmouth)	I. 8 II. 12	5	15	I. 6/8 II. 7/12	3/12	Best results with one seizure type, unilateral damage, IQ > 70
Marino and Ragazzo [4] (São Paulo Brazil)	20	20	—	Not given	—	Results predicted by interictal EEG. Three patients had large unilateral lesions. Intraoperative ECOG used to determine length of section. Eight out of 20 had "marked" improvement in absences and atonic seizures
Rayport *et al.* [5] (Medical College, Ohio)	9	1 (Posterior)	8	2/9 (akinetic)	5/9	Three out of 9 language difficulties, 1/9 severe "hemispheric competition"
Geoffroy *et al.* [6] (St Justin, Montreal)	9	—	9	6/9	1/9	All retarded children with severe epilepsy
Blume [7] (University of Western Ontario)	8	8	—	3/8	2/8	All improved patients had IQ > 64

Saint-Hilaire *et al.* and Bouvier *et al.* [8,9] (Notre Dame, Montreal)	10	10	—	9/10	1/10	Three simultaneous frontal resections. All CPS studied with depth electrodes
Gates *et al.* [10,11] (University of Minnesota)	24	—	24	17/17 (GTCS) 19/24 (atonic) 12/21 (CPS)	— 3/24 —	All had tonic/atonic seizures. IQ not documented
Spencer *et al.* [12] (Yale)	22	9	13	16/22 (GTCS) 9/22(CPS)	— 2/22 (CPS)	Seventeen out of 22 two-stage procedures, providing comparison of anterior and complete section
Purves *et al.* [13] (University of British Columbia)	24	24	—	4/8 (GTCS) 6/8 (akinetic) 13/21 (CPS)	1/8 1/8 4/21	Patients included frontal CPS without generalization. Overall 75% "improved"
Murro *et al.* [14] (Medical College, Georgia)	25	25	—	7/18 1/1 (akinetic) 3/13 (CPS)	2/18 — 2/13	Generalized or frontal CPS. Better outcome with normal IQ, infantile hemiplegia, seizure onset < 5 years
Garcia-Flores [15] (Monterrey, Mexico)	14	8	6	7/14	5/14	Many structural multifocal lesions. Better results in 8 adults than 6 children
Totals	185	110	75	82/126 (GTCS) 28/42 (akinetic, atonic/tonic) 37/77 (CPS)	24/168 (GTCS, atonic)	

ECoG, electrocorticography.

1960s Bogen and his colleagues began to report the results of their series [20,21] with most attention directed to the neuropsychologic consequences of the CC section with respect to lateralized hemispheric function in humans, but few details of seizure outcome. In 1970 Lussenhop *et al.* [22] reported excellent results with division of the CC, one fornix and the anterior commissure in a group of four children with seizures of unilateral hemispheric origin.

The report by Wilson *et al.* in 1977 [2] was the first with a detailed analysis of clinical seizure patterns and prolonged follow-up data. Wilson proposed a modification of the procedure to section only CC and underlying hippocampal commissures by a microsurgical approach without entering the ventricular system and without sectioning the anterior commissure or fornix. This resulted in a decisive drop in the incidence of infection and appeared to make the procedure safe without any loss in efficacy. It is this surgical approach that has been used in most subsequent series with modifications described by Roberts [23]; see also Chapter 8.

In 1971 Gordon *et al.* suggested that undesirable hemispheric disconnection effects of complete CC could be avoided by leaving the posterior CC intact without adversely affecting control of seizures [24]. Other centers [4,8,25] began to try anterior CC section alone. In 1982 Wilson *et al.* reported that two-stage callosotomy dramatically shortened the postoperative convalescence time by decreasing the severity of the acute disconnection syndrome which followed complete one-stage CC section. Their two-stage approach started with section of the posterior CC first [3]. But in subsequent reports of two-stage complete CC sections [5,11,12,16] the anterior callosotomy was usually done as the first stage, as it appeared to be more effective and caused less sequellae. Others have continued to restrict surgery in all cases to division of the anterior portion of callosum [4,7–9,13,14,17) in an attempt to limit the extent of surgery and avoid the possibility of disconnection syndromes. Most of these centers have focused on patients who are presumed to have frontal lobe epilepsy, but there have also been some generalized epilepsies treated in this way. The effectiveness of the anterior partial section compared to the complete section is discussed below.

Rationale

Rationale for division of the corpus callosum for control of generalized seizures is based on the premise that it is the major route of spread of the epileptic discharges from one hemisphere to the other. Erickson [26] first described this mode of spread in 1940. Subsequent experimental work has confirmed the critical role of the CC in the generation of 3 Hz spike and wave in animal models of generalized epilepsy [27], and in secondary spread from acute or chronic unilateral structural epileptic foci [28, 29]. In the kindling model Wada and colleagues [30–35] demonstrated that it was the anterior two-thirds of the CC that was critical for the development of generalized convulsive seizures after chronic amygdaloid stimulation.

The anatomy of the CC has been carefully studied in the primate by Pandya and Rosene [36] with both homotopic and nonhomotopic connections between the hemispheres demonstrated. They showed that the connections from frontal and cingulate regions cross in the anterior half of the CC, including rostrum, and some of the body. Connections originating in temporal lobes cross in the posterior part of the body as well as in the underlying hippocampal commissure. Parietal connections occupy the anterior part of the splenium with occipital fibres in the most posterior splenium. The human anatomy has been reviewed in further detail by Pandya and Yeterian [37]

Physiologic studies suggest only 30% of human temporal seizures studied with depth electrodes cross to contralateral temporal regions by hippocampal commissures [38,39]. The remaining temporal seizures spread to ipsilateral neocortex or subcortical structures. Propagation of seizure activity from frontal foci in humans has been much more difficult to delineate even with simultaneous bilateral depth electrode studies [9], suggesting rapid spread across anterior callosal pathways. Akinetic seizures, accompanied by generalized EEG ictal discharges are also thought to utilize the commissural pathways [10]. Saint-Hilaire *et al.* [8] observed a surprising improvement in a patient with partial seizures of frontal cingulate origin after CC section, leading to the hypothesis that bilateral frontal lobe involvement is necessary for clinical manifestations of some partial seizures. Others have extended this hypothesis [40].

While the CC appears to be the preferential pathway for bilateral synchrony in most circumstances, experimental evidence indicates that sufficiently intense seizure activity can spread by subcortical pathways in thalamus and midbrain [41]. The factors that determine the extent of subcortical spread or its importance in the individual patient are considered in Spencer's review but remain uncertain [42]. A clearer understanding of non-callosal interhemispheric pathways may help to predict in which patients the CC section will fail to stop the generalized seizures.

Criteria for patient selection

The selection of patients who will have a good outcome from this procedure remains a difficult problem, as does the decision of how much of the CC should be divided. While most centers agree on the ''negative'' criteria, i.e. that the patient is *not* medically controllable and *not* eligible for cortical resection, the importance of factors such as seizure type, age of onset of seizures, etiology of seizures, and degree if any of mental retardation remain uncertain. The presence of structural abnormalities and the criteria by which results are judged are also approached differently between centers. In both the summary undertaken for the preparation of Table 4.1, and the following discussion of these issues, selection and results of series reported after 1977 are considered. This period encompasses a group of patients who were all operated on using microsurgical technique or a modification of it as described by Wilson *et al.* in 1977 [2] without division of the anterior commissure and in most cases without entry into the ventricular system.

Seizure frequency and type

Seizure frequency has varied from one per week to many per day, and all authors have indicated that seizures must be clearly of a disabling type. Most patients have been on two or three medications and criteria of a minimum of 2–4 years of medical therapy have been suggested. In practice it appears that most patients have been medically intractable prior to surgery for many, many years.

The major seizure type targeted for treatment has also varied between centers, and many of the patients will have had more than one seizure type. No systematic analysis of the presence of multiple seizure types as a predictive factor has been done, but in our experience [13] these patients appear to have a less favourable outcome both in terms of reduction of the primary seizure type as well as the secondary ones.

The most common type of seizures

selected for treatment have been akinetic or atonic–tonic seizures resulting in frequent and disabling falls and injuries in patients with associated bilateral ictal and interictal EEG discharges. The Minnesota and Ohio series have been selected purely for this type of seizures [5,13], but at other centers this seizure type appears in 0–60% of patients. Not all centers have insisted on ictal video-EEG recordings to identify the exact type of seizures preoperatively. A good result (>50% seizure reduction) with complete CC section for this seizure type is reported by Spencer *et al.* [12] (8/8 patients), Gates *et al.* [11] (21/24 patients) and Rayport *et al.* [5] (5/8 patients) and in smaller numbers with anterior CC section by Purves *et al.* [13] (7/8 patients), Blume [7] (5/8 patients) and Murro *et al.* [14] (1/1 patient). The numbers remain too small to determine if complete CC section is more effective than anterior CC section for these attacks, but all of the larger series were using complete callosotomies.

Secondarily GTC seizures appear to respond in a favorable manner somewhat less predictably in most series, but patients with this seizure type are not selected and investigated in a uniform manner, making comparison of results difficult. Depth electrode studies are done preoperatively in some centers [9,12,16] although not necessarily in every patient, and CC section is confined to patients with bifrontal or unlateralized seizures after attempts to localize a single focus with depth electrodes have failed [9,12,16]. Determination of frontal origin complex partial seizures (CPS) at other centers [13,14] is made on the basis of scalp video-EEG ictal recordings. Purves *et al.* [13] have suggested that the anterior CC section can be used as an alternate strategy to lateralize the focus without placing intracranial electrodes in selected cases of frontal lobe epilepsy. They have reported four out of eight of patients with frontal CPS to be seizure-free after the CC section, and one patient who stopped having GTCS and underwent a subsequent successful focal resection of a lateral frontal focus. This had been identified by noninvasive EEG studies of a new clinical seizure pattern, which had emerged after the anterior CC section.

The surgical management of a patient with partial seizures suspected on the basis of noninvasive studies to originate from a frontal focus with spread to contralateral hemisphere during the clinical seizure will be based on a number of factors including the availability of invasive techniques and local experience. They may be a candidate for an anterior callosotomy (which is classified as a "palliative" procedure) or for intracranial recordings to localize a focus which can then be resected and more likely "cure" the condition. In the 1987 survey of Engel [43], including 16 centers and 197 patients for CC section, the results of extratemporal resection showed that a slightly higher number of patients had improved after callosotomy (76%) than after extratemporal resection (71%), but far less were seizure-free (5% vs. 43%). The patients from different centers may not have been strictly comparable, but the point that extratemporal resections carry a poorer prognosis of cure or improvement than temporal lobectomies (55% seizure-free and 83% improved) is important. Newer techniques being developed for assessment of patients for extratemporal resection such as subdural grid electrodes (see Chapter 3) may change these results but these invasive techniques are still very expensive, time consuming, and limited in availability. In situations when intracranial exploration is unavailable or impossible, anterior callosotomy may provide an alternative for lateralizing frontal lobe foci and improving the seizures in some patients without such invasive studies.

Both Spencer *et al.* [12] and Purves *et al.* [13] found that where it could be demonstrated that GTC seizures originated from a single focus, they responded better to CC division than those of multifocal origin. Purves *et al.* reported that repeated bouts of generalized status epilepticus were eliminated with anterior CC section and Geoffroy *et al.* [6] also reported improvement in near status with complete section in severely retarded children. Status epilepticus is not specifically mentioned in any of the other reports. Clearly identified primary generalized seizures have not been treated with this surgery.

Complex partial seizures are separately considered by some authors but still represent a very heterogeneous group. Complex partial seizures presumed of frontal or bifrontal origin have been improved in 12/21 [11], 13/21 [13], 17/25 [16] and 9/22 [12] patients in separate series, but the exact criteria used to define these are variable and sometimes unavailable.

Simple partial seizures are generally not improved by this procedure and have sometimes been made worse. More importantly they may appear *de novo* where the patient did not have them preoperatively. Gates *et al.* [11] showed that many of these new partial seizures appear to be the aborted onset of the patient's preoperative GTC seizure pattern, now confined to a simple partial seizure. Spencer *et al.* [12] identified three patients with more intense partial seizures and discussed mechanisms involved [44].

Selection in children

Spencer [42] reviewed the literature for results in children under 15 as compared with adults, and found that 84% of both adults and children had decreased or eliminated generalized seizures after callosotomy but more children [55%] than adults [29%] had partial seizures which had been made worse. The number of cases she found for calculation of these figures is unclear. Some of the series reported in Table 4.1 included children under 15 years (Garcia-Flores [15] 6/14; Geoffroy *et al.* [6] 9/9; Purves *et al.* [13] 2/24; and Spencer *et al.* [12] 2/22); but no one series has enough each of both adults and children to made useful comparisons within a center. Taking into account the theoretical considerations of the neuropsychologic effects of CC section (since the ability to learn new tasks requiring hemispheric integration could be impaired) great caution would be expected in choosing children. Only those so severely incapacitated by seizures as to make this an acceptable risk should be considered. However, many single-case reports document dramatic improvement in children's performance levels if seizures are stopped [6,45].

The presence of structural lesions

There is general agreement that patients who have generalized tonic–clonic or atonic seizures and clinical hemiparesis, hemiatrophy, or unilateral structural lesions visualized on computed tomography (CT) scans have a better result from CC section than patients with no structural lateralizing features. Some suggest that congenital lesions, or seizures beginning before the age of 5 years also indicate a better outcome than lesions acquired at a later age [3,12]. Two of Wilson's patients with good results had herpes encephalitis or failed temporal lobectomy, but in other series such patients with later onset of seizures had a poor result [13,14].

In the series studied by Spencer and colleagues [12,45], 17 out of 22 patients had some structural unilateral abnormality on CT scan, but it was only when the CT results were used with the clinical and intracarotid Amytal test results to establish a classification of patients with "moderate to severe lateralized CNS dysfunction" that a clear trend with a better outcome for this group appeared. Marino and Ragazzo's [4] group of three patients who had unilateral structural lesions are reported as one of their good outcome groups. Murro *et al.* [14] reported two patients with hemiparesis who both had an excellent result. Purves *et al.* [13] found excellent results (> 80% seizure reduction) in five patients with clinical evidence of lateralized function although one of these required subsequent excision because of worsening partial seizures with adversive motor phenomena. Three other patients in our series [13] with clinical hemiatrophy but other evidence of bilateral disease did not have such a good result. Garcia-Flores [15] reported that out of two children and five adults with unilateral pathology, three became seizure-free and four had substantial improvement. His report of a patient with bilateral lesions in right frontal and left parietal regions from a gunshot wound who became seizure-free after complete commissurotomy is of interest since Spencer *et al.* [12] and Purves *et al.* [13] have found bilateral, multifocal pathology usually results in poor outcome. Documentation of the ictal EEG onset is not provided in Garcia-Flores' patient however, raising the possibility that the seizures were only originating from one of these two lesions. This author also reports a successful outcome in a child with bilateral lesions due to tuberous sclerosis but no improvement in another patient with bilateral subcortical atrophy secondary to anoxia. Gates *et al.* [11] noted no improvement in a patient demonstrated to have bilateral frontal postradiation necrosis. These latter two cases would suggest that such bilateral diffuse structural disease due to anoxia or postradiation damage gives a prognosis for a poorer outcome but there are relatively few such cases in the literature at present.

Mental retardation

Most authors [3,7,13,14] who have addressed this question have found that mental retardation is associated with a poor outcome, with those with IQ scores >70 doing fairly well, and the group of patients with IQs <70 having a poorer percentage of successes in terms of major seizure reduction. Other series [6,12] have found this correlation with poor outcome only with much more severe retardation (IQ score <45). In our experience [13] the presence of unilateral structural damage and ictal pattern should be considered in conjunction with the IQ to predict the outcome. In the group of patients with hemiatrophy and secondarily generalized seizures demonstrated to originate from only the damaged hemisphere two patients with very low IQs still had an excellent outcome, but in the group of patients with suspected bilateral damage where anterior corpus callosotomy was used to treat partial complex seizures of presumed frontal lobe origin, the patients with an IQ score <70 had poorer results. In a third group of patients who all had an IQ score <70, the presence of ictal and interictal bilateral slow spike and wave in patients with tonic–clonic or atonic seizures (Lennox–Gastaut syndrome) appeared to correlate with a good result from the anterior callosotomy while complex partial seizures with or without secondary generalization did not improve very often in this group.

In conclusion, while the level of intellectual function should certainly be documented preoperatively (and, as will be discussed later, rarely changes postoperatively), it should probably be used as a predictive factor in conjunction with the presence of clear focal brain involvement and the type of seizures targeted for improvement. When the CC section is directed at a very specific seizure type with quite specific EEG abnormalities [11], IQ may not be as important a factor in patient selection.

EEG

The use of EEG in patient selection has been discussed in some detail by Spencer *et al.* [46]. Most patients have one of the following interictal EEG patterns: generalized spike and wave with or without a normal background, focal spikes with secondary bilateral synchrony, or multifocal spike or slow wave abnormalities with secondary generalization. Although no single pattern clearly carries a better prognosis of outcome, patients with multifocal, unilateral, or bilateral independent interictal EEG spike patterns had poorer seizure results in our series [13]. These patients were also identified to be at risk for developing more intense or frequent focal seizures by Spencer *et al.* [44]. All centers who report ictal EEG patterns indicate that they show bilateral spread of the seizure discharge and the rationale for treatment with CC section in these patients is based on this finding. Fiol and Gates [48] found the most favorable ictal pattern for a good outcome was epileptiform fast activity at onset. Postoperative EEG changes can be quite dramatic with desynchronization of the bilateral abnormal EEG patterns and emergence of clearer focal abnormalities sometimes seen [49].

Infantile hemiplegia

Corpus callosum section has been proposed as an alternative to hemispherectomy in patients with infantile hemiplegia [22,50] but some controversy remains [51]. A modified hemispherectomy holds the promise of complete seizure control for the majority of patients with severe hemiplegia [52,53,54] but is recommended only in patients with no useful finger movements. This procedure has a high rate of delayed complications. The modification called "functional hemispherectomy" by Rasmussen [54] which spares frontal and occipital cortex, but isolates them from both callosal and subcortical connections, has been used in an attempt to prevent the delayed complications of late hydrocephalus and superficial cerebral hemosiderosis, and appears to still stop the seizures. Corpus callosum section was initially proposed as an alternative treatment [22, 50] because of the high complication rate. The best discussions of results of the two procedures come from the reports of Goodman *et al.* [55] who documented five patients with infantile hemiplegia of varying severity undergoing CC section and Tinuper *et al.* [51], who reported 14 patients from the Montreal Neurological Institute who underwent modified hemispherectomy. Only 1/5 of the callosotomy patients was reported to be seizure-free, but the authors point out that the remaining seizures in 3/5 patients were minor in nature, and documented a good social outcome in this group. The number of seizure-free patients in the MNI hemispherectomy series (10/14) is higher. These patients had hemiplegia from a variety of etiologies. Only 4/14 patients had generalized seizures but all 14 had severe hemiparesis maximum in the upper limb. From these reports it appears that for patients with milder degrees of hemiplegia and preservation of the visual field, callosotomy holds the prospect of a cure from generalized seizures and a marked decrease in the partial complex seizures. For the more severely affected patients, a hemispherectomy may be considered despite the increased risk of complications because of the higher probability of having the patient completely seizure-free postoperatively.

Follow-up period and medications

The question of medications before and after callosotomy has not been widely discussed. Patients usually come to surgery on two or three drugs and in some centers a considerable reduction in the number and dosages of medications postoperatively has been possible. Whether there are specific groups of medications which can be targeted for reduction after callosal section remains to be delineated. Blume [7] has suggested that the patient's medication regimen should undergo a retrial since he or she may be more amenable to control postcallosotomy. No patients have been reported to be seizure-free off medication postcallosotomy, and this should be emphasized to the patient.

The duration and evolution of seizures in the postoperative period has been evaluated briefly in the reports of Spencer *et al.* [42] and Purves *et al.* [13]. They have found that the seizure pattern by 6–12 months postcallosotomy appears to be stable. There are no reports of significant worsening in frequency or severity of generalized seizures >1 year after surgery. A few patients may have seizures in the immediate postoperative weeks and then improve, but these also appear to stabilize by 6 months. Spencer *et al.* also report occasional worsening of partial seizures after the one year follow-up period [42]. These reports together suggest that a 6–12 month period of documentation after an anterior callosotomy would be appropriate before completion of the callosotomy is undertaken.

Neurologic consequences of callosotomy

Immediately after complete callosal section patients demonstrate an acute disconnection syndrome which varies widely in severity and usually resolves within a few days to weeks [56]. The acute disconnection syndrome (in right-handed patients operated on from the right side) is characterized by an akinetic state in which the patients lie quietly but will cooperate when stimulated to perform simple commands with the right limbs. They may be mute, but able to write short answers and have a left-sided apraxia for verbal commands which can be quite severe and mistaken for a left hemiplegia. There may also be weakness in the left leg thought to be due to retraction on the medial frontal lobe. Rarely transient urinary incontinence, bilateral grasp reflexes and bilateral Babinski reflexes are reported in this acute syndrome.

In anterior callosal sections these initial effects are a great deal milder. A reluctance to initiate speech and mild paresis of the non-dominant leg are usually noted in the first 2 days after surgery, but are so mild that they may go unnoticed as specific effects of the procedure unless looked for [13]. Speech disturbances may persist longer than the weakness in about 10% of the patients. These have always resolved within 1 month in our experience [57] but others have reported longer-term effects [46].

The long-term effects of complete CC section have been studied extensively in selected patients particularly those of the Dartmouth group [56,58,59]. Within a few months after an operation most patients become compensated to a remarkable degree and in personality and social situations appear much as before the surgery. By 1 year postoperative most groups report no significant difference in a wide variety of neuropsychologic tests including the standard intellectual measures of a WAIS-R IQ test [13,45,59,60]. Anecdotal clinical reports from the original series of Wilson *et al.* [3] indicate that 50% (5/10) had resumed their previous occupations. Sass *et al.* [46] using more functional measures have reported that 6/10 patients who had undergone one- or two-stage complete CC sections had neuropsychologic scores which were better than their preoperative ones, while four had experienced some decline in their level of function. Ferguson *et al.* [61], however, found 5/5 patients significantly impaired in activities of daily living due to sequellae of speech disturbance, hemispheric competition, memory loss or motor incoordination. Because of the wide variability in the incidence of sequellae from one series to another it is difficult to assess their overall frequency. Different surgical techniques leading to variable manipulation and trauma to the fornix, hippocampal commissures, third ventricular structures and anterior commissure may account for some of these differences and these factors should be carefully assessed when reviewing case reports from different centers.

The midline approach using microscopic techniques in experienced hands (see Chapter 8) minimizes trauma to this area. Reports of comprehensive neuropsychologic studies of series of patients studied pre- and postoperatively with two-stage callosal sections using such techniques are still unavailable in the literature.

Permanent effects in all patients of a complete or posterior CC section can be demonstrated using a lateralized input such as that provided with a tachistoscope for visual stimulation presented to one visual field or an object presented to one hand with the patient blindfolded. With these techniques isolation of the language hemisphere from tactile, visual and auditory information to the nonlanguage hemisphere can be documented. Thus the patient is unable to name, or if questioned verbally may even deny the existence of, stimuli in the left visual field. Unilateral tactile anomia of objects placed in the left hand and poor identification of words presented in a dichotic listening paradigm to the left ear are also seen. However since visual, auditory and tactile inputs are normally bilateral, this sensory disconnection is not usually a significant phenomenon in daily activities. However, it is critical to understand its mechanisms and have patients thoroughly tested preoperatively for any unilateral deficits of sensory input such as hemianopia, which would then predict a significant functional deficit from a complete callosotomy.

Speech disturbances of a permanent nature have occurred in patients but they appear to be rare. Comprehension is not affected but speech output can be absent or disturbed by severe stuttering [62–64]. Reviews of the topic [46,56,57] have suggested that the patients at risk are those with bilateral speech representation or crossed dominance as determined by intracarotid Amytal testing [65]. This suggests that patients should be carefully tested in this manner preoperatively. Patients with the above findings are then either excluded for surgery or at least considered to be at a very high risk for such problems.

Because the motor function in the nondominant hand is also disconnected from verbal commands it can sometimes function antagonistically to the dominant hand in a syndrome of "hemispheric competition." Two patients (of the 185 reported in Table 4.1) are vividly described as severely affected by this "split brain phenomenon" [2,5]. In most patients, however, this phenomenon is not seen or is only a transient and not an ongoing problem.

Deficits in motor coordination, including difficulty learning bimanual tasks, were reported in patients with a complete CC section (including anterior commissure via a transventricular approach) who had been operated on before 1977 [66–68]. Campbell *et al.* [68] have emphasized the need to interpret the postoperative findings in comparison with preoperative assessments particularly in patients with evidence of preoperative lateralized deficits. However Sass *et al.* [46] have found these patients to have a good outcome without increased functional deficit. Memory disturbances have also been described in some callosotomy patients [61,69,70] but others [46,60] found memory scores unchanged in most patients. It has been suggested the apparent memory problems are due to attention deficits [60]. The memory problems of the earlier cases may also be due to the lesions of fornix and trauma in the wall of the third ventricle rather than to the callosal division.

Permanent effects of anterior CC section appear to be less frequent and more difficult to detect than those reported for complete CC section [13,46,71]. Appearance or exacerbation of lateralized preexisting deficits are reported [45,68,72] and even in patients without neurologic deficits some loss in a complex bimanual task has been demonstrated [73]. In our testing [13], while the bimanual performance scores were the most significantly changed at one month postoperatively, at 1 year follow-up these scores had returned to preoperative levels.

In summary the neuropsychologic consequences of complete CC section are invariably some sensory disconnection, but as long as sensory inputs are normal bilaterally, this is compensated for in day-to-day living. In patients undergoing anterior callosotomy there is no sensory disconnection syndrome. Other significant sequelae of either procedure, including speech disturbance, bimanual coordination difficulties (particularly in learning new such tasks, memory and attention deficits), and a personality syndrome of interhemispheric competition, have been reported in individual cases, but their overall incidence with newer microsurgical techniques and our ability to predict their occurrence with preoperative testing is at present unclear and in need of further study.

The extent of section: partial or complete callosotomy?

This is an extremely important but still very difficult question to answer using the currently available literature. An important factor may be the problem of determining at surgery the full extent of the callosotomy, due to the difficulty of visualizing the entire callosum through the microscopic approach. A few recent studies have included magnetic resonance imaging (MRI), which provides a method of clearly assessing the extent of the postoperative section. The technique often demonstrates some remaining corpus callosum fibres in either the rostrum or splenium, depending on the surgical approach that was used. The number of reported patients assessed by MRI is very low [13,16,74].

The only study [12] which attempts to compare results of partial vs. complete section claims that the complete section was twice as effective as partial section for control of tonic–clonic seizures. Eight out of 17 patients who had undergone a partial section had continued to have seizures and underwent completion of the callosotomy. It is difficult to tell how many of these eight were helped by completion. Comparison between the overall outcome in the series which did anterior sections only [13,14] appears to show poorer results for the control of GTCS (an improvement in 5/8 and 9/18) as compared with those doing mostly complete CC sections [11,12] with 17/27 and 16/22 patients improved. However, with different patient groups at these centers such comparisons should be considered with caution. Only further studies of the effects of completion of an anterior CC section in the same patients will clarify the question of the need for this more extensive procedure and perhaps predict who should have it.

The recent MRI reports of the CC anatomy [75] would suggest that the shape and density of this structure is quite variable. Some assessment of the volume of CC sectioned, compared with the results of the procedure for seizure control, would be most interesting. In the Minnesota series [18] where the intention had been to perform a complete CC section, postoperative MRI in 6/15 patients documented that the splenium was intact. There is no evidence that these six patients did any worse than the overall group. A single case is reported [74] with persistent seizures postoperatively in a patient who had an MRI showing some corpus callosum still intact. The patient went on to a second operation to complete the section. This decreased but failed to stop the seizures despite a postoperative MRI scan demonstration of a now-complete CC section.

At most centers [12,16,76] complete callosotomy is now done as a two-stage procedure with an interval of at least 6 months between the two procedures in order to document whether the anterior section is adequate for seizure control. The remarkable decrease in the postoperative disconnection syndrome and resultant shortening of the convalescence time with the two-stage procedure would justify the two-stage approach on these merits alone. It will also provide the opportunity to determine with MRI scan documentation what percentage and which type(s) of patients achieve good seizure control with only the anterior half or two-thirds of the callosum sectioned.

Conclusions

Corpus callosum section appears to have an important role in treating the medically intractable seizure patients who are not eligible for focal resections. The severity of the seizures must be great enough to justify the risks of surgery but in many cases the patients are improved postoperatively, due to a reduction in the frequency and severity of seizures. The neuropsychologic sequellae of disconnection after complete CC section are rarely noted by the patient or his family in the activities of daily living and after anterior callosotomy there are not usually any easily detectable deficits by patient observation or with neuropsychologic testing.

It is important that patients are studied preoperatively so that a clear definition of their seizure type with ictal EEG is available, preferably including an attempt to delineate a focal onset with intracranial electrodes. Documentation of the preoperative neuropsychologic level of function, as well as detection of any lateralized deficits in sensory input, is essential. Patients also require structural studies including CT scans and MRI, and assessment of localization of language function by the intracarotid Wada Sodium Amytal test to detect mixed or crossed dominance.

The use of a two-stage procedure promises to provide useful data regarding the need for partial or complete callosotomies. There are clearly many who will benefit from the partial callosotomy only and those who will benefit from completion of the section remain to be defined.

The surgical procedure itself is a difficult one and some series report a considerable complication rate of 16–25% [2,3,10,13]. This suggests the need for specific experience with the procedure by the surgical team. It is not a procedure to be undertaken on a sporadic basis.

The selection of patients for this procedure remains a challenging topic. Technical developments such as MRI scans and better video-EEG systems along with a growing experience with carefully studied patients promises to help the epilepsy team when faced with the decision of offering this type of surgery to the individual medically intractable patient.

Acknowledgement

My thanks to my colleagues W.B. Woodhurst, J. Wada and G.B. Purves for helpful discussions and advice on this subject, and to Louise Kokotailo for manuscript preparation.

References

1 Williamson PD. Corpus callosum section for intractable epilepsy. In Reeves AG (ed) *Epilepsy and the Corpus Callosum*. New York, Plenum Press, 1985, pp 243–257.
2 Wilson DH, Reeves A, Gazzaniga M, Culver C. Cerebral commissurotomy for control of intractable seizures. *Neurology* 1977; **27**: 708–715.
3 Wilson DH, Reeves A, Gazzaniga M. Central commissurotomy for intractable generalized epilepsy: series two. *Neurology* 1982; **32**: 687–697.
4 Marino R Jr, Ragazzo PC. Selective criteria and results of selective partial callosotomy. In Reeves AG (ed) *Epilepsy and the Corpus Callosum*. New York, Plenum Press, 1985, pp 281–301.
5 Rayport M, Ferguson SM, Corrie WS. Outcomes and indications of corpus callosum section for intractable seizure control. *Appl Neurophysiol* 1983; **46**: 47–51.
6 Geoffroy G, Lassonde M, Delisle F, Decarie M. Corpus callosotomy for control of intractable epilepsy in children. *Neurology* 1983; **33**: 891–897.
7 Blume WT. Corpus callosum section for seizure control: rationale and review of experimental and clinical data. *Cleve Clin Quart* 1984; **51**: 319–332.
8 Saint-Hilaire JM, Giard N, Bouvier G, Labrecque R. Anterior callosotomy in frontal lobe epilepsies. In Reeves AG (ed) *Epilepsy and the Corpus Callosum*. New York, Plenum Press, 1985, pp 303–314.
9 Bouvier G, Mercier C, Saint-Hilaire JM, Giard N, Labrecque R, Weique RA. Anterior callosotomy and chronic depth electrode recording in the surgical management of some intractable seizures. *Appl Neurophysiol* 1983; **46**: 52–56.
10 Gates JR, Leppik IE, Yap J, Gumnit RJ. Corpus callosotomy: Clinical and electroencephalographic effects. *Epilepsia* 1984; **25**: 308–316.
11 Gates JR, Rosenfeld WE, Maxwell RE, Lyons RE. Response of multiple seizure types to corpus callosum section. *Epilepsia* 1987; **28**: 28–34.
12 Spencer SS, Spencer DD, Williamson PD, Sass K, Novelly RA, Mattson RH. Corpus callosotomy for epilepsy: I. seizure effects. *Neurology* 1988; **38**: 19–24.
13 Purves SJ, Wada JA, Woodhurst WB, Moyes PD, Strauss E, Kosaka B, Li D. Results of anterior corpus callosum section in 24 patients with medically intractable seizures. *Neurology* 1983; **38**: 1194–1201.
14 Murro AM, Flanigin HF, Gallagher BB, King DW, Smith, JR. Corpus callosotomy for the treatment of intractable epilepsy. *Epil Res* 1988; **2**: 44–50.
15 Garcia-Flores E. Corpus callosum section for patients with intractable epilepsy. *Appl Neurophysiol* 1987; **50**: 390–397.
16 Roberts DW, Reeves A. Effect of commissurotomy on complex partial epilepsy in patients without a resectable seizure focus. *Appl Neurophysiol* 1987; **50**: 398–400.
17 Marino R. Selective partial micro surgical callosotomy for intractable multiform seizures: Criteria for clinical selection and results. *Appl Neurophysiol* 1985; **48**: 404–407.
18 Maxwell RE, Gates JR, McGeachie R. Magnetic resonance imaging in the assessment and surgical management of epilepsy and functional neurological disorders. *Appl Neurophysiol* 1987; **50**: 369–373.
19 Van Wagenen WP, Herren RY. Surgical division of commissural pathways in the corpus callosum: Relation to spread of an epileptic attack. *Arch Neurol Psychiat* 1940; **44**: 740–759.
20 Bogen J. Cerebral commissurotomy. A second case report. *JAMA* 1965; **194**: 1328–1329.
21 Bogen JE, Sperry RW, Vogel PJ. Commissural section and propagation of seizures. In Jasper H. (ed) *Basic Mechanisms of the Epilepsies*. Little, Brown, Boston, 1969, pp 439–440.

22 Lussenhop AJ, Dela Cruz TE, Fenichel GM. Surgical disconnection of the cerebral hemispheres for intractable seizures. *JAMA* 1970; **213**: 1630.

23 Roberts DW. Corpus callosotomy: surgical technique. In Reeves AG (ed) *Epilepsy and the Corpus Callosum*. Plenum Press, New York, 1985, pp 259–267.

24 Gordon HW, Bogen JE, Sperry RW. Absence of deconnexion syndrome in two patients with partial section of the neocommissures. *Brain* 1971; **94**: 327–336.

25 Wada JA. New surgical treatment through experimental models. In Wada JA, Penry K (eds) *Advances in Epileptology*. Raven Press, New York, 1980, pp 195–213.

26 Erickson TE. Spread of the epileptic discharge: an experimental study of the after discharge induced by electrical stimulation of the cerebral cortex. *Arch Neurol Psychiatr* 1940; **43**: 429–452.

27 Musgrave J, Gloor P. The role of the corpus callosum in bilateral interhemispheric synchrony of spike and wave discharge in feline generalized penicillin epilepsy. *Epilepsia* 1980; **21**: 369–378.

28 Marcus EM. Generalized seizure models and the corpus callosum. In Reeves AG (ed) *Epilepsy and the Corpus Callosum*. Plenum Press, New York, 1985, pp 131–206.

29 Kopeloff N, Kennard MA, Pacella DL, Kopeloff LM, Chusid JG. Section of corpus callosum in experimental epilepsy in the monkey. *Arch Neurol Psychol* 1950; **63**: 719–727.

30 Wada JA, Sato M. Generalized convulsive seizure state induced by daily electrical stimulation of the amygdala in split brain cats. *Epilepsia* 1975; **16**: 417–430.

31 Wada JA, Nakashima T, Kaneko Y. Forebrain bisection and feline amygdaloid kindling. *Epilepsia* 1982; **23**: 521–531.

32 Wada JA, Mizoguchi T, Komai S. Cortical motor activation in amygdaloid kindling: observations in non-epileptogenic rhesus monkeys with the anterior 2/3 callosal bisection. In Wada JA (ed) *Kindling 2*. Raven Press, New York, 1981, pp 235–248.

33 Wada JA, Komai S. Effect of anterior two-thirds callosal bisection upon bisymmetrical and bisynchronous generalized convulsions kindled from amygdala in epileptic baboon, *Papio papio*. In Reeves AG (ed) *Epilepsy and the Corpus Callosum*. Plenum Press, New York, 1985, pp 75–97.

34 Wada JA, Mizoguchi T. Limbic kindling in forebrain bisected photo-sensitive baboon, *Papio papio*. *Epilepsia* 1984; **25**(3): 278–287.

35 McCaughran JA Jr, Corcorcan ME, Wada JA. Facilitation of secondary site amygdaloid kindling following bisection of corpus callosum and hippocampal commissure in rats. *Exper Neurol* 1977; **57**: 132–141.

36 Pandya DN, Rosene DL. Some observations on trajectories and topography of commissural fibres. In Reeves AG (ed) *Epilepsy and the Corpus Callosum*. Plenum, New York Press 1985, pp 21–40.

37 Pandya DN, Yeterian EH. Hodology of limbic and related structures: cortical and commissural connections. In Weiser HG and Elger CE (ed) *Presurgical Evaluation of Epileptics*. Springer-Verlag, Berlin, 1987, pp 3–14.

38 Spencer SS, Williamson PD, Spencer OP, Mattson RH. Human hippocampal seizure spread studies by depth and subdural recording the hippocampal commissure. *Epilepsia* 1987; **28**: 479–489.

39 Leib JP, Hogue K, Skomer CE, Sung X. Interhemispheric propagation of human mesial temporal seizures: a coherence phase analyses. *EEG Clin Neurophysiol* 1987; **67**: 101–119.

40 Waterman K, Purves SJ, Kosaka B, Strauss E, Wada JA. An epileptic syndrome caused by mesial frontal lobe seizure foci. *Neurology* 1987; **37**: 577–582.

41 Ottino CA, Meglio M, Rossi GF, Tercero E. An experimental study of the structures mediating bilateral synchrony of epileptic discharges of cortical origin. *Epilepsia* 1971; **12**: 299–311.

42 Spencer, SS. Corpus callosum section and other disconnection procedures for medically intractable epilepsy. *Epilepsia* 1988; **29** (Suppl 2): 585–599.

43 Engel J. Outcome with respect to epileptic seizures. In Engel J (ed) *Surgical Treatment of the Epilepsies*. Raven Press, New York, 1987, pp 553–571.

44 Spencer SS, Spencer DD, Glaser GH, Williamson PD, Mattson RH. More intense focal seizure types after callosal section: The role of inhibition. *Ann Neurol* 1984; **16**: 686–693.

45 Wylie E. Corpus callosotomy for intractable generalized epilepsy. *J Pediatrics* 1988; **113**: 255–261.

46 Sass KJ, Spencer DD, Spencer SS, Novelly RA, Williamson PD, Mattson RH. Corpus callosotomy for epilepsy. II. Neurologic and neuropsychological outcome. *Neurology* 1988; **38**: 24–28.

47 Spencer SS, Gates JR, Reeves AG, Spencer DD, Maxwell RE, Roberts D. Corpus callosum section. In Engel J Jr (ed) *Surgical Treatment of the Epilepsies.* Raven Press, New York, 1987, pp 425–444.

48 Fiol ME, Gates JR. EEG studies and corpus callosotomy results. *EEG Clin Neurophysiol* 1984 **58**: 34.

49 Gates JR, Maxwell R, Leppik JE, Fiol M, Gumnet RJ. Electrographic and clinical effects of total corpus callosotomy. In Reeves AG (ed) *Epilepsy and the Corpus Callosum.* Plenum Press, New York, 1985, pp 315–328.

50 Wilson DW, Culver C, Waddington M, Gazzinaga M. Disconnection of the cerebral hemispheres: an alternative to hemispherectomy for the control of intractable seizures. *Neurology* 1975; **25**: 1149–1153.

51 Tinuper P, Andermann F, Villemerre JG, Rasmussen T, Quesney L. Functional hemispherectomy for treatment of epilepsy associated with hemiplegia: rationale, indications, results and comparisons with callosotomy. *Ann Neurol* 1988; **24**: 27–34.

52 Verity CM, Strauss EH, Moyes PD, Wada JA, Dunn HG, Lapointe, JS. Long term follow-up after cerebral hemispherectomy: neurophysiologic, radiologic and psychological findings. *Neurology* 1982; **32**: 629–639.

53 Ignelzi RJ, Bucy PC. Cerebral hemidecortication in the treatment of infantile cerebral hemiatrophy. *J Nerv Ment Dis* 1968; **147**: 14–30.

54 Rasmussen T. Hemispherectomy for seizures revisited. *Can J Neurol Sci* 1983; **10**: 71–78.

55 Goodman RN, Williamson PD, Reeves AG, Spencer S, Spencer DD, Mattson RH, Roberts DW. Interhemisphere commissurotomy for congenital hemiplegics with intractable epilepsy. *Neurology* 1985; **35**: 1351–1354.

56 Bogen JE. Physiological consequences of complete or partial commissural section. In Apuzzo MLJ (ed) *Surgery of the Third Ventricle.* Williams & Wilkins, Baltimore, 1987, pp 175–194.

57 Woodhurst WB, Wada JW, Purves SJ. Speech disturbances after anterior callosal section. *Epilepsia* 1989; **30**: 677–8.

58 Gazzaniga MS, Risse GL, Springer SP, Clark E, Wilson DH. Psychologic and neurologic consequences of partial and complete cerebral commissurotomy. *Neurology* 1975; **25**: 10–15.

59 Ferrell RB, Culver CM, Tucker GJ. Psychosocial and cognitive function after commissurotomy for intractable seizures. *J Neurosurg* 1983; **58**: 374–380.

60 Beniak TE, Gates JR, Risse GL. Comparison of selected neuropsychological test variables pre- and post-operatively on patients subjected to corpus callosotomy. *Epilepsia* 1985; **26**: 534.

61 Ferguson SM, Rayport M, Corrie WS. Neuropsychiatric observations on behavioral consequences of corpus callosum section for seizure control. In Reeves AG (ed) *Epilepsy and the Corpus Callosum.* Plenum Press, New York, 1985, pp 501–514.

62 Ross MK, Reeves AG, Roberts DW. Post commissurotomy mutism. *Ann Neurol* 1984; **16**: 14.

63 Sussman NM, Gur RC, Gur RE, O'Connor M. Mutism as a consequence of callosotomy. *J Neurosurg* 1983; **59**: 514–519.

64 Rayport M, Ferguson SM, Currie WS. Mutism after corpus callosum section for intractable seizure control. *Epilepsia* 1984; **25**: 665.

65 Wada J, Rasmussen T. Intracarotid injection of Sodium Amytal for the lateralization of cerebral speech dominance. Experimental and clinical observations. *J Neurosurg* 1960; **17**: 266–282.

66 Preilowski BFB. Possible contribution of the anterior forebrain commissures to bilateral motor coordination. *Neuropsychologia* 1972; **10**: 167–177.

67 Zaidel D, Sperry RW. Some long-term motor effects of cerebral commissurotomy in man. *Neuropsychologia* 1977; **15**: 193–204.

68 Campbell AL, Bogan JG, Smith A. Disorganization and reorganization of cognitive and sensorimotor functions in cerebral commissurotomy. *Brain* 1981; **104**: 493–511.

69 Ledoux JE, Risse GL, Springer SP, Wilson DW, Gazzaniga MS. Cognition and commissurotomy. *Brain* 1974; **100**: 87–104.

70 Zaidel E, Sperry RW. Memory impairment after commissurotomy in man. *Brain* 1974; **97**: 263–272.

71 Harbaugh RE, Wilson DH, Reeves AG, Gazzaniga MS. Forebrain commissurotomy for epilepsy. Review of 20 consecutive cases. *Acta Neurochir (Wien)* 1983; **68**: 263–275.

72 Novelly RA, Lifrak MD. Forebrain commissurotomy reinstates effects of pre-existing hemisphere lesions: an examination of the hypothesis. In Reeves AG (ed) *Epilepsy and the Corpus Callosum.* Plenum Press, New York, 1985 pp 467–500.
73 Jeeves MA, Silver PH, Jacobsen I. Bimanual coordination in callosal agenesis and partial commissurotomy. *Neuropsychologia* 1988; **26**: 833–850.
74 Gates JR, Mireles, R, Maxwell R, Sharbrough F, Forbes G. Magnetic resonance imaging, electroencephalogram and selected neuropsychologic testing in staged corpus callosotomy. *Arch Neurol* 1986; **43**: 1188–1191.
75 Reinarz SJ, Coffman CE, Smoker WRK, Godersky JC. MRI imaging of the corpus callosum: normal and pathologic findings and correlation with CT. *Am J Neuroradiol* 1988; **9**: 649–656.
76 Maxwell RE, Gates JR, Gumnit RJ. Corpus callosotomy at the University of Minnesota. In Engel J, Jr (ed) *Surgical Treatment of the Epilepsies.* Raven Press, New York, 1987, pp 659–666.

Comment

Susan S. Spencer

Corpus callosum section is a palliative surgical approach to patients with secondarily generalized (tonic–atonic/tonic–clonic) seizures who are not candidates for focal resection. It usually results in near or complete cessation of generalized seizures, at the expense of persistent partial seizures (50%), worsening partial seizures (25%), and neurologic or neuropsychologic sequelae in motor, language, or cognitive spheres (20%). To some degree, the same patients are at risk for significant neurologic sequelae and diminished seizure response, making strict criteria for patient selection doubly important.

Unfortunately, strict patient selection criteria are not available. The difficulties have been pointed out in this chapter. Thus, although nonresponders usually have low IQ and/or multifocal seizure onset, some such patients will respond. Conversely, focal CNS pathology is usually but not always associated with good responses and lack of sequelae. Early seizure onset and lateralized deficit of moderate–severe degree are predictive in general of minimal neurologic sequelae, and crossed dominance or prior mild neurologic impairment may predict language or motor deficits. Neither scenario, however, is without its exceptions. At present, cognitive and behavioral sequelae are poorly defined as are the *a priori* indications for partial sections.

Some comments on patient and family expectations after corpus callosum section should be made. Although rare individuals have a marked decrease in seizure frequency as well as cessation of generalized seizures, most successful candidates will have their satisfactory response manifested only by elimination of generalized seizures with persistent and sometimes more intense or more frequent partial seizures. Despite extensive patient and family counselling on these predicted results, the hope for a cure persists, and when it does not occur the operation is often judged to be a failure. The application of a palliative procedure for treatment of uncontrolled epilepsy with multiple seizure types is thus a very difficult proposition and one which requires more than the usual lengthy preoperative patient and family counselling.

It is understood that most patients will be counselled as to the unpredictability of exact response to partial or total section because of the lack of previously well documented candidates and guidelines. We require more data on this approach to surgical epilepsy treatment, which emphasizes the need for careful and continued pre- and postoperative evaluation at all centers involved in such operations. Such data will be important to analyze with respect to the differences in response at different ages, since minimal information is available in this regard. The literature has been well reviewed by Dr Purves and our comments serve only to consolidate our viewpoints and put issues in perspective.

chapter 5

Epilepsy Surgery: Special Considerations for Children

Elaine Wyllie, Hans Lüders, and A. David Rothner

Introduction

There are now several reports of epilepsy surgery in children, with consistently good results [1–10]. The most frequent operation is temporal lobectomy, but many children have also benefited from frontal lobectomy, other extratemporal resections, hemispherectomy [11–18], or corpus callosotomy [19–30]. It has become clear that children as well as adults may benefit from early epilepsy surgery, yet it remains usual for patients to be referred for surgical evaluation only after their childhood-onset seizures have continued well into adulthood.

This delay in performing surgery for childhood-onset epilepsy was illustrated in a recent series of patients who had temporal or extratemporal resection [10]. The mean duration of seizures prior to operation for adult patients was 15.9 years, and for children operated before age 18 was 7.5 years [10]. The two age groups had similar frequency of good outcome after surgery, so it is not clear that there was any benefit from prolonged waiting. On the contrary, there may have been a medical, psychological, and social price to pay for the extra years of intractable seizures.

These issues have raised questions about the optimum age at which epilepsy surgery should be performed. This review will consider some special aspects of epilepsy surgery in children.

Focal cortical resection in children

The major criteria for focal cortical resection in children and adults include the following: (1) a clearly established diagnosis of localization-related (partial, or focal) epilepsy; (2) location of seizure onset in a relatively "silent" area of the brain which could be removed with a low risk of neurologic deficit; and (3) intractable, handicapping seizures for at least 2 or 3 years. The first two of these criteria are based on results of an intensive presurgical evaluation, usually at a specialized center for epilepsy surgery. The third criterion is more relative, based to a great degree on the clinician's judgement.

A clearly established diagnosis of localization-related epilepsy

In the current classification system of the International League Against Epilepsy [31], the partial or focal epilepsies are called "localization-related" epilepsies. For a solid diagnosis of localization-related epilepsy, the child's episodes should be consistent with the clinical profile of partial seizures, and the ictal or interictal EEG should show focal spikes or sharp waves. The following are aspects of these criteria which are specific to children.

Because complex partial seizures (*with* impairment of consciousness [32]) are the typical seizure type in temporal lobe epilepsy, and because temporal lobe epilepsy is the most common problem leading to epilepsy surgery, it is important to be aware of the special EEG and clinical aspects of complex partial seizures in children. Simple partial seizures (*without* impairment of consciousness [32]), which are more commonly seen in extratemporal epilepsy, are described elsewhere [33]).

Clinical manifestations of complex partial seizures in children The clinical features of complex partial seizures have been well-defined in adults [34–40] but there is less detailed information about these seizures in infants and young children [33,41]. The available data indicate that there are some differences between age groups. Most of these differences lead to increased difficulty in recognition of complex partial seizures in young children.

Auras have been reported for the majority of adult patients with temporal lobe epilepsy [35,37,38,40] but for less than one-third of children [42,43]. It is possible that more children actually have an aura, but cannot describe the feeling. Sometimes an aura can be suspected because the child always comes to a parent for help just before the development of altered consciousness.

Impairment of consciousness is more difficult to assess in infants and children than in adults, and this sometimes complicates the identification of seizures as complex partial. An arrest or activity, decreased responsiveness, or a blank stare may be all that occurs with altered awareness, and these signs may be difficult to appreciate in an infant or young child. In addition, the infant or young child will not be able to explain that he "blacked out." It may be difficult to determine whether the child had amnesia for ictal events, but amnesia is very helpful in determining whether unresponsiveness is due to impairment of consciousness, aphasia, oromotor phenomena, or strong and distracting sensory phenomena. In addition, because the International Classification [32] requires amnesia to define ictal unconsciousness, it is especially difficult to apply this classification system to younger patients, and to group them for scientific study.

Automatisms have been reported to be equally frequent during complex partial seizures in children [43–45] and adults [35,38, 46] but the features of automatisms may differ in the youngest patients. Children and adolescents may have automatisms consisting of a wide range of poorly coordinated semipurposeful activity, similar to those seen in adults [43,45]. Infants most often have just alimentary automatisms, such as chewing, swallowing, or lip smacking [44,45]. Gestural automatisms, such as fumbling with nearby objects or picking at clothes or bedsheets, are infrequent in infants [44, 45], perhaps because babies, unlike older children or adults, do not yet have a large repertoire of coordinated, purposeful hand movements as part of their normal behavior. Some infants may also have other types of motor phenomena during videotaped complex partial seizures, such as "hooking" or "boxing" movements of the arms, loss of neck muscle tone, or posturing resembling an asymmetric tonic neck response [44]. The exact significance of these more unusual motor phenomena is unclear.

Because automatisms may also occur during the seizures of childhood absence epilepsy (petit mal) [47], especially during longer attacks, it is important to rule out this diagnosis during the presurgical evaluation. Clinically, the absence seizures of childhood absence epilepsy tend to differ from the complex partial seizures of temporal lobe epilepsy in the following ways: (1) they are usually brief, lasting only seconds; (2) they tend to be very frequent, occurring many times each day; and (3) they tend to resolve suddenly, without a significant period of postictal confusion. The key to diagnosis is EEG, which shows bursts of generalized spike and slow-wave complexes, usually with 3-frequency. Children with childhood absence epilepsy are not candidates for cortical resection.

Electroencephalographic manifestations of complex partial seizures in children If the interictal EEG shows focal spikes or sharp waves from the temporal lobe, then there is strong supportive evidence for a diagnosis of complex partial seizures in the proper clinical setting. However, some patients with complex partial seizures have normal interictal EEGs, and this may be especially true for infants [45] and children [42]. In this situation, if the history is suggestive, and initial medical treatment is ineffective, then it is appropriate to consider additional prolonged EEG recording to confirm the diagnosis [48,49]. The chance of recording a seizure may be increased by weaning the antiepileptic medication.

It must be remembered that children of 2–16 years of age may have the centrotemporal spikes of benign childhood epilepsy. Although these discharges are clearly epileptiform, they frequently occur in normal children: it has been estimated that only 8.8% of children with these EEG discharges actually ever have a seizure [50]. In addition, among children with these centrotemporal spikes who do have seizures, the type is usually generalized tonic–clonic or simple partial with focal motor phenomena, not complex partial [51]. In a child with staring spells and benign centrotemporal spikes, it is likely that the two phenomena are unrelated. If there is a strong clinical suspicion for complex partial seizures, it is important to record an attack on EEG, because it is possible that the child has temporal lobe epilepsy and coincidental benign centrotemporal spikes.

In children with complex or simple partial seizures due to extratemporal epilepsy, the key EEG findings are focal spikes or sharp waves from frontal, parietal, or occipital regions. The relationship of these findings to the plans for surgery in children have been discussed in detail elsewhere [52], and are beyond the scope of this review.

Location of seizure onset in a relatively "silent" area of the brain

In most cases, it is unacceptable to purposefully trade seizures for another postsurgical disability such as aphasia or hemiparesis. However, some patients may choose to suffer certain postoperative deficits in exchange for relief of seizures. For example, some patients with severe intractable seizures arising from one occipital lobe may elect surgery despite near-certain postoperative hemianopsia. Another example might be a patient with severe debilitating epilepsia partialis continua who might elect resection of rolandic areas despite the postoperative hemiplegia. Usually, however, it is imperative to avoid postoperative deficit. This involves determination of the precise location of seizure onset in relation to eloquent cortex, and requires intensive EEG evaluation.

The cornerstone of localization of the epileptogenic area continues to be the surface EEG evaluation [48,52]. For precise mapping of focal ictal and interictal epileptiform discharges, it is helpful to record from closely spaced electrodes over the area of interest in addition to the standard electrodes of the International 10–20 system [48,57]. Also helpful in recording from mesial temporal regions are sphenoidal electrodes, but they are painful to insert. To permit comfortable insertion of sphenoidal electrodes in younger patients, it is helpful to use bedside intravenous sedation with medication combinations such as meperidine and midazolam [58].

Even after the epileptogenic region has been identified with detailed surface recording, it may still be necessary in certain cases to gain further information with invasive neurophysiologic techniques. Such techniques are used widely in adult patients [55,56,59–66] but they have been less frequently used in children. A few reports of epilepsy surgery in children have included intraoperative electrocorticography [2,4,6,9] or extraoperative EEG from subdural [10,67,68] or epidural [7] electrodes. There has not yet been a large reported series of children who had depth electrodes, although some predominantly adult series have included younger patients. There may be a greater reluctance to use invasive neurophysiologic techniques in children than in adults, but when some of these techniques were compared in pediatric and adult patients, there was equal efficacy and safety [10].

The authors feel that if invasive neurophysiologic techniques are needed to further define the epileptogenic area and surrounding eloquent cortex prior to surgery, then these procedures should be performed, regardless of age. In some cases, this may require special tailoring of techniques to suit younger patients. A key feature is that cortical stimulation and EEG recording should be extraoperative, because children can have difficulty tolerating operation under local anesthesia. For this reason, chronically implanted epidural, subdural, depth, or foramen ovale electrodes may often be more useful in children than intraoperative EEG and cortical electrical stimulation.

Intracarotid amobarbital (Wada) testing [69,70] is another presurgical localization technique which is helpful for determination of cerebral dominance for language and memory in adults, but which may be difficult to use in children. Insertion of the arterial catheter is painful, even with local anesthesia. Systemic analgesics, anxiolytics, and sedatives may have an adverse effect on cognitive function and compromise the test. If the child is mature enough to tolerate placement of the catheter under local anesthesia, then he or she is likely to be able to cooperate with the rest of the test. In our experience, it has been difficult to perform Wada testing in children under about 8 years old.

Intractable, handicapping seizures

This is the most difficult and controversial of the criteria for epilepsy surgery, especially in children. There are three questions which must be answered to satisfy this criterion. Here we will review the aspects of these questions which pertain to children.

Are the seizures truly intractable? This depends on the degree to which the medical management has been aggressive. A strategy for medical management of intractable partial seizures has been described elsewhere in detail [33,41,71]. The general principles of this strategy are similar for adults and children, but its exact implementation requires a detailed understanding of the use of antiepileptic medications in pediatric patients.

Are the seizures sufficiently handicapping to warrant a surgical procedure? In young children, compared with adults, it may be more difficult to appreciate the adverse impact of the epilepsy or lifestyle. For children the seizures do not result in loss of employment or driving privileges, but the child has the special problem of having to deal with the epilepsy while developing a sense of self [72–74]. The unpredictable, recurrent nature of the attacks may cause anxiety, depression, and poor self-esteem [75,76] and in children especially this may lead to a sense of decreased competency and independence. Compounding this is a tendency for the parents of children with epilepsy to be overprotective [77,78] as well as the tendency for social ostracism by peers [79]. By the time these children reach early adulthood, they may already have significant psychosocial difficulties which limit their education, social, and vocational potential. It has been suggested that earlier epilepsy surgery may help prevent these long-term problems [1,9,80–82].

The same type and severity of seizures may mean a different degree of disability to two different children. For example, two or three complex partial seizures a month may have a serious adverse effect on the lifestyle of a high school student who is active in sports and social activities, learning to drive, and preparing for college and a career. On the other hand, two or three complex partial seizures a month may be acceptable to a more limited youngster who lives in a supervised home and is training for a job in a sheltered workshop. These differences must be appreciated when epilepsy surgery is considered.

For every epilepsy surgery candidate, there should be specific identifiable goals for surgery based on realistic expectations for an improved lifestyle after a decrease in seizures. In patients with high intellectual functioning, the goal is a normal, independent life; in patients with mental retardation, the goals may be more limited, such as increased social functioning, decreased physical injury from secondary generalized tonic–clonic seizures, or qualification for placement in a sheltered home with less extensive medical supervision.

Another reason for timely epilepsy surgery is to avoid chronic exposure to high doses of antiepileptic medications. Each of the drugs may have serious side effects [83], especially when used at high doses. If surgery is delayed until adulthood in a patient with early childhood-onset epilepsy, there may be a decade or so of unnecessary exposure to these agents.

Is there any realistic chance that the seizures will remit spontaneously? A major concern about early surgery in children is that until adulthood it may be difficult to be sure that the child will not outgrow the seizures. It has not been clearly demonstrated, however, that childhood-onset complex partial seizures have higher rates of spontaneous remission than adult-onset seizures. Recently reported remission rates in children with partial seizures have ranged from 10% to 62% (Table 5.1) [40,84–93], but most reports have had limitations. Several were based on clinical criteria only, so some patients may have had childhood absence epilepsy or psychogenic

TABLE 5.1 Rates of spontaneous remission in series of children with complex partial seizures. Only the series by Harbord and Manson [84] and Kotagal *et al.* [85] were limited to children with firm EEG evidence of localization-related epilepsy, and specifically excluded patients with benign focal epilepsy with centrotemporal spikes. (Modified and reprinted with permission [41].)

Report	All patients had focal EEG sharp waves	No patient had benign focal epilepsy	% of patients seizure-free at follow-up
Glaser 1967 [86]	—	—	29
Currie *et al.* 1971 [40]	—	—	32
Lindsay *et al.* 1979 [87]	—	—	33
Iemolo *et al.* 1981 [88]	—	Yes	20
Sofijanov 1982 [89]	Yes	—	36
Loiseau *et al.* 1983 [90]	—	Yes	48
Sillanpää 1983 [91]	—	—	29
Schmidt *et al.* 1983 [92]	—	—	62
Deonna *et al.* 1986 [93]	—	Yes	24
Harbord and Manson 1987 [84]	Yes	Yes	10
Kotagal *et al.* 1987 [85]	Yes	Yes	18*

*None was off antiepileptic medication

seizures, and several included patients with benign childhood epilepsy with centrotemporal spikes. The possible inclusion of these other groups might have falsely raised the remission rate.

Only two reports have been limited to children with EEG-demonstrated temporal lobe epilepsy, and in these the remission rates were only 10% [84] and 18% [85]. In addition, in one of these series [85] remission was defined as seizure-free on medications; not one of these patients was seizure-free off medications. These data suggest that temporal lobe epilepsy is frequently intractable in children as well as adults, and that spontaneous remission is unlikely.

Results of cortical resection in children

The results of cortical resection in children are comparable to those in adults. The definition of good outcome after cortical resection has varied between reports, but in general it includes being seizure-free, with auras only, or with a very marked decrease in seizure frequency. The overall reported rate of good outcome in pediatric series has ranged from 57% to 100% of patients, with most centers reporting good outcome for about three-quarters of operated children (Table 5.2) [1–10]. These rates are comparable to those reported in adult series. It has become clear that children as well as adults with localization-related epilepsy may benefit from early surgery.

The timing of cortical resection in children

The authors feel that if there is clear EEG and clinical evidence of localization-related epilepsy, with rigorous exclusion of childhood absence epilepsy and benign childhood epilepsy with centrotemporal spikes, and if the seizures are truly intractable and disabling despite aggressive medication trials for

TABLE 5.2 Results of epilepsy surgery in pediatric series. (Modified and reprinted with permission [41].)

Report	No. of patients	Ages at operation (years)	Resected areas	% of patients with good outcome
Davidson and Falconer [1]	40	2–34	Temporal	60
Rasmussen [2]	77	6–15	Temporal	73
Jensen and Vaernet [3]	12	3–15	Temporal	83
Green [4]	32	2–18	Temporal	93
Polkey [5]	40	<15	Temporal	57
Whittle [6]	8	5–18	Temporal	62
Goldring and Gregorie [7]	29	0.5–14	Temporal or extratemporal	62
Lindsay *et al.* [8]	13	7–36	Temporal or hemispheric	100
Meyer *et al.* [9]	50	7–18	Temporal	78
Wyllie *et al.* [10]	23	3–18	Temporal or extratemporal	70

2 or 3 years, then it is appropriate to consider epilepsy surgery, even in young children. At the Cleveland Clinic Foundation, the average time between the onset of seizures and the performance of epilepsy surgery has been 15 years, and it appears that in many cases this wait resulted in unnecessary medical and psychosocial difficulties during childhood and adolescence. It is becoming increasingly clear that early epilepsy surgery is appropriate in carefully selected cases.

Several pediatric operative series have included patients as young as 1 or 2 years old [1,3,4,7,10,67,94,95]. The increasing use of EEG monitoring in infants is broadening our understanding of localization-related epilepsy in this age group [44,45,49] and, in selected cases, operation may be helpful. However, in all but the most severe cases, it usually takes several years for the diagnosis to become clear and for exhaustive medication trials to be completed. Even in patients with onset of seizures in infancy, the selection criteria are usually not fulfilled before at least the early school-age years.

If a focal intracranial structural lesion is found on neuroimaging, then the patient may be operated earlier because of a concern that the lesion is neoplastic [2,5,10]. This is especially true when the lesion is seen to enlarge on serial magnetic resonance imaging (MRI) or computed tomography (CT) scans, although even apparently static lesions may be slow-growing gliomas. In one recent series [10] 39% of patients operated upon in childhood had a structural lesion shown by CT scans, compared to 10% of adults, and this difference appeared to be due to earlier operation in the patients with structural lesions.

It has also been suggested that a structural

lesion seen on CT scans or MRI may indicate an increased chance that the seizures are truly intractable and unlikely to remit spontaneously [5]. In addition, if the focal structural lesion is in the same region as the epileptiform discharges on EEG, then the finding may give added confidence that the EEG localization is correct and that epilepsy surgery would be effective [1]. For all of these reasons, a focal structural lesion seen on neuroimaging may make it appropriate for a child to be evaluated early for epilepsy surgery, even if the usual intractability criteria are incompletely satisfied.

Hemispherectomy

Hemispherectomy is a very effective form of epilepsy surgery in selected patients, because it involves essentially complete removal of all epileptogenic tissue as long as the focus is one-sided. Previously, there were problems with the operation. In recent years, there has been a resurgence of interest in the procedure.

Hemispherectomy first became an established type of epilepsy surgery after the report by Krynauw of 12 patients [11]. Between 1950 and 1968, there were many reports of excellent results, including a review of 420 cases [12]. The standard operation was complete hemispherectomy, with sparing only of basal ganglia. Candidates were patients with the following features: (1) intractable seizures arising from widespread areas of one damaged hemisphere; (2) dense hemiplegia since before 4 years of age; (3) no functional hand use on the weak side of the body; and (4) homonymous hemianopia. Most of the patients were children or adolescents, and essentially all had childhood-onset epilepsy. Dramatic improvement in seizure control and behavior was reported in 70–100% of patients, with rare worsening of neurologic deficits. In one report [16] 12% of 50 patients had worse speech function after hemispherectomy, and a few had to relearn walking, but other reports have not included patients with worsened function after operation.

By the late 1960s, 17–35% of patients had serious late complications after hemispherectomy [15,16,95]. Among patients who developed late complications, the mortality was 44% [15]. Problems appeared 1–20 years postoperatively: patients had an initial problem-free period followed by a progressive slow neurologic deterioration, often ending in death. Signs and symptoms included increased intracranial pressure, ataxia, dementia, brainstem dysfunction, and red blood cells or increased protein in the cerebrospinal fluid. Pathologic findings included obstructive hydrocephalus and superficial hemosiderosis of the cerebral hemisphere, cerebellum, and brainstem. One theory about etiology is that the problems are caused by repeated low-grade bleeding into the huge subdural hemispherectomy cavity [13,15, 96], but this remains controversial. One problem in our understanding of these complications is that they were reported before the advent of CT scanning or MRI.

In an attempt to reduce these late complications without sacrificing the benefits of hemispherectomy, there have been modifications of the original operating technique [13–15,17]. Current operations include the following: (1) subtotal hemispherectomy, with sectioning of the remaining white matter [15, 17]; (2) complete hemispherectomy, with suturing of the dura to reduce the size of the subdural space [13]; and (3) the traditional complete hemispherectomy [97] with frequent neuroimaging for early detection and management of complications. Long-term results from these different operations are not yet available, but preliminary data suggest that the incidence of late complications may be much reduced.

Some centers now also include patients for hemispherectomy who are not totally hemiplegic but who have progressive devastating illness such as Rasmussen's chronic focal encephalitis [97]. Children with this chronic focal encephalitis have intractable focal-onset seizures or epilepsia partialis continua, progressive atrophy of the affected hemisphere, and progressive neurologic deficit [98,99]. The mortality rate is significant, but if patients survive for several years, their seizures may gradually remit. However, the end result of Rasmussen's chronic encephalitis most often includes hemiplegia. For this reason, it has been suggested that complete hemispherectomy is appropriate at the time of definite diagnosis, even in the face of only minimal hemiparesis [96].

Hemispherectomy has also been performed on infants who have intractable focal-onset seizures and large unilateral congenital structural lesions [100] or focal areas of hypometabolism on position emission tomography (PET) [101], even if there is not a dense hemiplegia. However, few cases have been reported, and further data are required to define the selection criteria for hemispherectomy in infants.

Corpus callosotomy

In recent years, corpus callosotomy has gained recognition as a safe and effective treatment for selected patients with intractable, debilitating, secondarily generalized seizures, especially atonic or myoclonic "drop attacks" [26,102]. Results from recent operative series have been encouraging: 62–100% of patients have had significant improvement in the frequency of generalized seizures, and serious complications have been rare [19–30]. Division of all or part of the corpus callosum is thought to give its resultant benefit by interfering with the spread of epileptic discharges from one cerebral hemisphere to the other [103,104].

The early, more radical commissurotomy operations were found to have serious complications, resulting in the development of modified, safer techniques. Modern series involve section only of all or part of the corpus callosum and hippocampal commissure with sparing of the anterior commissure, massa intermedia of the thalamus, and fornix. With newer microsurgical techniques, there have been few serious operative complications.

Patient selection criteria for corpus callosotomy have not been completely defined. Current indications include the following: (1) at least a 3 year duration of daily or weekly intractable, debilitating secondary generalized tonic–clonic, atonic, tonic, or myoclonic seizures; (2) specific identifiable social or vocational goals for surgery based on realistic hopes for an improved lifestyle; and (3) EEG findings that rule out a single resectable epileptogenic focus. Because a large number of severely affected individuals fulfill these basic criteria, there is a need to further identify the subgroups that are most likely to benefit from surgery. Investigations are underway at several epilepsy surgery centers to address these issues.

There are no specific age restrictions for corpus callosotomy. Most patients have been teenagers or young adults at the time of operation, but recent series have also included children as young as 5 and 6 years old [20,24,28–30]. Potentially, more patients could be operated upon early in childhood, because the epilepsy is typically intractable and severe from a very early age. Reports of large pediatric series will be important to further define the optimum age for this operation.

References

1 Davidson S, Falconer MA. Outcome of surgery in 40 children with temporal-lobe epilepsy. *Lancet* 1975; **2**: 1260–1263.

2 Rasmussen TB. Surgical aspects. In Wise G (ed) *Topics in Child Neurology.* Spectrum, Englewood Cliffs, NJ, 1977, pp 143–153.

3 Jensen I, Vaernet K. Temporal lobe epilepsy. Follow-up investigation of 74 temporal lobe resected patients. *Acta Neurochir (Wien)* 1977; **37**: 173–200.

4 Green JR. Surgical treatment of epilepsy during childhood and adolescence. *Surg Neurol* 1977; **8**: 71–80.

5 Polkey CE. Selection of patients with intractable epilepsy for resective surgery. *Arch Dis Child* 1980; **55**: 841–844.

6 Whittle IR, Ellis HJ, Simpson DA. The surgical treatment of intractable childhood and adolescent epilepsy. *Aust NZ J Surg* 1981; **51**: 190–196.

7 Goldring S, Gregorie EM. Surgical management using epidural recordings to localize the seizure focus: review of 100 cases. *J Neurosurg* 1984; **60**: 457–466.

8 Lindsay J, Glaser G, Richards P, Ounsted C. Developmental aspects of focal epilepsies of childhood treated by neurosurgery. *Dev Med Child Neurol* 1984; **26**: 574–587.

9 Meyer FB, Marsh WR, Laws ER, Sharbrough FW. Temporal lobectomy in children with epilepsy. *J Neurosurg* 1986; **64**: 371–376.

10 Wyllie E, Lüders H, Morris HH, Lesser RP, Dinner DS, Hahn J, Estes ML, Rothner AD, Erenberg G, Cruse R, Friedman D. Subdural electrodes in the evaluation for epilepsy surgery in children and adults. *Neuropediatrics* 1988; **19**: 80–86.

11 Krynauw R. Infantile hemiplegia treated by removing one cerebral hemisphere. *J Neurol Neurosurg Psychiatr* 1950; **13**: 243–267.

12 Ignezi RJ, Bucy PC. Cerebral hemidecortication in the treatment of infantile cerebral hemiatrophy. *J Nerv Ment Dis* 1968; **147**: 14–30.

13 Adams CBT. Hemispherectomy — A modification. *J Neurol Neurosurg Psychiatr* 1983; **46**: 617–619.

14 Goodman R. Hemispherectomy and its alternatives in the treatment of intractable epilepsy in patients with infantile hemiplegia. *Dev Med Child Neurol* 1986; **28**: 251–258.

15 Rasmussen T. Hemispherectomy for seizures revisited. *J Canad Sci Neurol* 1983; **10**: 71–78.

16 Wilson PJE. Cerebral hemispherectomy for infantile hemiplegia. *Brain* 1970; **93**: 147–180.

17 Tinuper P, Andermann F, Villemure MG, Rasmussen TB, Quesney LF. Functional hemispherectomy for treatment of epilepsy associated with hemiplegia: rationale, indications, results, and comparison with callosotomy. *Ann Neurol* 1988; **24**: 27–34.

18 Rasmussen T, Villemure JG. Cerebral hemispherectomy for seizures with hemiplegia. *Cleve Clin J Med* 1989; **56**: 562–568.

19 Wilson DH, Reeves AG, Gazzaniga MS. "Central" commissurotomy for intractable generalized epilepsy: series two. *Neurology* 1982; **32**: 687–697.

20 Geoffroy G, Lassonde M, Delisle F, Decarie M. Corpus callosotomy for intractable epilepsy in children. *Neurology* 1983; **33**: 891–897.

21 Gates JR, Leppik IE, Yap J, Gumnit RJ. Corpus callosotomy: clinical and electroencephalographic effects. *Epilepsia* 1984; **25**: 308–316.

22 Murphy JV, Meyer GA, Harrington GJ, Hammeke TA, Newby RF. Corpus callosum resection in five patients with intractable seizures and mental retardation. *Ann Neurol* 1986; **20**: 388.

23 Spencer S, Spencer D, Glaser GH, Williamson PD, Mattson RH. More intense focal seizure types after corpus callosum section: the role of inhibition. *Arch Neurol* 1984; **116**: 686–693.

24 Rayport M, Corrie WS, Ferguson SM. Corpus callosum section for control of clinically and electroencephalographically classified intractable seizures. In Reeves AG (ed) *Epilepsy and the Corpus Callosum.* Plenum Press, New York, 1985, pp 329–340.

25 Rayport M, Corrie WS, Ferguson SM. Corpus callosum section for control of clinically and electroencephalography classified intractable seizures. In Reeves AG (ed) *Epilepsy and the Corpus Callosum.* Plenum Press, New York, 1985, pp 329–340.

26 Gates JR, Rosenfeld WE, Maxwell RE, Lyons

RE. Response of multiple seizure types to corpus callosum section. *Epilepsia* 1987; **28**: 28–34.

27 Bouvier G, Mercier C, St. Hilaire JM, Giard N, Labrecque R, Beique RA. Anterior callosotomy and chronic depth electrode recording in the surgical management of some intractable seizures. *Appl Neurophysiol* 1983; **46**: 52–56.

28 Marino R. Selective partial microsurgical callosotomy for intractable multiform seizures: criteria for clinical selection and results. *Appl Neurophysiol* 1985; **48**: 404–407.

29 Murro AM, Flanigan HF, Gallagher BB, King DW, Smith JR. Corpus callosotomy for the treatment of intractable epilepsy. *Epil Res* 1988; **2**: 44–50.

30 Spencer SS, Spencer DD, Williamson PD, Sass K, Novelly RA, Mattson RH. Corpus callosotomy for epilepsy. I. Seizure effects. Neurology 1988; **38**: 19–24.

31 Commission on Classification and Terminology of the International League Against Epilepsy. Proposal for classification of epilepsies and epileptic syndromes. *Epilepsia* 1985; **26**: 268–278.

32 Commission on Classification and Terminology of the International League Against Epilepsy. Proposal for revised clinical and electroencephalographic classification of epileptic seizures. *Epilepsia* 1981; **22**: 489–501.

33 Wyllie E, Rothner AD, Lüders H. Partial seizures in children, and surgical consideration. *Ped Clin North Am* 1989; **36**: 343–364.

34 Sharbrough RW. Complex partial seizures. In Lüders H, Lesser RP (eds) *Epilepsy: Electroclinical Syndromes.* Springer-Verlag, New York, 1987, pp 279–302.

35 Delgado-Escueta AV, Bascal RE, Treiman DM. Complex partial seizures on closed-circuit television and EEG: a study of 691 attacks in 79 patients. *Ann Neurol* 1982; **11**: 292–300.

36 Delgado-Escueta AV, Walsh GO. Type I complex partial seizures of hippocampal origin: excellent results of anterior temporal lobectomy. *Neurology* 1985; **35**: 143–154.

37 Gupta A, Jeavons PM, Hughes RC, *et al.* Aura in temporal lobe epilepsy: clinical and electroencephalographic correlation. *J Neurol Neurosurg Psychiatr* 1983; **46**: 1079–1083.

38 King DW, Ajmone-Marsan C. Clinical features and ictal patterns in epileptic patients with EEG temporal lobe foci. *Ann Neurol* 1977; **2**: 138–147.

39 Wieser HG. *Electroclinical Features of the Psychomotor Seizure.* Butterworths, New York. 1983, pp 30–110.

40 Currie S, Heathfield KWG, Henson RA, *et al.* Clinical course and prognosis of temporal lobe epilepsy: a survey of 666 patients. *Brain* 1971; **94**: 173–190.

41 Wyllie E, Lüders H. Complex partial seizures in children: clinical manifestations, and identification of surgical candidates. *Cleve Clin J Med* 1989; **56**: S43–S52.

42 Holmes GL. Partial complex seizures in children: an analysis of 69 seizures in 24 patients using EEG FM radiotelemetry and videotape recording. *EEG Clin Neurophysiol* 1984; **57**: 13–20.

43 Holmes GL. Partial seizures in children. *Pediatrics* 1986; **77**: 725–731.

44 Duchowny MS. Complex partial seizures in infancy. *Arch Neurol* 1987; **44**: 911–914.

45 Yamamoto N, Watanabe K, Negoro T, Takaesu E, Aso K, Furune S, Takahashi I. Complex partial seizures in children: ictal manifestations and their relation to clinical course. *Neurology* 1987; **37**: 1979–1982.

46 Theodore WH, Porter RJ, Penry JK. Complex partial seizures: clinical characteristics and differential diagnosis. *Neurology* 1983; **33**: 1115–1121.

47 Penry JK, Porter RJ, Dreifuss FE. Simultaneous recording of absence seizures with videotape and electroencephalography: a study of 374 seizures in 48 patients. *Brain* 1975; **98**: 427–440.

48 Lesser RP, Dinner DS, Lüders H, Morris HH. Differential diagnosis and treatment of intractable seizures. *Cleve Clin Q* 1984; **51**: 227–240.

49 Duchowny MS. Intensive monitoring in the epileptic child. *J Clin Neurophysiol* 1988; **2**: 203–219.

50 Lüders H, Lesser RP, Dinner DS, Morris HH. Benign focal epilepsy of childhood. In Lüders H, Lesser RL (eds) *Epilepsy: Electroclinical Syndromes.* Springer-Verlag, New York, 1987, pp 303–346.

51 Holmes GL. Partial seizures. In *Diagnosis and Management of Seizures in Children. Major Problems in Clinical Pediatrics,* Vol. 30. WB Saun-

ders, Philadelphia, 1987, pp 125–161.

52 Lüders H, Dinner DS, Morris HH, Wyllie E, Godoy J. EEG evaluation for epilepsy surgery in children. *Cleve Clin J Med* 1988; **56**: S53–S61.

53 Wyllie E, Lüders H, Morris HH, Lesser RP, Dinner DS, Hahn J, Estes ML, Rothner AD, Erenberg G, Cruse R, Friedman D. Clinical outcome after complete or partial cortical resection for intractable epilepsy. *Neurology* 1987; **37**: 1634–1641.

54 Lüders H, Lesser RP, Dinner DS, Morris HH, Hahn JF, Friedman L, Skipper G, Wyllie E, Friedman D. Chronic intracranial recording and stimulation with subdural electrodes. In Engel J (ed) *Surgical Treatment of the Epilepsies*. Raven Press, New York, 1987, pp 297–321.

55 Spencer DD, Spencer SS. *Surgery for Epilepsy*. Neurological Clinics of North America. WB Saunders, Philadelphia, 1985, pp 313–330.

56 Spencer SS. Depth electroencephalography in selection of refractory epilepsy for surgery. *Ann Neurol* 1981; **9**: 207–214.

57 Morris HH, Lüders H. Electrodes. In Gotman J, Ives JR, Gloor P (eds) Long-term monitoring in epilepsy (EEG Suppl No. 37). Elsevier, New York, 1985, pp 3–26.

58 Wyllie E, Wyllie R, Kanner A, Kotagal P. A technique for comfortable insertion of sphenoidal electrodes in children and adolescents. *Epilepsia* 1988; **29**: 656.

59 Bancaud J. Surgery of epilepsy based on stereotactic investigations — the plan of SEEG investigations. *Acta Neurochir (Wien)* 1980; **30** (Suppl 1): 25–34.

60 Cahan LD, Sutherling W, McCullough MA, *et al.* Review of the 20-year UCLA experience with surgery for epilepsy. *Cleve Clin Q* 1984; **51**: 313–318.

61 Delgado-Escueta AV, Treiman DM, Walsh GO. The treatable epilepsies (second of two parts). *New Eng J Med* 1983; **308**: 1576–1584.

62 Engel J, Rausch R, Lieb JP, Kuhl DE, Crandall P. Correlation of criteria for localizing epileptic foci in patients considered for surgical therapy of epilepsy. *Ann Neurol* 1981; **90**: 215–224.

63 Rasmussen T. Surgical treatment of patients with complex partial seizures. In Penry JK, Daly DD (eds) *Advances in Neurology* Vol. 11. Raven Press, New York, pp 415–442.

64 Walter RD. Tactical considerations leading to surgical treatment of limbic epilepsy. In Brazier MAB (ed) *Epilepsy: Its Phenomenon in Man*. Academic Press, New York, 1973, pp 99–121.

65 Walter RD. Principles of clinical investigation of surgical candidates. In Purpura DP, Penry JK, Walter RD (eds) Neurosurgical management of the epilepsies. *Adv Neurol* 1975; **8**: 49–58.

66 Wieser HG, Bancaud J, Talairach J, Bonis A, Szikla G. Comparative value of spontaneous and chemically and electrically induced seizures in establishing lateralization of temporal lobe seizures. *Epilepsia* 1979; **20**: 47–59.

67 Duchowny MS, Alvarez LA, Resnick TJ, Morrison G. Surgery in infancy for partial seizures. *Cleve Clin J Med*, 1989; **56**: 5275.

68 Resnick TJ, Duchowny MS, Deray MJ, Alfonso I. Subdural electrode recording in the preoperative evaluation of partial seizures in children. *Ann Neurol* 1987; **22**: 415.

69 Branch C, Milner B, Rasmussen T. Intracarotic Sodium Amytal for the lateralization of cerebral speech dominance: observations in 123 patients. *J Neurosurg* 1964; **21**: 399–405.

70 Milner B, Branch C, Rasmussen T. Study of short-term memory after intracarotid injection of Sodium Amytal. *Trans Am Neurol Assoc* 1962; **87**: 224–226.

71 Theodore WH. What is uncontrolled epilepsy, and who should be referred for surgery? In Spencer SS, Spencer DD (eds) *Surgery for Epilepsy* Blackwell Scientific Publications, Boston, 1990, pp 3–17.

72 Holmes GL. Psychosocial factors in childhood epilepsy. In *Diagnosis and Management of Seizures in Children. Major Problems in Clinical Pediatrics*, Vol. 30. WB Saunders, Philadelphia, 1987, pp 112–124.

73 Ziegler RG. Impairments of control and competence in epileptic children and their families. *Epilepsia* 1981; **22**: 339–346.

74 Viberg M, Blennow G, Polski B. Epilepsy in adolescence: implications for the development of personality. *Epilepsia* 1987; **28**: 542–546.

75 Hoare P. Does illness foster dependency? A study of epileptic and diabetic children. *Dev Med Child Neurol* 1984; **26**: 3–13.

76 Matthews WS, Barabas G, Ferrari M. Emotional concomitants of childhood epilepsy. *Epilepsia* 1982; **23**: 671–681.

77 Long CG, Moore JR. Parental expectations for their epileptic children. *J Child Psychol Psychiatr* 1970; **23**: 80–89.

78 Ross EM, Peckham CS. School children with epilepsy. In Parsonage M, Grant RHE, Craig AG (eds) *Advances in Epileptology: XIVth Epilepsy International Symposium.* Raven Press, New York, 1983, pp 215–220.

79 Caveness WF, Gallop GH. A survey of public attitudes toward epilepsy in 1979 with an indication of trends over the past thirty years. *Epilepsia* 1980; **21**: 509–518.

80 Falconer MA. Place of surgery for temporal lobe epilepsy during childhood. *Brit Med J* 1972; **2**: 631–635.

81 Lindsay J, Ounstead C, Richards P. Long-term outcome in children with temporal lobe seizures. V: Indications and contraindications for neurosurgery. *Dev Med Child Neurol* 1984; **26**: 25–32.

82 Rasmussen T. Cortical resection in children with focal epilepsy. In Parsonage M, Grant RHE, Craig HG (eds) *Advances in Epileptology: XIVth Epilepsy International Symposium.* Raven Press, New York, 1983, pp 249–254.

83 Holmes G. Pharmacology of antiepileptic drugs. In *Diagnosis and Management of Seizures in Children. Major Problems in Clinical Pediatrics,* Vol. 30. WB Saunders, Philadelphia, 1987, pp 72–111.

84 Harbord MG, Manson JI. Temporal lobe epilepsy in childhood: a reappraisal of etiology and outcome. *Pediatr Neurol* 1987; **3**: 263–268.

85 Kotagal P, Rothner AD, Erenberg G, Cruse R, Wyllie E. Complex partial seizures of childhood onset: a five-year follow-up study. *Arch Neurol* 1987; **44**: 1177–1180.

86 Glaser GH. Limbic epilepsy in childhood. *J Nerv Ment Dis* 1967; **114**: 391–397.

87 Lindsay J, Ounsted C, Richards P. Longterm outcome in children with temporal lobe seizures: I. Social outcome and childhood factors. *Dev Med Child Neurol* 1979; **21**: 285–298.

88 Iemolo F, Farnarier G, Serbanescu T, Menendez P. Étude longitudinale des épilepsies survenant dans l'adolescence. *Rev EEG Neurophysiol* 1981; **11**: 502–508.

89 Sofijanov NG. Clinical evolution and prognosis of childhood epilepsies. *Epilepsia* 1982; **23**: 61–69.

90 Loiseau P, Dartiques JF, Pestre M. Prognosis of partial epileptic seizures in the adolescent. *Epilepsia* 1983; **24**: 472–481.

91 Sillanpää M. Social functioning and seizure status of young adults with onset of epilepsy in childhood. *Acta Neurol Scand* 1983; **68**: 8–77.

92 Schmidt D, Tsai JJ, Janz D. Generalized tonic–clonic seizures in patients with complex partial seizures: natural history and prognostic relevance. *Epilepsia* 1983; **24**: 43–48.

93 Deonna T, Ziegler AL, Despland PA, *et al.* Partial epilepsy in neurologically normal children: clinical syndromes and prognosis. *Epilepsia* 1986; **27**: 241–247.

94 Chugani HT, Shewmon DA, Peacock WJ, Shields WD, Mazziotta JC, Phelps ME. Surgical treatment of intractable neonatal-onset seizures: the role of positron emission tomography. *Neurology* 1988; **38**: 1178–1188.

95 Nespeca M, Wyllie E, Lüders H, *et al.* EEG recording and functional localization studies with subdural electrodes in infants and young children. *J Epilepsy*, in press.

96 Oppenheimer DR, Griffith HB. Persistent intracranial bleeding as a complication of hemispherectomy. *J Neurol Neurosurg Psychiatr* 1966; **29**: 229–240.

97 Dalos N, Vining EPG, Carson B, *et al.* Rasmussen's encephalitis: clinical recognition and surgical management. *Ann Neurol* 1986; **20**: 434.

98 Rasmussen T, McCann W. Clinical studies of patients with focal epilepsy due to "chronic encephalitis." *Trans Am Neurol Assoc* 1968; **93**: 89–94.

99 Gupta PC, Rapin I, Houroupian DS. Smoldering encephalitis in children. *Neuropediatr* 1984; **15**: 191–197.

100 Vining EPG, Freeman JM, Carson BS, Long DM. "Bilateral" epileptic abnormalities: a unilateral cure. *Ann Neurol* 1987; **22**: 412.

101 Chugani HT, Shielda WP, Shewman DA, Olson DM, Phelps ME, Peacode WJ. Infantile Spasm: I. PET identifies focal cortical dysplasia in cryptogenic cases for surgical treatment. *Ann. Neurol* 1990; **27**: 406–413.

102 Wyllie E. Corpus callosotomy for intractable generalized epilepsy. *J Pediatr* 1988; **113**: 255–261.

103 Blume WT. Corpus callosotomy section: rationale and review of experimental and clinical data. *Cleve Clin Q* 1984; **51**: 319–332.

104 Spencer SS, Gates JR, Reeves AR, *et al.* Corpus callosum section. In Engel J, Jr (ed) *Surgical Treatment of the Epilepsies.* Raven Press, New York, 1987, pp 425–444.

Comment

Susan S. Spencer

This chapter emphasizes that epilepsy surgery is an appropriate option for treatment of uncontrolled seizures in children. The question of possible remission is most critical for the younger population. However, risk factors which make remission exceedingly unlikely have been identified (see Chapter 1). Other special aspects of patient selection include the presence of benign or primary (petit mal) epilepsies which must be diagnosed accurately, since these patients are not candidates. The difficulty of establishing the aura and its characteristics and the unusual behaviors associated with infantile seizures are additional difficulties in patient selection in this age group.

Patient evaluation is complicated in children by degree of cooperation with Amytal tests (usually not possible under the age of 6) and with invasive monitoring (although children as young as 5 years old have been successfully studied with depth, subdural, or epidural electrodes).

Surgical results with respect to seizure control are equivalent to those in adults and some studies suggest psychosocial improvement is even more dramatic [4,9]. Thus, much the same approach to children as to adults with uncontrolled partial seizures can yield quite gratifying results.

Dr Wyllie indicated that epilepsy surgery is frequently delayed for unnecessary lengths of time in children. The editors agree and propose that with appropriate scrutiny of the history, seizure type, and risk factors, and with appropriate flexibility and attention in the approach to patient evaluation, young children could be increasingly considered surgical candidates. Furthermore, we feel that the age at which patients should undergo operation for epilepsy is more appropriately in childhood, as soon as the criteria for surgical selection have been satisfied, and before devastating emotional, psychological, and neurologic consequences of recurrent seizures occur. Although slow to be accepted, this viewpoint is rapidly being adopted by the majority of epilepsy surgery centers in this country.

part *II*

Surgery

chapter 6

Temporal Lobectomy

Anatomy of the temporal lobe

Richard A. Bronen

Surface anatomy

The temporal lobe has a lateral surface which is delineated superiorly by the lateral sulcus (Sylvian fissure) and posteriorly by an imaginary line extending from the parieto-occipital sulcus to the preoccipital notch [1] (Fig. 6.1). Three parallel gyri are present, the superior, middle, and inferior temporal gyri. The superior temporal sulcus separates the superior and middle temporal gyri while the inferior temporal sulcus (formerly the middle temporal sulcus) separates the middle from the inferior temporal gyrus. The gyri and sulci extend the length of the temporal lobe in the anterior–posterior direction [2,3].

The inferior surface of the anterior temporal lobe resides within the middle cranial fossa. The most anterior portion of the temporal lobe, the temporal pole, may be formed by one or several of the temporal lobe gyri. As one moves just posterior to the temporal pole but still within the anterior temporal lobe, the inferior surface is formed by the lateral occipitotemporal gyrus (LOTG) (fusiform gyrus) laterally, and the parahippocampal gyrus (PHG) medially (Fig. 6.2). The occipitotemporal sulcus (formerly the inferior temporal sulcus) separates the inferior temporal gyrus from the lateral occipitotemporal gyrus. The collateral sulcus forms the medial margin of the LOTG, separating the LOTG from the PHG. The uncus is that portion of the PHG which hooks medially at the level of the suprasellar cistern. The rhinal sulcus separates the uncus and PHG from the temporal pole. The rhinal sulcus sometimes continues posteriorly to become continuous with the collateral sulcus. Superior to the PHG is the hippocampal sulcus or fissure (Fig. 6.3). Surrounding the hippocampal fissure is the hippocampal formation, which constitutes the medial temporal lobe. Structures within the hippocampal formation and their relationship to the limbic system will be reviewed later. In the posterior temporal lobe, the me-

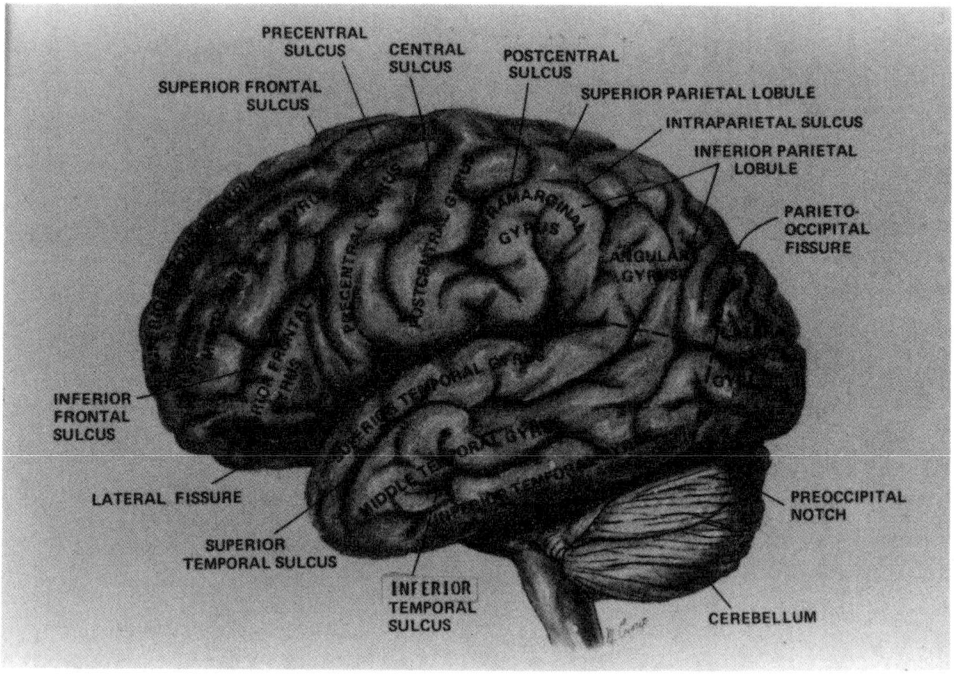

FIGURE 6.1 Lateral surface of the brain. From Gelman and Newman [1].

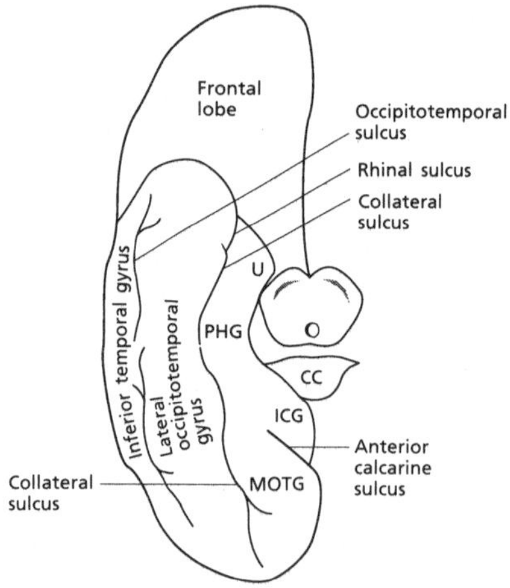

FIGURE 6.2 Basal view of the right cerebral hemisphere. Key: U, uncus; ICG, isthmus of the cingulate gyrus; CC, splenium of corpus callosum; MOTG, medial occupitotemporal gyrus; PHG, parahippocampal gyrus.

dial occipitotemporal gyrus (MOTG) insinuates itself between the LOTG laterally, and the PHG which becomes continuous with the isthmus of the cingulate gyrus, medially. The collateral sulcus which separates the LOTG from the PHG anteriorly now lies between the LOTG and MOTG posteriorly. The anterior portion of the calcarine sulcus separates the MOTG from the more medial PHG and isthmus of the cingulate gyrus [2,3].

Hippocampus and limbic system

"Limbic lobe" is a term which was coined by Broca in 1878 to describe a series of gray and white matter tracts on the medial hemisphere which arc around the brainstem, diencephalon and corpus callosum. These are phylogenically old and functionally related. The limbic lobe consists of the subcallosal area, cingulate gyrus, PHG, and hippocampal formation (Fig. 6.3). Although there is some disagreement over terminology, the "limbic system" is a more inclusive term which includes in addition to the limbic lobe, the amygdala nuclei, septal nuclei, anterior thalamic nuclei, hypothalamus, epithalamus, and midbrain. Some authors also include the olfactory pathways. The hippocampal formation is a composite structure. Its components include Ammon's horn (hippocampus or cornu ammonis), subiculum, dentate gyrus, subsplenial gyrus, supracallosal gyrus, alveus, fimbria, and fornix [3, 4].

The hippocampal formation and limbic lobe are complex because in addition to the "C"-shaped arcuate pathway, there is also an infolding of gray matter along this curve [3, 4]. A coronal slice of the medial temporal lobe clearly reveals this complex anatomy [2] (Fig. 6.4). The PHG is transformed from a six-layered cortex to a three-layered cortex along its superior surface, just under the hippocampal fissure. This transition area is known as the subiculum. On the surface of the subiculum is a layer of white matter, the superficial medullary lamina. As the subiculum curves laterally around the hippocampal fissure it is known as Ammon's horn which continues superioriomedially. Ammon's

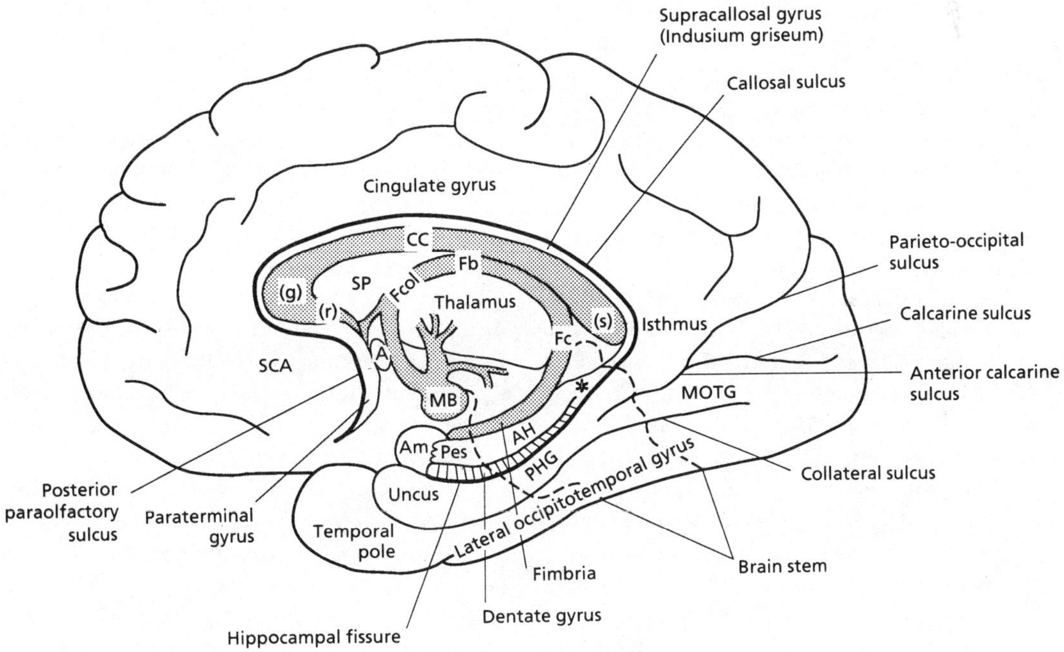

FIGURE 6.3 Medial view of the brain without the brainstem. Schematic representation of limbic lobe structures. Note the "C"-shaped arch formed by the (1) uncus, PHG gyrus, isthmus of the cingulate gyrus, and subcallosal area; (2) hippocampal fissure, callosal sulcus, and posterior paraolfactory sulcus; (3) dentate gyrus, subcallosal gyrus, supracallosal gyrus, and paraterminal gyrus; (4) fimbria and fornix (shaded): Key: SCA, subcallosal area; (r), rostrum, (g), genu, (s) splenium of corpus callosum, CC; Fcol, columns, Fb, body, Fc, crus of fornix; SP, septum pellucidum; A, anterior commissure; MB, mammillary body; Am, amygdala; Pes, pes hippocampi; AH, Ammon's horn; *subsplenial gyrus. After Williams and Warwick [4].

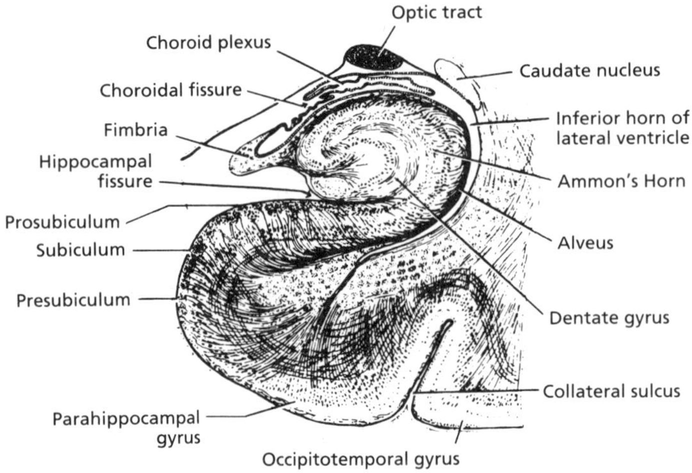

FIGURE 6.4 Coronal section through the medial temporal lobe and hippocampal formation. Carpenter and Sutin [3].

horn is a three-layered cortex. An infolding of gray matter immediately above the hippocampal fissure is known as the dentate gyrus. The hippocampal formation protrudes into the medial surface of the temporal horn. The temporal horn is separated from the circummesencephalic cistern by the choroidal fissure which is found on the superior surface of the hippocampal formation.

The strict definition of the choroidal fissure is the space between the two pial layers which unite laterally to form the choroidal plexus in the medial temporal horn. A loose usage of the term "choroidal fissure" includes the portion of circummesencephalic cistern superior to the alveus and fimbria [5]. The PHG and subiculum have been further divided into the following sections proceeding from the PHG toward Ammon's horn: the parasubiculum, presubiculum, subiculum, and prosubiculum [4]. The zones are related to differences in the cytoarchitectural pattern. Ammon's horn can also be divided into several zones. One method uses the cornu ammonis fields CA1 to CA4 of Lorente de No [7]. Another method proposed by Rose is not limited to Ammon's horn but includes the prosubiculum and subiculum, the hippocampal fields H1 to H5 [8]. The alveus is a collection of white matter fibers on the lateral and superior surfaces of Ammon's horn. The alveus is found adjacent to the ependyma of the medial surface of the temporal horn. As the alveus converges along the superiomedial aspect of the hippocampal formation, it becomes the fimbria.

One can approach the complex topography of the limbic lobe as a series of "C"-shaped arcs of gray matter, white matter, and cerebrospinal fluid (CSF) which change name with location [2–6] (Fig. 6.3). These arcs, which are relatively more laterally in the medial temporal lobe, swing medially as they course over the diencephalon [6,9] (Fig. 6.5).

One can begin with the CSF arc central to the hippocampal formation (Fig. 6.3). This sulcus is known as the hippocampal fissure in the temporal lobe. It is superior to the subiculum (PHG), inferior to the dentate gyrus, and medial to Ammon's horn. As it sweeps around the corpus callosum, the name changes to the cingulate sulcus. It separates the more superior cingulate gyrus from the supracallosal gyrus and corpus callosum in-

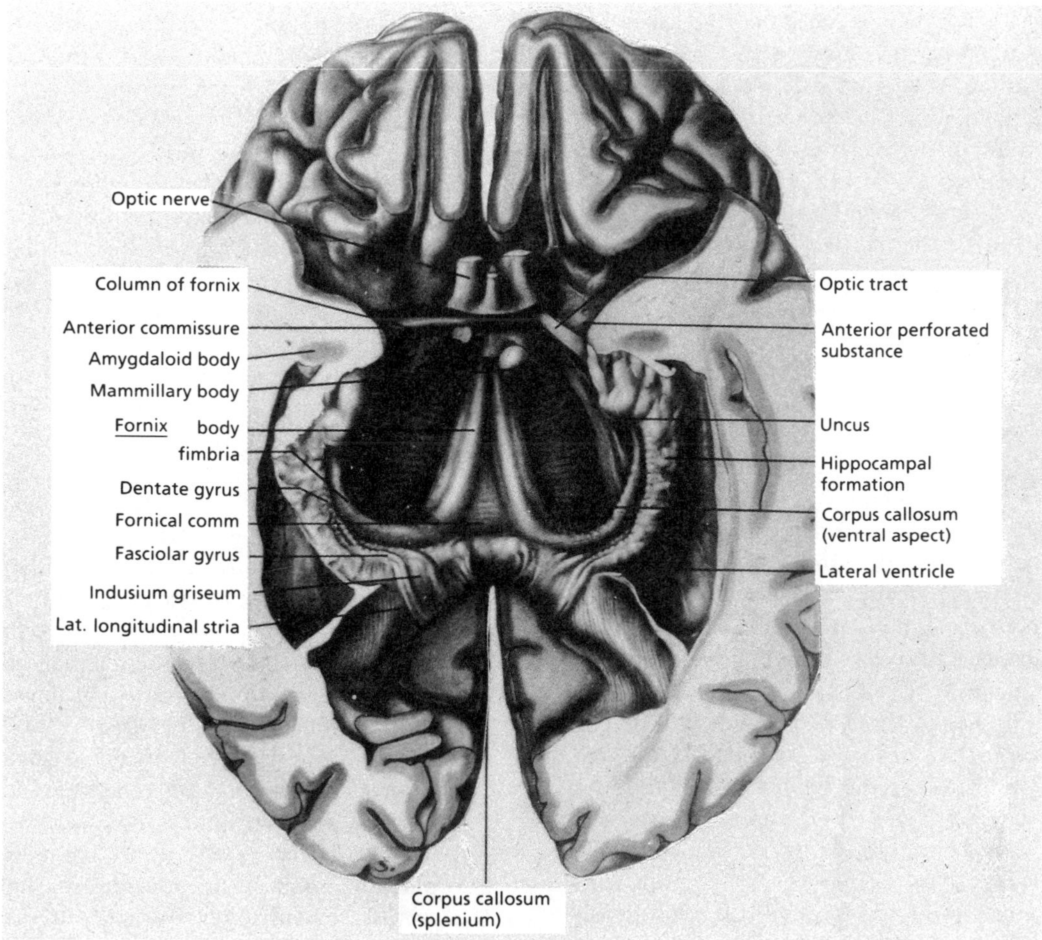

FIGURE 6.5 Basal view of dissected brain with removal of brain stem, diencephalon, and inferior cerebral surface. Note the curvature of the hippocampal formation, fornix, and ventricles. From Carpenter and Sutin [3] — originally in Mettler [9].

feriorly. Anteriorly this sulcus swings inferiorly and becomes continuous with the posterior paraolfactory sulcus. The subcallosal area is anterior to this sulcus [2,6].

A "U"-shaped layer of gray matter surrounds the CSF arc on its inferior, lateral and superior aspects (the superior and inferior cortices form the arms of the "U" which is rotated 90°). This "U"-shaped cortex of hippocampal formation is well developed in the temporal lobe (Fig. 6.4), but becomes progressively smaller as the arc passes around the corpus callosum. The gray matter on the outer aspect of the CSF arc is known as the subiculum in the temporal lobe. The subiculum is part of the PHG. As the cortex of the subiculum and PHG pass posterior to the splenium, it is renamed the isthmus of the cingulate gyrus. This gyrus sweeps around the splenium. At it continues above the corpus callosum, it is called the cingulate gyrus. Anteriorly, this gray matter tract merges with the subcallosal area (paraolfactory area) anterioinferior to the rostrum of the corpus callosum, between the anterior and posterior paraolfactory sulci [2–6].

The gray matter forming the lateral cap of tissue on the CSF arc is known as Ammon's horn in the temporal lobe. The most anterior portion, the pes hippocampi, is enlarged and lobulated (digitated "foot of hippocampus"). As the hippocampal formation ascends around the splenium, the lateral strip of cortex is called the retrosplenial gyrus [5,6].

The ribbon of gray matter located on the inner aspect of the CSF crescent is called the dentate gyrus in the temporal lobe (Figs 6.3 & 6.5). If forms the superior border of the hippocampal fissure. The dentate gyrus is a notched strip of cortex which starts in the uncus. As it sweeps around the splenium, the dentate gyrus fuses with a medial strip of gray matter, the fasciolar gyrus. In this vertical portion of the "C"-shaped arc, the dentate gyrus together with the fasciolar gyrus and retrosplenial gyrus are known collectively as the subsplenial gyrus. The subsplenial gyrus curves anteriorly over the corpus callosum and the name changes to the supracallosal gyrus or indusim griseum. This gyrus is markedly attenuated compared to its counterpart in the temporal lobe. The vestigial supracallosal gyrus is found inferior to the callosal sulcus (along the inner aspect of the CSF arc) and superior to the corpus callosum. Anteriorly, as the supracallosal gyrus travels around the genu of the corpus callosum, it becomes continuous with the paraterminal gyrus. The paraterminal gyrus is a thin strip of gray matter between the posterior paraolfactory sulcus and the lamina terminalis. The paraterminal gyrus and subcallosal area form the septal area [2–6].

Several white matter tracts are associated with the hippocampus. The cingulum is an association fiber bundle found within the subcortical white matter of the PHG and cingulate gyrus. Thus it also follows a similar semicircular route. The fornix along with its components, the alveus and fimbria, is the major efferent white matter pathway of the hippocampal formation. The thin white matter layer on the surface of Ammon's horn, the alveus, is composed of axons primarily from Ammon's horn en route to the fimbria. The fimbria is the most medial segment of the alveus, situated above the dentate gyrus and below the choroidal fissure of the temporal horn [2–6].

The fornix forms a "C"-shaped arc of white matter (Figs 6.3 & 6.5). The fimbria (and alveus) extend from the uncus posteriorly to the splenium. The fibers arch superiorly toward the splenium to form the crus of the fornix, which is affixed to the anterior surface of the splenium. The crura and fimbria form the medial walls of the atria. The two crura curve anteriomedially below the body of the corpus callosum, adjacent to the inferior surface of the corpus callosum. Transverse fibers connect the crura as they merge forming the commissure of the fornices (hippocampal commissure, psalterium, lyre of David). The two crura join anteriorly to form the bilobed body of the fornix. The body of the fornix is found below the septum pellucidum, in the medial floor of the body of the lateral ventricles. It is attached to the roof of the third ventricle. At the level of the foramen of Monroe, the fornices diverge into two bundles, the columns of the fornix. The columns arch anteriorly above and around the interventricular foramena. The columns turn inferior, anterior to the interventricular foramen, and course toward the anterior commissure. At the anterior commissure the columns split into an anterior component, the precommissure fornix, and a posterior

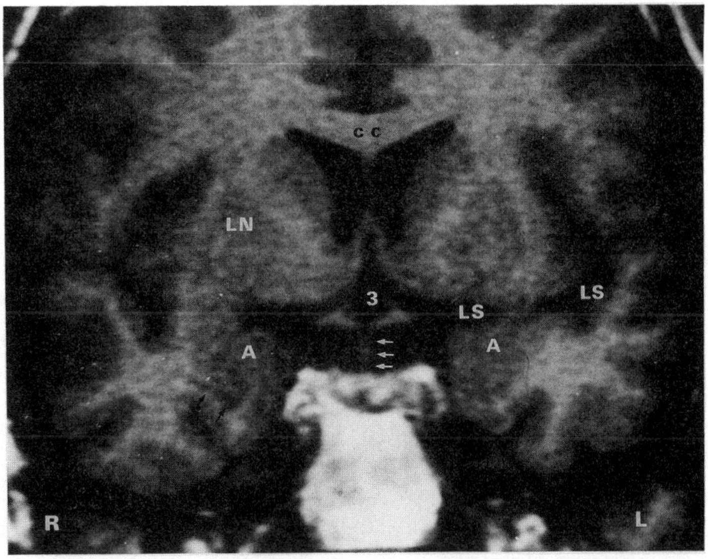

FIGURE 6.6 Coronal T1W. PPS. The amygdala (A) on the left is imaged in a slightly more anterior section than the right amygdala because of mild head rotation. The right amygdala is superior to the tip of the temporal horn (black arrows). Superior to the amygdala is the lateral sulcus (LS) and lentiform nucleus (LN). cc, corpus callosum; 3, third ventricle; white arrows, pituitary stalk.

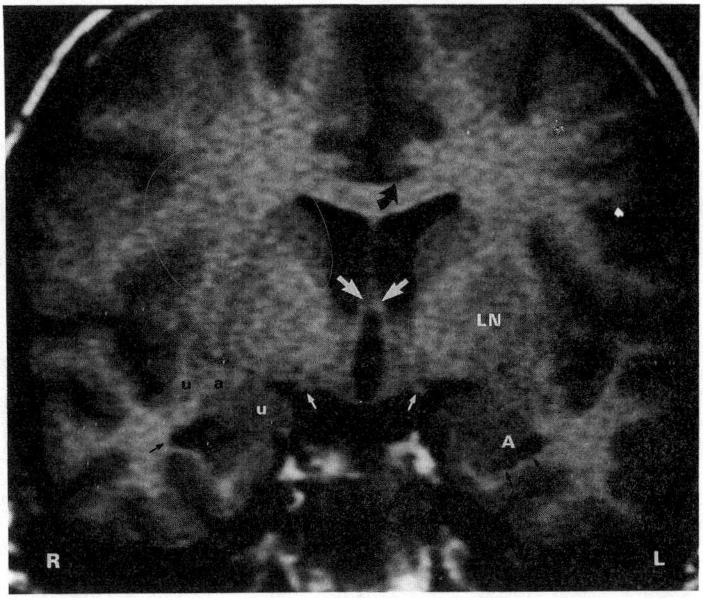

FIGURE 6.7 Coronal T1W. SSS. Left amygdala (white "A") is superior to anterior temporal horn (small black arrows). Adjacent white matter consists of anterior commissure (black "a") medially, and uncinate fasciculus (black "u") more laterally. On the right, the temporal horn (small single black arrow) swings lateral to the gray matter, indicating that this gray matter is the beginning of the hippocampal formation. The gray matter of the amygdala is inseparable from that of the medial uncus (white "u"). The thin supracallosal gyrus cannot be separated from the callosal sulcus (curved black arrow) superior to the corpus callosum. LN, lentiform nucleus; small white arrows, optic tracts; large white arrows, columns of the fornix, just anterior to foramen of Monro.

component, the retrocommissure fornix. The retrocommissure fornix courses to the anterior thalamus and mammillary body. The precommissure fornix courses to the septal region. In addition to the major pathway just described, a small segment of fibers from the fimbria separate from the main bundle of the fornices inferior to the splenium. These fibers course over the splenium and join the supracallosal gyrus [2–6].

The lateral ventricle is also "C"-shaped. The anterior tip of the temporal horn is sloped such that the amygdala forms its anterior and superior surfaces. The medial wall of the temporal horn is indented by the alveus and hippocampal formation.

The amygdala (amygdaloid body or nucleus) is found anteriosuperior to the temporal horn tip (Figs 6.6 & 6.7). Structures located adjacent to the superior surface of the amygdala include the anterior perforated substance, middle cerebral artery, innominate substance, putamen and globus pallidus. Immediately medial to the amygdala is the uncus (uncinate gyrus). The medial portion of the lateral fissure and the optic tract are superiomedial to the uncus and amygdala. Proceeding lateral and slightly superior from the amygdala one encounters the anterior commissure, then the uncinate fasciculus (the association tract connecting the anterior temporal lobe to the orbital frontal gyri) and claustrum, and finally the insular cortex.

Cross-sectional anatomy – revisited with MRI

Magnetic resonance imaging (MRI) has revolutionized *in vivo* imaging of the brain. This

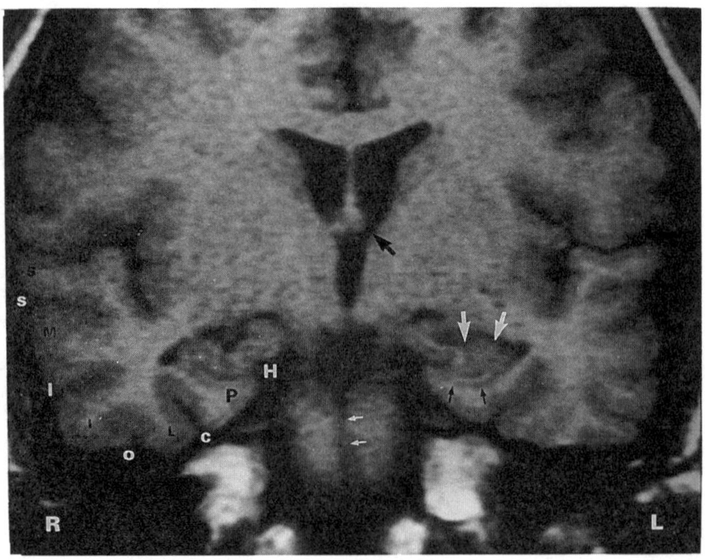

FIGURE 6.8 Coronal T1W. BAS. The sulci (white letters) and gyri (black letters) of the temporal lobe are easily identified. The right collateral sulcus (c) points to the temporal horn. The medial gray matter of the PHG (P) bends laterally to become the subiculum (small black arrows) beneath the hippocampal fissure (H). The gray matter above the hippocampal fissure is the pes hippocampi (white arrows), named for the digitations (lobulations) which are seen protruding into the temporal horn on the right. Small white arrows, signal void of the basilar artery; large black arrow, foramen of Monro. Gyri: S, superior temporal gyrus; M, middle temporal gyrus; I, inferior temporal gyrus; L, lateral occipitotemporal gyrus. Sulci: s, superior temporal sulcus; I, inferior temporal sulcus; o, occipitotemporal sulcus.

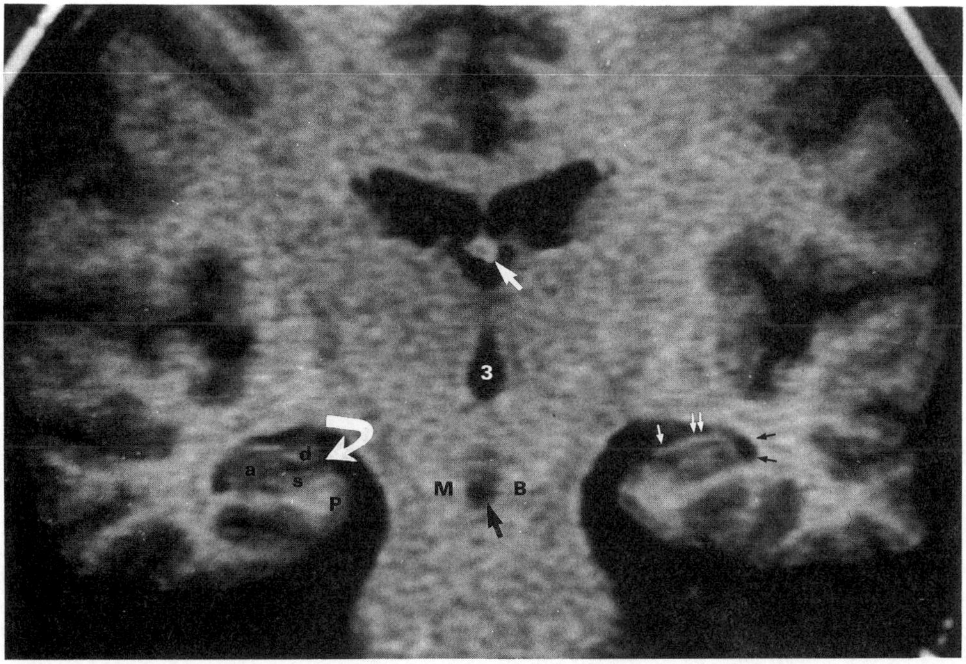

FIGURE 6.9 Coronal T1W. RNS. The red nucleus, which is easily seen on T2W images, is poorly seen on T1W scans. The gray matter of the hippocampal formation appears as an oval. This oval is actually a "U"-shaped cortex rotated and oriented around the horizontal hippocampal fissure (curved white arrow). The "U" consists of the subiculum (s) inferiorly, Ammon's horn (a) superiolaterally, and dentate gyrus (d) superiomedially and centrally. The white alveus (double small white arrows) and fimbria (single small white arrow) are clearly seen on the surface of the gray oval, capped by CSF from the temporal horn (small black arrows), the choroidal fissure superiorly, and the circummesencephalic cistern medially. The body of the fornix (large white arrow) is bilobed. P, PHG; MB, midbrain; 3, third ventricle; large black arrow, interpeduncular cistern.

is especially true of the temporal lobes which are imaged suboptimally by computed tomography (CT) scanning. Magnetic resonance images can be acquired by either T1-weighted (T1W) or T2-weighted (T2W) spin echo sequences. It is important to remember that on T1W images, gray matter is hypointense compared to white matter, or gray is gray and white is white. CSF is hypointense or dark compared to brain (Figs 6.6–6.10). On T2W scans, gray matter is white and white matter is gray. CSF is hyperintense or extremely white compared to brain (Fig. 6.11). Anatomic detail is best appreciated on T1W images.

Coronal sections

The coronal plane is the most optimal plane for imaging the temporal lobe and hippocampal formation [10]. We have divided the temporal lobe into nine coronal sections approximately 5 mm thick. Two additional sections anterior and posterior to the nine sections are also defined. Because of the importance of the hippocampus in epilepsy, we have land-

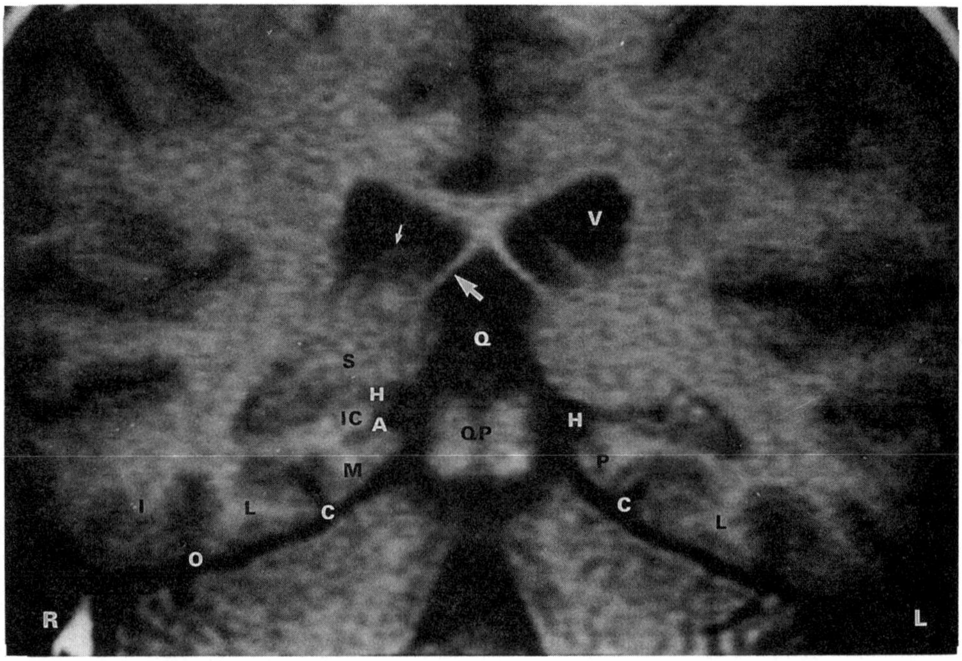

FIGURE 6.10 Coronal T1W. ICS. The right side is more posterior than the left. The hippocampal formation on the right has begun to sweep vertically around the splenium and become the subsplenial gyrus (S). The PHG (P) becomes the isthmus of the cingulate gyrus (IC). The MOTG (M) has insinuated between the isthmus of the cingulate gyrus (IC) and the LOTG (L). The crus of the fornix (large arrow) forms the medial border of the atrium (V). The choroid plexus (small white arrow) arises from the pia of the fornix. Q, quadrigeminal plate cistern; QP, inferior colliculis of the quadrigeminal plate; H, hippocampal fissure; A, anterior calcarine sulcus; C, collateral sulcus; I, inferior temporal gyrus; o, occipitotemporal sulcus.

marked our coronal slices to structures at the same craniocaudal level as the hippocampal formation. Thus the same coronal section of hippocampus can be referred to regardless of obliquity (within reason). The landmarks for the 11 sections are: (1) temporal lobe anterior to the anterior clinoid (anterior temporal section, ATS); (2) optic chiasm, pituitary gland, middle or anterior cerebral artery (anterior pituitary section, APS); (3) posterior pituitary lobe, infundibulum, dorsum sella (posterior pituitary section, PPS); (4) suprasellar cistern, amygdala (suprasellar section, SSS); (5) basilar artery, prepontine cistern (basilary artery section, BAS); (6) interpeduncular cistern, anterior brainstem (interpeduncular section, IPS); (7) red nuclei, very small portion of the interpeduncular cistern (red nuclei section, RNS); (8) midbrainstem with no visualization of the interpeduncular cistern nor the colliculi (mid brain stem section, MBS); (9) superior collicular section, (SCS); (10) inferior collicular section (ICS); and (11) posterior to the colliculi (posterior collicular section, PCS). Since comparison of left–right hippocampus and temporal lobe is important, we assess acoustic nerve symmetry to determine the amount

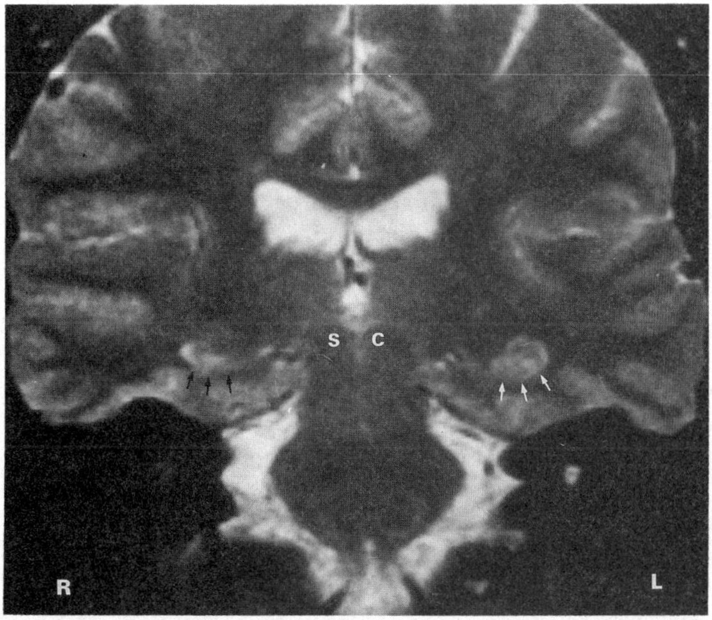

FIGURE 6.11 Coronal T2W. SCS. CSF is very white, while the gray matter is lighter (hyperintense) compared to white matter (which is darker or hypointense). Magnetic resonance imaging exquisitely demonstrates the atrophic hyperintense hippocampal formation (black arrows) on the right in this patient with surgically proven right mesial temporal sclerosis. The associated hyperintensity is partial volume averaging of the CSF in the slightly dilated right temporal horn. Computed tomography cannot routinely identify mesial temporal sclerosis and was normal in this patient. The normal sized oval of hippocampal gray is seen on the left (white arrows). SC, superior colliculli. From Am J Neurorad [11]

of head rotation. An abnormal hippocampal formation is imaged in Fig. 6.11.

The coronal anatomy of the temporal lobe is fairly uniform in the first two sections, ATS and APS. The Sylvian fissure defines the superior surface. The lateral surface is formed by the superior, middle, and inferior temporal gyri and the superior and inferior temporal sulci. The inferior surface contains LOTG, the beginning of PHG, the occipitotemporal sulcus and the collateral sulcus. The collateral sulcus often points to, or is adjacent to, the temporal horn (Fig. 6.8 identifies the sulci and gyri) [5,6].

The next two sections, at approximately the posterior pituitary and suprasellar levels, define the PHG more clearly as it hooks medially to form the uncus (Figs 6.6 & 6.7). The gray matter lateral to the uncus is the amygdala. Note that the gray matter of the amygdala is superior to the temporal horn tip. More posteriorly at the BAS, the gray matter is now located medial and inferior to the CSF in the temporal horn and choroidal fissure (Fig. 6.8). This indicates that the amygdala has ended and this is the pes hippocampi, the anterior portion of the hippocampal formation. The pes hippocampi is the most bulbous portion of the hippocampal formation. The notched surface is sometimes visible on MRI. The medial aspect of the hippocampal fissure can be seen on MRI. The lateral extension of the hippocampal fissure is obliterated *in utero* [5].

The next three to four sections (IPS, RNS, MBS, SCS) are best for evaluating the hippocampal formation (Fig. 6.9). The cortex of PHG along the medial temporal lobe turns lateral to become continuous with gray matter in an oval shape. This oval is composed of the subiculum, Ammon's horn, dentate gyrus and obliterated hippocampal fissure. Although the components cannot be individually resolved, their locations can be approximated. A sliver of white matter forming the lateral and superior aspects of this gray matter oval is often seen. This is the alveus and fimbria. The fimbria may project a free edge medially into the perimesencephalic cistern. The temporal horn is seen as a small crescent of CSF lateral and superiolateral to the hippocampal formation, adjacent to the alveus. The choroidal fissure and circummesencephalic cistern are seen as a small rim of CSF superior to the alveus and fimbria. With gadolinium-DTPA, an MRI contrast agent, there is enhancement of the choroid plexus [5,12].

As the hippocampal formation thins and sweeps vertically around the splenium (at the SCS, ICS, PCS) the anatomy becomes more complex in the coronal plane (Fig. 6.10). The MOTG begins to insinuate itself between the LOTG and PHG here. This is also where the PHG becomes the isthmus of the cingulate gyrus, and the hippocampal formation becomes the subsplenial gyrus. Tracing a coronal section from lateral to medial starting with the LOTG we find: LOTG, collateral sulcus, MOTG, anterior portion of the calcarine sulcus, PHG becoming the isthmus of the cingulate gyrus, hippocampal fissure surrounded by the subsplenial gyrus, splenium of corpus callosum and quadrigeminal plate cistern. Lateral to the subsplenial gyrus and splenium is the atrial–posterior temporal horn complex, whose medial wall is formed by the alveus inferiorly and crus of the fornix superiorly [5,6].

The superior portion of the "C"-shaped arc

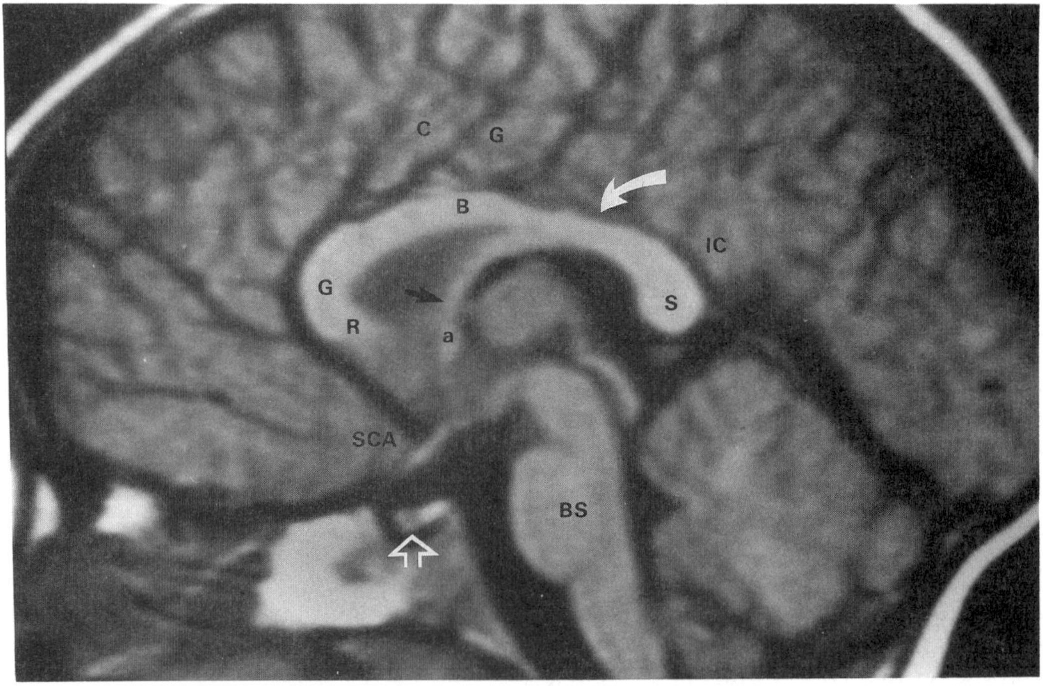

FIGURE 6.12 Midline sagittal T1W. Corpus callosum consists of the rostrum (R), genu (G), body (B), and wide splenium (S). Curved white arrow points to callosal sulci and supracallosal gyrus coating the superior surface of the corpus callosum. SCA, subcallosal area; CG, cingulate gyrus; IC, isthmus of cingulate gyrus; black arrow, column of fornix; a, anterior commissure; BS, brain stem; open arrow, pituitary.

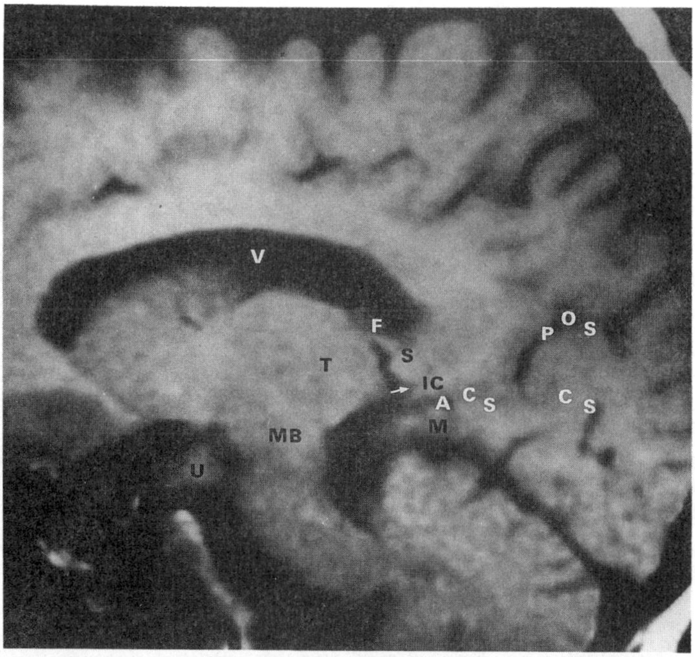

FIGURE 6.13 Paramedian sagittal T1W. The anterior calcarine sulcus (ACS) separates the MOTG (M) from the isthmus of cingulate gyrus (IC). The hippocampal fissure (white arrow) separates the isthmus from the splenium (S). The circummesencephalic cistern separates the thalamus (T) from the splenium and isthmus. The fornix (F) is attached to the undersurface of the splenium (S). The uncus (U) is imaged as a discontinuous portion of brain because of its curved surface. V, lateral ventricle; MB, midbrain; POS, parieto-occipital sulcus; CS, calcarine sulcus.

of the limbic lobe is evaluated on more anterior slices. The crus of the fornices unite to form the body of the fornix, located on the roof of the third ventricle, floor of the septum pellucidum, and medial inferior aspect of the lateral ventricles (Fig. 6.9). The roof of the lateral ventricles is formed by the body of the corpus callosum. On the superior surface of the corpus callosum is a sliver of gray matter inferior to the callosal sulcus, the supracallosal gyrus (Fig. 6.7). The callosal sulcus and supracallosal gyrus may be difficult to resolve on MRI. However, the cingulate gyrus, the gray matter superior to the callosal sulcus and along interhemispheric fissure, is easily discerned [5,6].

Sagittal sections

Midline sagittal sections show the four regions of the centrally located corpus callosum, the rostrum, genu, body, and splenium (Fig. 6.12). The cingulate gyrus, seen superior to the corpus callosum, becomes continuous with the isthmus of the cingulate gyrus posterior and with the subcallosal area anteriorly. Inferior to the corpus callosum the fornix is seen coursing rostrally and inferiorly toward the anterior commissure [5,6].

A paramedian section shows the isthmus of the cingulate gyrus is separated from the more inferiolaterally related MOTG by the anterior calcarine sulcus (Fig. 6.13). The circummesencephalic cistern separates the isthmus of the cingulate gyrus and PHG from the diencephalon. The uncus is seen separately [5,6].

The hippocampal formation is better visualized more laterally (Fig. 6.14). Because of the curve of the medial temporal lobe and hippocampal formation (see Fig. 6.5), the circummesencephalic cistern is seen between discontinuous portions of the hippocampal formation (Fig. 6.14) and lateral ventricle (Fig. 6.15). The diencephalon is super-

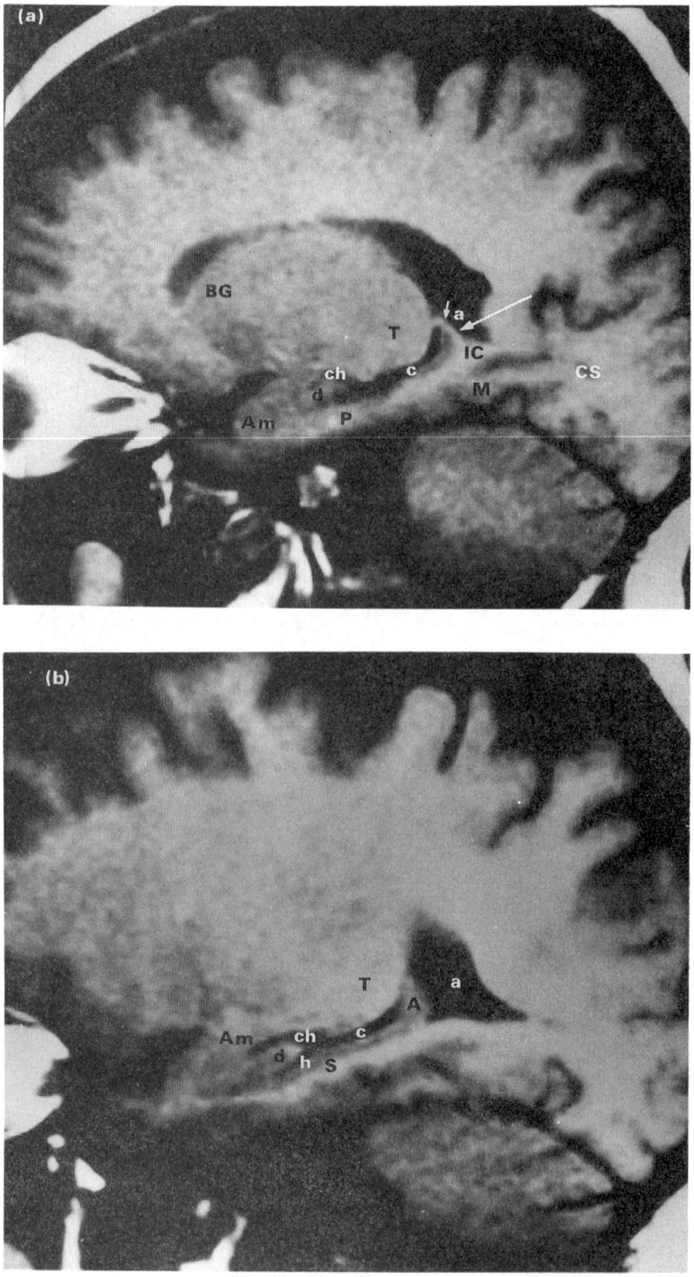

FIGURE 6.14 Sagittal T1W. (a) Lateral to Fig. 6.13. (b) Lateral to (a). The circum-mesencephalic cistern (c) forks anteriorly into the choroidal fissure (ch) and hippocampal fissure (h) with the dentate (d) in between. Amygdala (Am) forms the anterior border of the temporal horn tip which is continuous with the choroidal fissure posteriorly. Subiculum (S) forms the inferior border of the circummesencephalic cistern, becoming Ammon's horn (black "A") posteriorly and anteriorly. Alveus (long arrow) separates Ammon's horn from atrium (white "a") and becomes the fimbria (small arrow). BG, basal ganglia; T, thalamus; P, PHG; IC, isthmus of cingulate gyrus; M, MOTG; CS, calcarine sulcus.

ior to the circummesencephalic cistern while the subiculum and PHG is inferior. Anteriorly the cistern forks into two CSF components separated by the gray matter of the dentate gyrus. The inferior fork is the hippocampal fissure, with the subiculum forming the inferior bank, the dentate gyrus the superior bank, and Ammon's horn the anterior border. The superior CSF fork is formed by the choroidal fissure and temporal horn. The anterior tip of the temporal horn can sometimes be seen as a sliver of CSF coursing anterioinferiorly, separating the amygdala from the hippocampal formation. Posteriorly, the circummesencephalic cistern is capped by the gray matter of Ammon's horn and the dentate gyrus. A small layer of white matter, the alveus and fimbria, surrounds this gray matter. The alveus forms the anterior border of the atrium [5,6].

Proceeding more laterally, but still medial to most of the temporal horn, CSF in the choroidal fissure is seen above a strip of gray matter (Fig. 6.15). The upper border of gray is the dentate gyrus while the lower border is Ammon's horn. The CSF at both the anterior and posterior ends of the choroidal fissure becomes the temporal horn and atrium, respectively. The surface anatomy is demonstrated on the most lateral images (Fig. 6.16) [5,6].

Axial sections

The uncus is the medial protuberance of the PHG at the level of the suprasellar cistern. The amygdala is the gray matter lateral to the uncus, anterior to the temporal horn. The gray matter of the amygdala and uncus is continuous. Depending on the slice level and orientation, the medial temporal lobe is composed of either the PHG or hippocampal

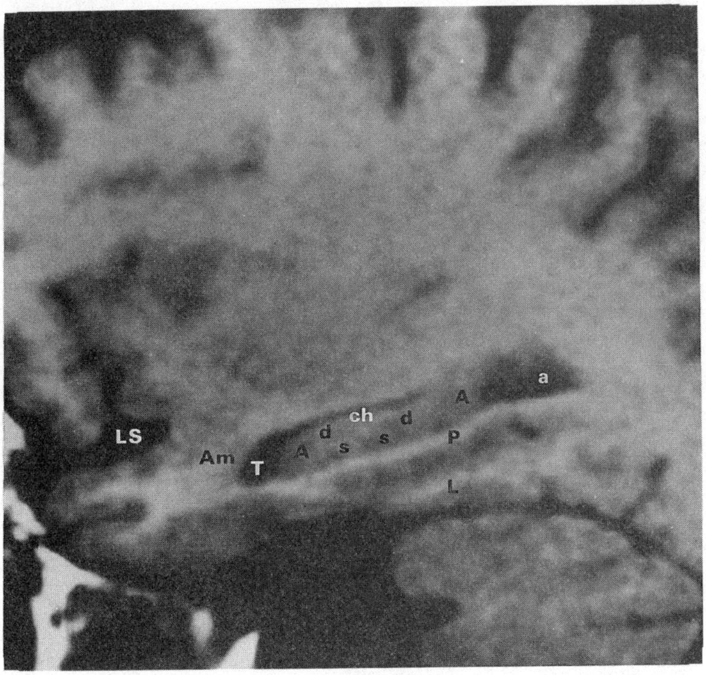

FIGURE 6.15 Sagittal T1W. Lateral to Fig. 6.14b. The dentate gyrus (d) is inferior to the choroidal fissure (ch). Subiculum (s) is inferior to the dentate gyrus and hippocampal fissure (not visualized). Ammon's horn and pes hippocampi (black "A"s) connect the dentate to the subiculum cortex around the hippocampal fissure. LS, lateral sulcus; Am, amygdala; T, temporal horn tip; a, posterior temporal horn becoming atrium of the lateral ventricle; P, PHG; L, LOTG.

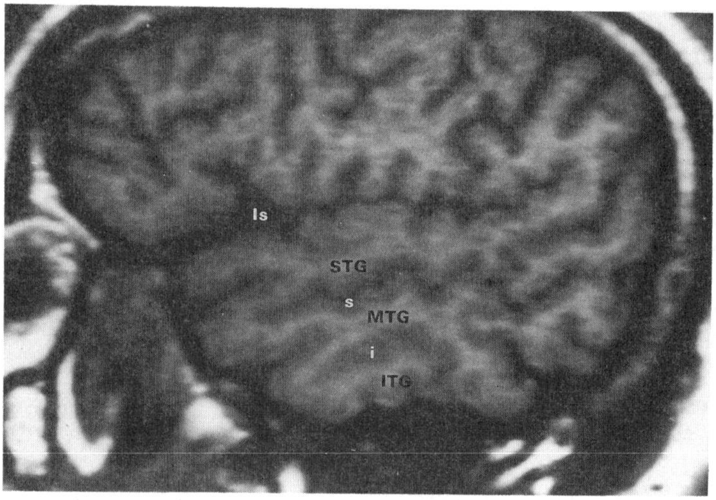

FIGURE 6.16 Sagittal T1W. Surface anatomy of the temporal lobe. STG, superior temporal gyrus (and white matter); MTG, middle temporal gyrus; ITG, inferior temporal gyrus; ls, lateral sulcus; s, superior temporal sulcus; i, inferior temporal gyrus.

formation. A sliver of CSF from the temporal horn is sometimes seen lateral to the hippocampal formation. Behind the midbrain, the PHG swings medial to become the isthmus of the cingulate gyrus bulging medially into the quadrigeminal plate cistern (Fig. 6.17) [5,6,13].

Standard *en bloc* anterior temporal lobectomy

Paul H. Crandall

This operation for temporal lobe epilepsy was developed by Falconer and his colleagues at the Maudsley Unit of Guy's Hospital, London [14,15]. It is clear that his interest was focused on the hippocampal formation rather than the temporal neocortex, in contrast to others at the time. The first large series of temporal lobectomies by Penfield and Flanigin was based on the presence of gross pathological lesions (atrophy, traumatic scars, microgyria and neoplasms), as well as the distribution of interictal discharges found on electrocorticography and the effects of electrical stimulation on patients under local anesthesia to locate the inferior motor strip, to elicit possible auras and to detect the language areas on the dominant lobe [16]. The extent of excisions was quite variable, sometimes including the insula. Penfield noted the high incidence of atrophic lesions (39/68 cases). "The abnormal sclerotic area of cortex, which must be removed in all cases, lies in the deepest, the most inferior and mesial portion of the lobe where it is adjacent to the midbrain." [17]. In his operations he used suction excision and followed the sclerosis from the anterior superior temporal gyrus to the PHG. He tried to avoid opening the ventricle. He removed the hippocampus in only two cases. However, others found that the majority of patients with temporal lobe epilepsy did not have visible, macroscopic pathology. Gibbs *et al.* described psychomotor epilepsy and showed that this condition was associated with EEG evidence of focal interictal discharges in one or both "low temporal areas" [18]. This focal

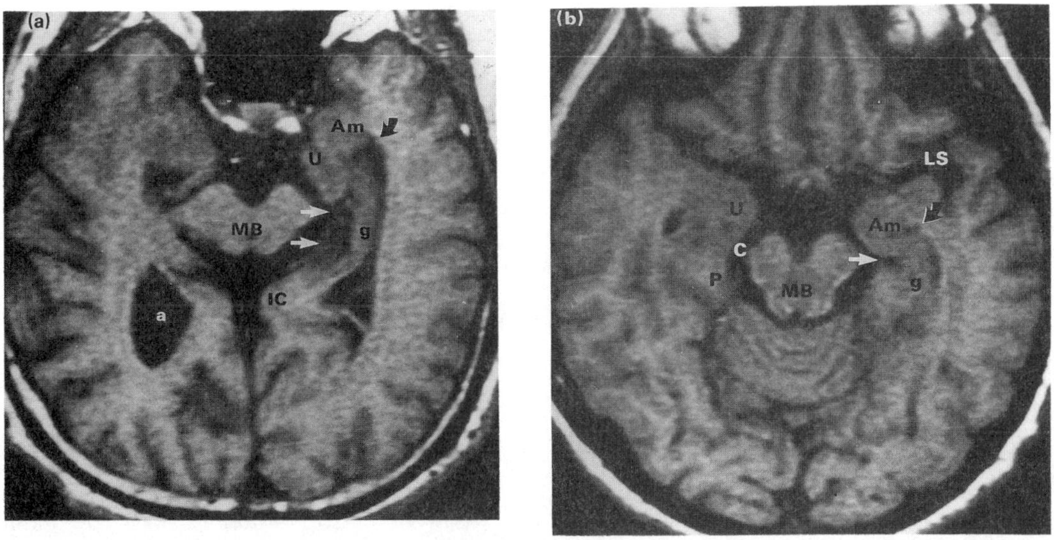

FIGURE 6.17 Axial T1W. Plane parallel to the length of the hippocampal formation, with head hyperextended. The entire length of the temporal horn and hippocampal formation (g) can be imaged on a single slice. Routine axial, head is not extended. Only portions of the temporal horn and hippocampal formation can be seen on a single slice. Black arrow, tip of temporal horn; white arrows, hippocampal fissure; Am, amygdala; U, uncus; g, gray matter of the hippocampal formation; IC, isthmus of cingulate gyrus; MB, midbrain; a, atrium; LS, lateral sulcus; C, circummesencephalic cistern; P, PHG.

EEG activity was most easily shown during natural or induced sleep. They suggested that, in view of the frequent lack of control of these seizures by medication, surgical excision should be based on the EEG evidence in severe cases. Bailey and Gibbs carried out various temporal gyrectomies and removals of the temporal pole sparing the insula and hippocampal formation. They recommended temporal lobectomy back to the level of the central sulcus and noted some success in controlling seizures [19]. Microscopic study of the cortex removed at operation did not reveal frequent pathologic alterations. In their first report of an operation, Falconer *et al.* took note of Penfield's observations but regretted that the deeper parts of the temporal lobe were removed by suction, "...thus precluding their detailed histological study." [14]. Their express intention was "...also to secure the affected tissue for histological study." As a result they disclosed a microscopic pathologic substrate to be present in the majority of patients with no visible lesions (50% hippocampal sclerosis, 25% minute hamartomas, tumors or vascular lesions) [15]. In addition, there was found to be a relationship between the presence and type of pathology and the prognosis.

After the efficacy of the standardized *en bloc* resection was established it was adopted at the UCLA Medical Center and carried out in 225 patients, between 1960 and 1987. Our program has been one of clinical research combined with clinical care. The principal aim of clinical research has been the demonstration of the efficacy of electrophysiologic techniques in identifying epileptogenic brain sites with maximal precision. Standardized arrays of depth electrodes bilaterally implanted in homotopic temporal lobe sites roughly matched standardized *en bloc* anterior temporal lobectomies. This approach has permitted: (1) the scientific assessment of intact tissue; (2) assessment of surgical outcome which is free from the confounding variations which are introduced by highly tailored resections; (3) scientific studies of surgically induced changes relevant to cognition, language, memory and psychosocial function; (4) validation of the importance of preoperative surgical criteria; and (5) the significance of tissue changes in the introduction and scientific assessment of new criteria such as positron emission tomography (PET) and computerized processing of EEG data. Our technique of standardized *en bloc* anterior temporal lobectomy differs little from that of Falconer [20] except that it is carried out more externally (e.g. opening the Sylvian fissure) and involves a more posterior removal of hippocampal formation as well as limiting the suction removal of tissue.

The operation

The UCLA operation has been "standard" from 1960 to 1987, during which anterior temporal lobectomy followed stereoencephalography (SEG) in 154 patients, without SEG in 23 patients and for treatment of small focal tumors in 48 patients.*

Operations are commonly conducted under a general anesthetic unless there is an important reason for defining language areas by electrical stimulation. Steroids, antibiotics and diuretics are used. The patient is positioned in a head clamp with the vertex slightly depressed, the shoulder raised and the table adjusted so that the head is above the level of the heart. The question-mark incision for a low temporal craniotomy is used. Burr holes are placed behind the frontal process of the zygoma and above the root of the zygoma. The sphenoid ridge is removed deeply as well as temporal bone to allow access directly at the middle fossa floor to behind the ear. The dura mater flap is hinged upward above the Sylvian fissure and the dural edges are tacked up. Throughout the operation hemostasis is most important as staining of the tissue will obscure important landmarks. It is also important to develop the dissection to an equal depth in all areas in order that good exposure is ultimately provided in the depth. Dissection is done with optical magnification, bipolar coagulation, microsurgical instruments, and a narrow-bore sucker which is adjusted to remove fluid only.

Stage I. Three anatomic landmarks: uncus; insula; and posterior temporal horn

The cortical incision is tentatively outlined (Fig. 6.18) measuring to a point 6 cm behind the temporal tip along the middle temporal gyrus on the nondominant lobe or 4.5 cm on the dominant one. More of the superior temporal gyrus is spared to avoid the primary auditory cortex lying on the supratemporal plane of the lobe and/or nearby language cortex. This second incision is slanted forward about 45°. On the dominant side the inferior incision can be slanted also posteriorly through the inferior temporal gyrus to reach the same point as would be used on the nondominant side, i.e. 7–8 cm from the temporal tip.

The Sylvian fissure is opened above the anterior superior temporal gyrus. If this gyrus

*The majority were performed by the author; but between 1980 and 1986 some were done by L.D. Cahan; and between 1986 and 1987 by M. Levesque.

is gently lifted off of the insula the plane of cleavage is clearly seen and the middle cerebral arteries will be relatively undisturbed. The fissure is opened anteriorly parallel to the sphenoid ridge down to the floor of the middle fossa and directed posteriorly to the anterior uncus. In this process three to four branches of the M-1 and M-2 segments of the middle cerebral artery to the temporal pole will be interrupted.

When the temporal operculum is lifted the insula is exposed and appears as a conical mound, the apex of which is directed forward and downward, the limen insulae or threshold of the insula (Fig. 6.19). Below the gyrus longus, the single long gyrus of the insula, is the lower circular sulcus. This thin cortex recurves to become the deep cortex of the temporal operculum. Beneath it is the white matter of the uncinate fasciculus which needs to be divided and thinned as it overlies the temporal horn of the ventricle but this should not be opened at this point.

The posterior cortical incision is carried through the three temporal gyri to the inferotemporal cortex which is divided directly medially until the incision passes through the fusiform gyrus to reach the collateral sulcus. A vertical incision with the use of two brain retractors is made towards the midline

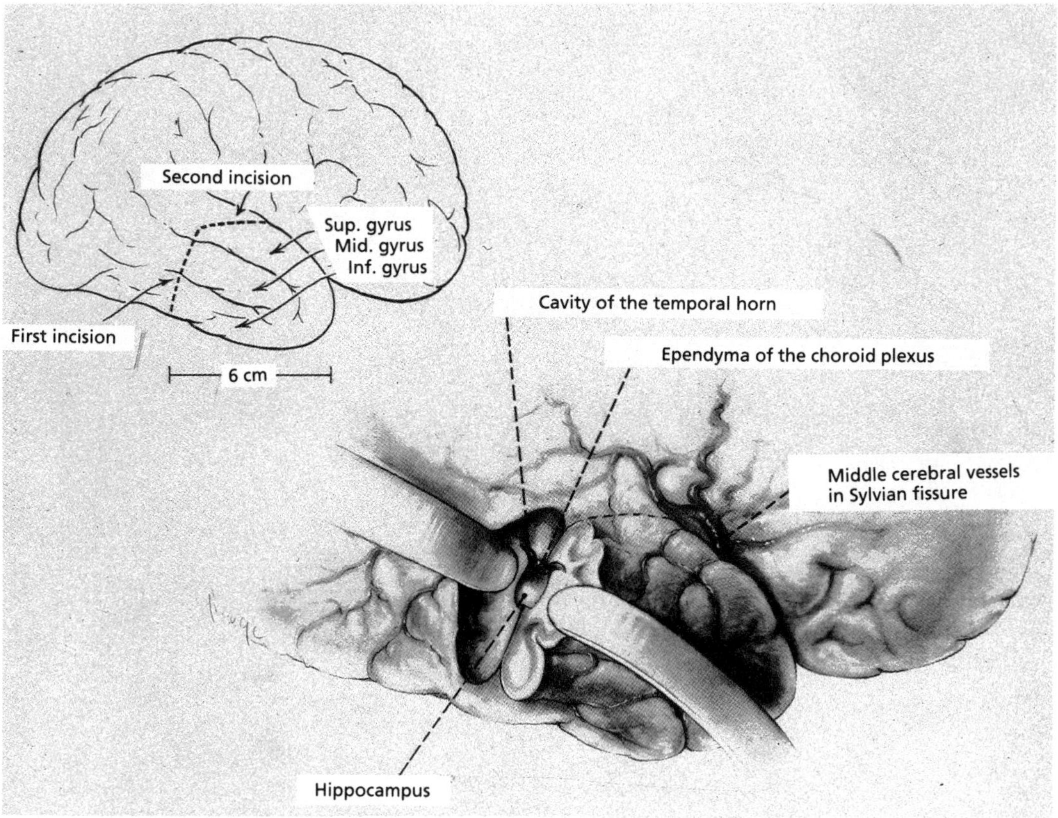

FIGURE 6.18 Illustration of initial cortical incisions and exposure of the hippocampal formation.

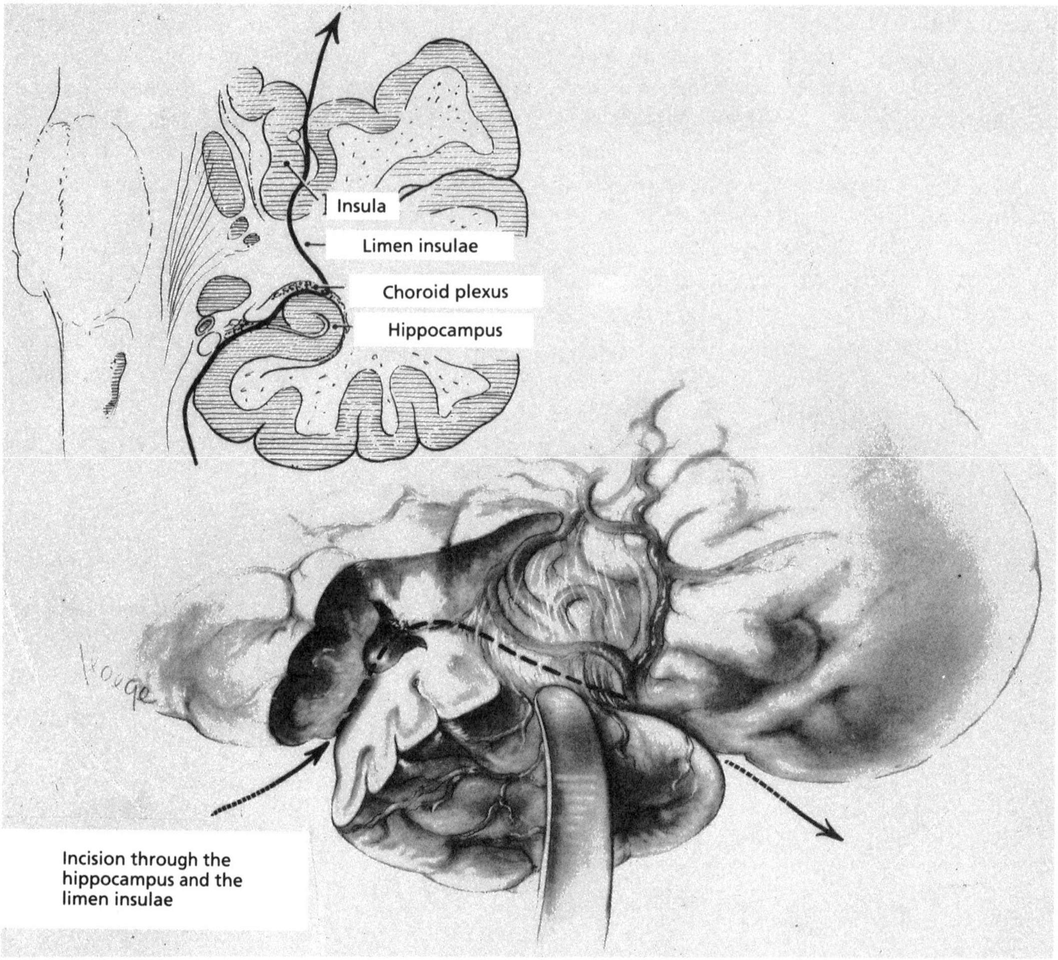

FIGURE 6.19 Opening the Sylvian fissure, exposure of the insula, incision through the temporal stem and completion of posterior cortical incision.

through the white matter of the temporal lobe. For orientation it is directly medial to the middle temporal gyrus. The ependyma may be ballotable. When it is opened, there is a gush of CSF and the choroid plexus emerges, confirming that it is the temporal horn. Immediately a microcottonoid should be placed within the temporal horn for use later.

Stage II. Exposure and detachment of the hippocampal body

The ependymal roof of the temporal horn is lifted, coagulated and divided moving forward until the glistening white pes hippocampi is fully exposed to the tip of the ventricle (Fig. 6.20). Medial and superior to this is the rounded amygdala. The incision is carried through the amygdala separating the basolateral portion from the corticomedial portion which fuses with the uncus. At that point one reaches the middle fossa floor and the junction of the former incision from Stage I.

It is helpful to insert a self-retaining retractor at this point. The retractor is directed posteromedially to open the temporal horn and retract the choroid plexus. Care should be taken that there is no retractor pressure on the insula or the brain stem as the choroid plexus attaches to the brain stem and optic tract. The hippocampus is attached to the brain stem just below the choroid plexus by the taenia fimbria. The hippocampus is then detached by dividing through the thin edge of the curved fimbria from behind forward. This exposes the superior surface of the PHG (Fig. 6.21). Posteriorly the hippocampus and PHG are transected in a coronal direction 3.0–3.5 cm behind the tip of the pes hippocampi. The PHG is lifted and transected until the edge of the tentorium is reached.

Stage III. Detachment of the PHG

The *en bloc* specimen now remains only attached by the PHG from the uncus to the posterior medullary cistern. This is the most risky part of the operation but complications are avoidable, i.e. by anatomic knowledge of the structures in the nearby ambient and crural cisterns. Figure 6.22 is a dissection diagram showing the relationships of the location of the hippocampus and PHG to the

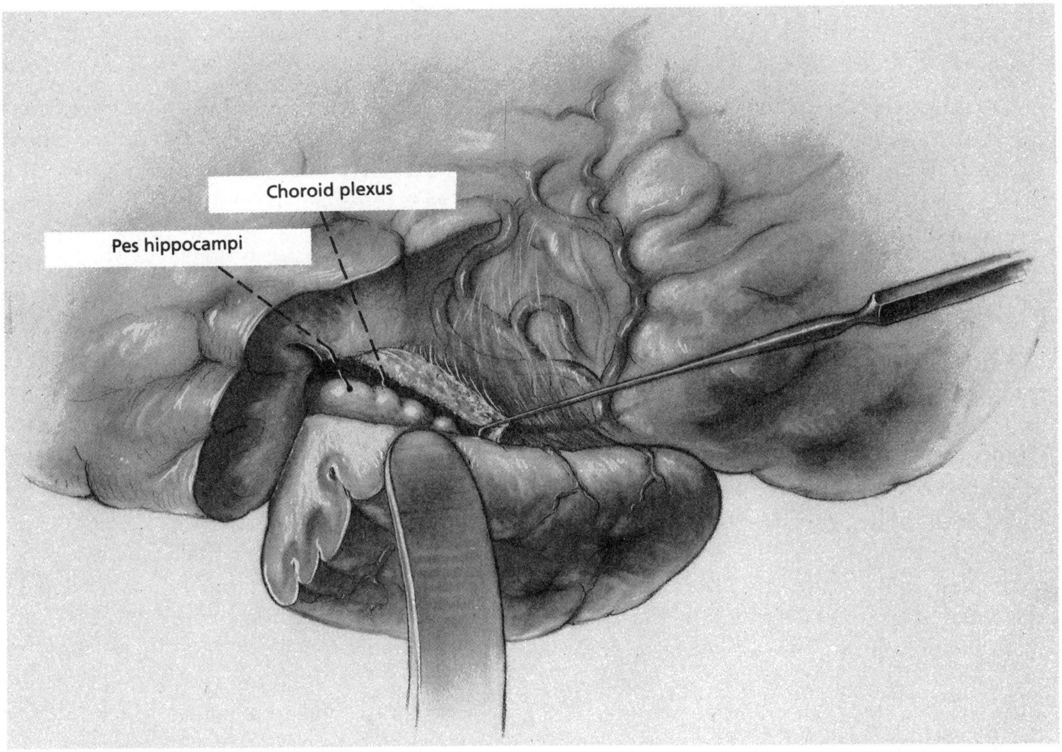

FIGURE 6.20 Exposure of the pes hippocampi. Hook indicates position of amygdalar incision.

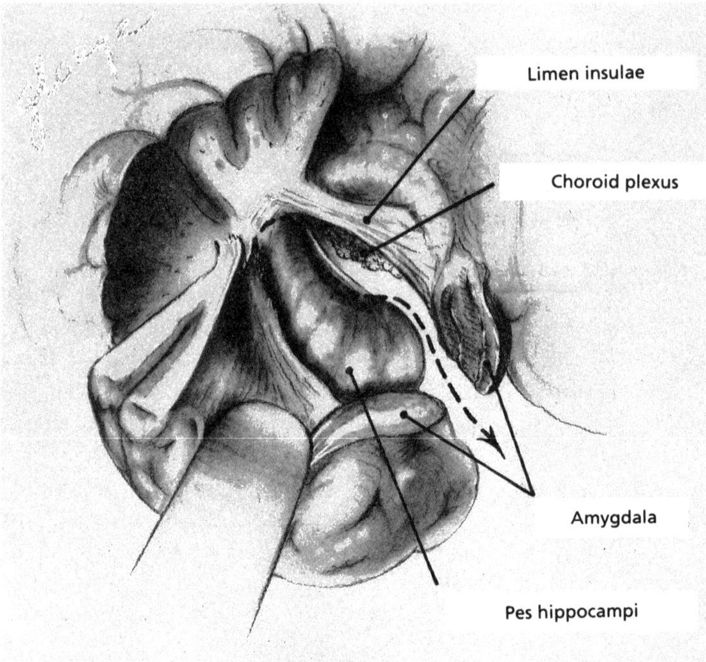

FIGURE 6.21 Completion of amygdalar incision and initial detachment of hippocampus by dividing the fimbria of the fornix.

important vascular and CNS structures. Damage to the anterior choroidal trunk may result in contralateral hemiparesis; to the P-2 segment posterior cerebral artery, in hemiparesis and hemianopsia; and to the third or fourth cranial nerves, in diplopia. The structures in the cisterna ambiens shown in Fig. 6.22 are not normally exposed in this operation because they remain protected by a transparent curtain of the medial pial and arachnoid membranes of the parahippocampal gyrus, following subsequent subpial dissection. The branches of these vessels will be interrupted as they pass over the edge of the tentorium.

The best guide to the safe preservation of the cisternal structures is to follow the edge of the tentorium and progressively to strip the medial pial wall of the PHG and doubly coagulate and divide the inferior pial membrane of the PHG just lateral to the tentorial edge. Beginning anteriorly at the level of the uncus the edge of the tentorium is identified. The lateral branches of the anterior choroidal artery, which supply the anterior one-third of the PHG and uncus, are divided. This spares the medial branches to the optic tract, peduncle, internal capsule, thalamus and choroid plexus. Moving posteriorly one progressively strips the inferior pial membrane, dividing *ca.* four to five "Ammon's horn arteries." These arteries mainly come from the P-2 segment, just proximal to the origin of the posterolateral choroidal artery which is usually behind the level of resection (Fig. 6.22). It is not advisable to interrupt the inferolateral branch of the posterior cerebral artery, just behind, because it supplies the important inferotemporal branches passing further posteriorly (inferoposterior, inferotemporooccipital), but there may be branches of this artery passing forward through the collateral sulcus which must be interrupted there. The posterior transverse incision through the PHG will have been reached and the specimen will be free except

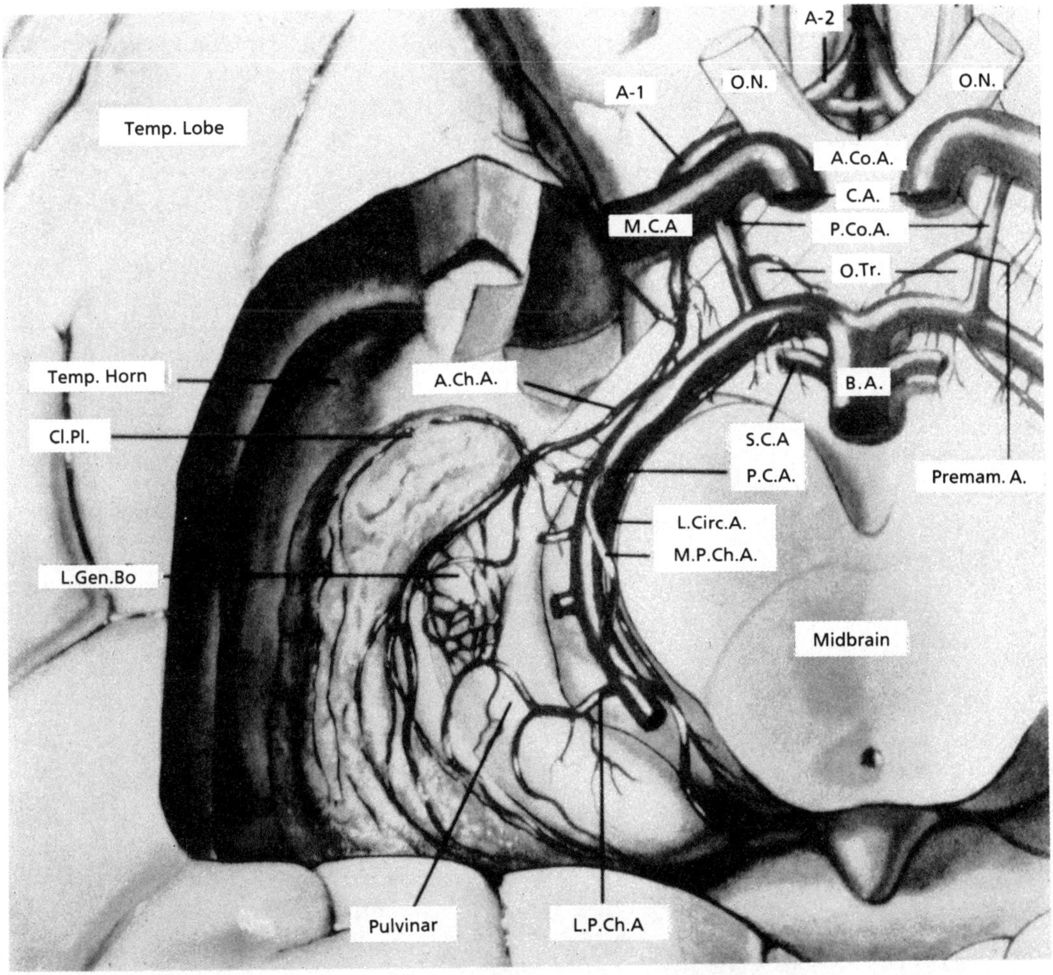

FIGURE 6.22 Dissection diagram showing relationships between the medial temporal lobe structure and important vessels, the thalamus and the midbrain. A. Ch. A., anterior choroidal artery; P.C.A., posterior cerebral artery; L.P. Ch.A., lateral posterior choroidal branches of the posterior cerebral artery; L. Gen. Bo., lateral geniculate body — note the optic tract anteriorly; M.P. Ch. A., medial posterior choroidal artery. From Rhoton *et al.* [21].

for possible veins on the inferior surface (Fig. 6.23).

Variations from standard *en bloc* anterior temporal lobectomy

One might suppose that the principal reason for extending the resection of an operation would be to include more lateral temporal neocortex. Since the more accurate definition of epileptogenic foci by means of stereotaxic implanted electrodes and video-EEG analysis of spontaneous seizures there have been found to be few sites of epileptogenesis in the posterior lateral temporal neocortex. In the UCLA series of 200 explorations by SEG, only four examples were found using both surface skull electrodes and multilead depth electrodes, and two were related to surface tumors. Wieser in Zurich reported three in 51 patients [22]. In a more extensive evaluation by the group at Yale–West Haven Medical Center, which included bilateral monitoring of medial temporal structures by anterior and temporal multilead implanted electrodes and several flexible subdural electrodes wrapped around the inferior and lateral temporal lobe surfaces, it was found that in 11 patients with 55 seizures recorded, four had had a simultaneous onset in the neocortex and the hippocampus, and 51 had had an onset in the unilateral hippocampus. None of the seizures had originated solely in the temporal neocortex [23]. It must be concluded that the interictal electrocorticographic discharges observed for so long on the lateral temporal lobe represented secondary propagated activity from the depth in almost all cases. Consequently the distribution of these interictal discharges cannot be considered to be an indication for further resection of temporal neocortex except when the pathology is obvious on the surface of the temporal lobe.

An important indicator of the presence of a pathologic substrate in this type of epilepsy is a zone of hypometabolism in one temporal lobe seen in interictal positron PET with 18-fluorodeoxyglucose [24]. The degree of relative hypometabolism on scans seems to correlate well with the severity of the pathologic lesion ($p < 0.02$). When related to tumors, angioma, or focal heterotopia it has

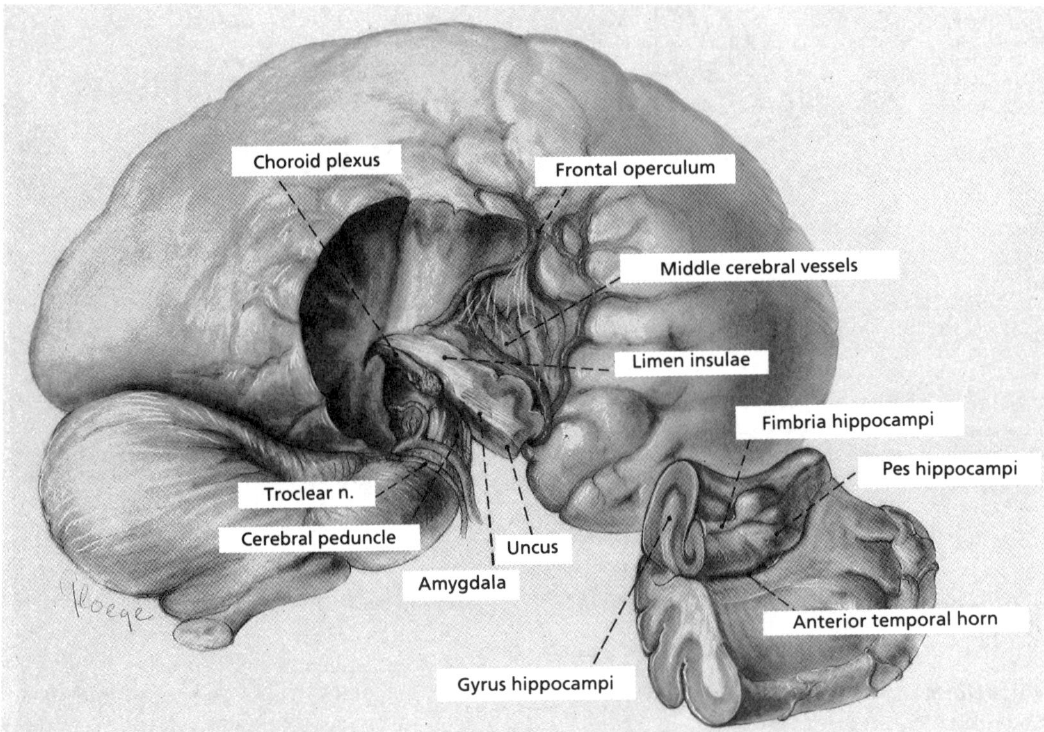

FIGURE 6.23 Final *en bloc* specimen freed from posterior PHG.

generally been focal to the lesion site. However, the majority of patients have hippocampal sclerosis of varying severity. In this condition the hypometabolic region is much larger than the extent of the underlying sclerosis defined by light microscopy. This may be accounted for in *ca.* one-third of patients by dual pathologies, e.g. dysplasias, microdysgenesis, nonspecific gliosis, or isolated large single neurons found within the lateral portion of the temporal lobes [25]. In the remaining cases there is apparent hypometabolism without structural change. This has been attributed to either functional inactivation of neuronal elements associated with the epileptogenic lesion, or to structural abnormalities below the resolution of present histopathologic study (e.g. loss of synapses). In the majority of patients who were later demonstrated to have hippocampal sclerosis in the lobectomy specimens, the extent of the temporal lobe hypometabolism corresponded closely with the extent of the anterior temporal lobectomy. In a smaller group the hypometabolism was confined to the mesial temporal region. No cases of isolated posterolateral temporal lobe hypometabolism have been encountered except for those in the presence of a small surface tumor. Until proven otherwise, this large interictal volume of anterior temporal lobe hypometabolism must be considered to reflect altered cerebral function associated with partial epilepsy. This supports the continued use of anterior temporal lobectomy to the extent described here. We have not encountered cases in which the standard operation had to be extended further because of the hypometabolism.

The lesions associated with hippocampal sclerosis have been defined in much more precise quantitative and topographic distribution since the introduction of volumetric neuronal density studies [26,27]. There may be at least two types of hippocampal sclerosis. Most common is "primary" temporal lobe epilepsy in which spontaneous seizures onset (as determined by depth electrodes) and neuronal cell loss is maximal in the anterior hippocampal formation. The EEG pattern is "focal type onset." It has been associated with a long duration of seizures beginning in children under 3 years of age, early onset of generalized or complex partial seizures and, in several surgical series, has had the best prognosis after temporal lobectomy for complex partial seizures. There appears to be a direct link between the extent of cell loss in Ammon's horn and nearby seizure genesis [26]. A less well defined and diffuse type of hippocampal sclerosis has been found in patients with ⩾ 50% "regional type" or posterior hippocampal seizure onsets. These patients tended to have a diffuse loss of pyramidal cells in the resected hippocampal formation, i.e. pyramidal cell loss extended both anteriorly and posteriorly in the hippocampus as well as seizure onsets occurring along the entire anteroposterior axis of the hippocampal formation in depth electrode analyses [26]. In these patients the age of seizure onset is possibly later. It has been associated with a less favorable outcome after anterior temporal lobectomy. In this series both anterior focal and regional epileptogenesis were associated with abnormal cytology in the mesial, not the lateral, temporal lobe.

At the Yale–West Haven Medical Center approximately 20% of patients with unilateral temporal lobe epilepsy had an abnormal electrical focus identified by depth electrodes in the posterior hippocampus, i.e. caudal to the usual limits of temporal lobectomy [28]. This led to the development of a new surgical approach which permitted access to the posterior temporal horn of the lateral ventricle with preservation of the most functional lateral temporal cortex. This operation is equally effective and with no greater consequences to the optic radiations. It therefore meets the need to cope with posterior medial seizure onsets and/or pathologic lesions.

In at least one-quarter of patients with temporal lobe epilepsy there are focal lesions of a developmental, malformative or neoplastic nature: vascular malformations, gliomas, gangliogliomas, dysplasias, tubers, and ectopias. Many of these are detected on CT or MRI scans. In previous series these lesions had been discovered in lobectomy specimens, since they were not demonstrable on conventional neuroradiologic examinations. When patients have had refractory partial seizures for many years, associated with a small mass lesion in any cerebral lobe, the prognosis for the control of seizures and the mass are generally excellent [29]. However, the small intracerebral tumors associated with temporal lobe epilepsy may represent a special biology. Small astrocytomas, oligodendrogliomas, mixed glial tumors and epidermoids have been found in lobectomy specimens in the UCLA series (48 patients). These tumors were entirely contained within the lobectomy specimens with subsequent seizure-free outcome and no recurrence of tumor. The exception has been the tuber, which has the potential to become neoplastic, is multicentric in origin and part of a neurocutaneous, inherited disorder. Patients with small temporal lobe masses should be closely examined preoperatively for these cutaneous features and genetic counseling is important when this disorder is found.

The possibility of complete removal of these small masses can be evaluated by preoperative MRI scans using a grid. The limits of resection can be extended to include the mass in many instances, depending on the position. Posterior and medial extension has already been discussed. When the lateral neocortex must be removed to include tumors the resection is coronally cut, rather than obliquely. As measured along the middle temporal gyrus from the temporal tip, a coronal cut anterior to or at 4.5 cm on either side is not likely to result in a permanent visual field defect. There is general agreement that the more posterior the damage or excision of a temporal lobe beyond 5.5–6.0 cm, the greater the field defect will encroach on the lower quadrant of vision. Contralateral superior quadrant homonymous defects begin to occur at this level. All visual field deficits are incongruous with the greater deficit using the eye ipsilateral to the lobectomy. Ipsilateral temporal retinal projections proceed through the temporal lobe more anteriorly and ventrally than the crossed nasal retinal projections from the same point in the visual field. There is considerable individual variability in this course and a deviant detour of the geniculostriate pathway may not be predictable without visual evoked potentials recorded from depth electrodes [30]. This variability is greatly reduced as the optic fibers converge toward the occipital lobe. Falconer and Wilson cautioned that "... with removals of more than 8 cm more and more fibers are cut as they begin to pass obliquely beneath the ventricle, and so the severity of the field defects tends to increase ...," i.e. contralateral homonymous hemianopsia [31].

In conclusion the standard *en bloc* anterior temporal lobectomy has served well as a safe and effective treatment for the control of temporal lobe epilepsy. Also it has led to the removal of unsuspected neoplasms which have not required further treatment.

Acknowledgments

Paul H. Crandall wishes to thank Gwynne Gloege for medical illustrations and Sasha LaHaye for preparation of his manuscript. The research at the UCLA School of Medicine was supported by United States Public Health Service NS 02808.

Anteromedial temporal lobectomy: directing the surgical approach to the pathologic substrate

Dennis D. Spencer

Rationale

Since 1825, when Bouchet and Cazauvieilh described palpably abnormal hippocampi in the autopsied brains of patients with "alienation" epilepsy, debate on the role of the hippocampus in epilepsy has continued [32]. The hippocampus has been variously ignored, described as secondarily injured by seizures [33, 34], or implicated as the epileptogenic focus created by another mechanism such as ischemia [35].

The resection of the hippocampal formation with other medial temporal lobe structures has undergone a similar debate. Anterior temporal lobectomy has enjoyed variable success in alleviating seizures thought to originate in a single temporal lobe. The two factors that seem to predict this success have been the ability to make the proper choice of candidates with unilateral temporal lobe epilepsy, and then to ascertain what portion of the temporal lobe constitutes the focus and what must be removed to optimize seizure control (and minimize neurologic and cognitive deficit).

In the early days of temporal lobectomy, resection of only the lateral temporal neocortex controlled some patients, but many partly or completely uncontrolled patients benefited from reoperation and resection of medial structures including the anterior hippocampus [19,36,37]. Over the last two decades, data from chronic invasive electrophysiologic monitoring have shown that the majority of ictal events in temporal lobe epilepsy appear to originate in the medial temporal lobe, if not clearly in the hippocampus [28]. Likewise, a predominance of neuronal loss, gliosis and histochemical changes are identified in the hippocampal formation of the excised temporal lobe structures in those patients most often cured of temporal lobe epilepsy [26]. Interictal spikes can be recorded from the surface of the temporal lobe and, up to 1980, our center occasionally performed electrocorticography which equated interictal spikes recorded from the surface of the neocortex with potential epileptic foci. We were discouraged, however, by the poor correlation of this activity with any pathology in the lateral neocortical tissue. Since seizures began almost exclusively in the hippocampus, where pathologic changes were frequent, interictal spikes emerging from histologically normal temporal neocortex could hardly be used to outline an excision of a potential epileptogenic zone. It remained unclear how much of the parahippocampus, amygdala, entorhinal cortex, and hippocampus should be identified as the sufficient epileptic region. Intraoperative hippocampal recording is not capable of providing an answer because of surgical disruption of pathways and the absence of ictal activity in this setting.

Thus, several convergent factors prompted us to tailor the temporal lobectomy to our noninvasive predictors of hippocampal pathology and to chronic EEG recording of ictal events rather than to intraoperative interictal recordings. If ictal events are most often recorded from the medial structures and the predominant neuropathologic features are seen in the hippocampus, a more medial temporal resection should remove the majority of the epileptogenic substrate. How much of the medial temporal lobe needs to be removed for control of anteromedial temporal lobe epilepsy? Initially, we attempted to tailor the length of the hippocampal resection to the ictal onset as determined by depth electrodes that study the anteroposterior axis of the hippocampus for approximately 3 cm of its length. Very rarely, however, is there a distinct segment of hippocampus that initiates the seizure and shows isolated neuronal loss and gliosis. In the majority of cases, the electrical and pathologic abnormalities are demonstrated throughout the body of the hippocampus. Our preliminary data indicated that a radical resection of the medial temporal structures would control seizures in approximately 85% of patients and could be accomplished with no additional neuropsychologic or neurologic morbidity. Anteromedial resection including most of the hippocampal formation then became the standard temporal lobectomy when a medial temporal lobe focus was identified [26]. The extent of lateral temporal resection was limited to the temporal pole to provide access to the medial structures unless lateral ictal events were recorded or a lateral lesion was imaged preoperatively.

Two advantages accrue from this approach. Firstly, operations under local anesthesia are not necessary since electrocorticography and language mapping would not be performed unless chronic electrical recordings or imaging implicated the neocortex of the dominant temporal lobe as the seizure focus. That is an unusual circumstance; when it occurs, one has the choice of intraoperative language mapping or implantation of subdural grids which can be used to map language and better defined the ictal area of the neocortex by chronic recording.

Many patients can tolerate craniotomy under local anesthesia with appropriate support. However, children, intellectually impaired patients, or patients with behavior problems cannot easily undergo such awake operations. Operations under local anesthesia are difficult for even the most cooperative and tolerant of individuals, since all patients suffer pain from coagulating and dissecting along the middle fossa dura and vessels.

The second advantage to this approach is the uniform preservation of the visual fields, since a lateral temporal incision of <3.5–4.0 cm should never give more than an upper quadrant field defect (save for an unexpected vascular injury). In fact, our experience would indicate that much less than a superior quadrant is lost with a temporal pole resection, as opposed to a somewhat more variable risk of a homonymous hemianopsia beyond 5–6 cm of lateral resection. We also hypothesized that a less radical lateral resection would reduce the risk of compromising the specific cognitive function of the temporal lobe. This appears to be true for visual spatial testing in the nondominant temporal lobe but no clear cognitive advantages are seen when resecting within the dominant lobe.

Prior to MRI, depth and/or subdural recordings were the mainstay in our decision-making. These recordings were used with noninvasive criteria derived through the history, neurologic examination, cognitive testing, and in conjunction with the intracarotid Amytal test. Following the 1.5 T MRI demonstration of hippocampal atrophy, especially in individuals with a history of childhood febrile seizures, an exceptionally strong correlation was noted between this image abnormality, medial temporal lobe ictal events and hippocampal cell loss on pathologic examination. Patients with a concurrence of all focal epileptogenic phenomena including temporal lobe specific cognitive deficits, appropriately diminished memory shown by the intracarotid amobarbital perfusion for language and memory lateralization (Wada Sodium Amytal test), scalp ictal and interictal activity, and MRI hippocampal atrophy are now offered an anteromedial resection without invasive study.

We are not, however, recommending the anteromedial temporal lobectomy for all patients with temporal lobe epilepsy. There are certainly patients with what appears to be unilateral temporal lobe epilepsy but whose boundaries of epileptogenicity are not well defined by present measuring devices. However, the largest subset of temporal lobe epilepsy patients have a syndrome that is probably initiated by a childhood injury, often heralded by a febrile seizure, and despite what may be broad etiologically, results in a specific injury to one hippocampus more than the other. It is this group to whom we have chosen to offer an operation directed specifically to the medial structures. Figure 6.24 is an abbreviated decision tree which points out our method of selection of patients for the preoperative tailored anterior medial temporal lobectomy.

Technique

The operation is performed under general anesthesia. The patient is supine, a blanket roll under the appropriate shoulder, and the head turned laterally in three-point fixation with the anterior zygoma at an angle of *ca.* 10° above a line parallel with the floor. (This slight angle along with tilting the table allows for an unobstructed microscopic line of sight along the length of the temporal horn and hippocampus during the later stages of

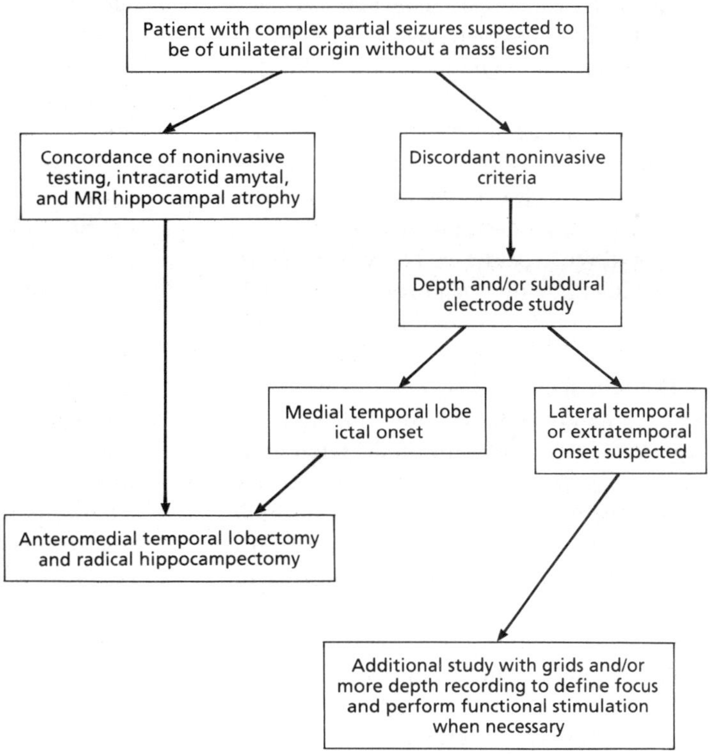

FIGURE 6.24 Selection methods for anterior medial temporal lobectomy — an abbreviated decision tree.

the operation.) The skin incision is begun on the superior aspect of the zygoma 1.5 cm anterior to the tragus and carried superiorly over the·ear to the mastoid vertex line where it curves gently just superior to the temporal squamosa and may stop at the hairline or extend medially along the hairline to the midline. The temporalis muscle is dissected from the temporal bone and turned in one piece with the skin flap anteriorly. A free frontotemporal bone flap is then fashioned. Its anterior–posterior axis should extend at least 6 cm along the temporal bone. The superior boundary of the bone flap should be designed to expose the orbital frontal region and the temporal bone should be rongeured as close to the floor of the middle fossa as possible without violating the mastoid air cells. The dura is tented and opened with the midline as a base and incised towards the temporal tip. The surface of the temporal lobe is inspected and particular attention is directed to the venous drainage system which should not be interrupted save for those veins at the anterior temporal tip and the inferior aspect of the inferior temporal gyrus and occipitotemporal gyrus. The remainder of the operation consists of taking two or three separate resective specimens, depending upon the shallowness of the middle fossa and the extent of temporal lobe atrophy.

The first stage consists of marking a line which extends 3–3.5 cm from the tip of the temporal lobe, along the middle temporal gyrus (Figs 6.25 & 6.26). This incision line should then curve inferiorly across the middle and inferior temporal gyri and may variably stop at the occipitotemporal gyrus or include a greater portion of this gyrus. The arachnoid along this line is coagulated with a bipolar forceps and this inferior portion of the temporal pole is resected *en bloc*. The superior margin of this resection is the inferior arachnoid of the superior temporal gyrus which is not violated. The depth of the resection is approximately 3 cm, designed to approach the temporal horn but not enter it, thus creating a block of tissue measuring approximately 3 cm^3. This cube of tissue is then submitted for histologic examination and the second stage of the procedure begins.

All exposed surfaces of the brain are covered with a collagen sponge and two self-retaining retractors are positioned, one to retract the superior temporal gyrus, and the second retractor placed on the cut surface of the middle and inferior temporal gyri (Fig. 6.27).

The ultrasonic aspirator is then placed on a setting of three vibration and two suction, the white matter overlying the temporal horn is dissected, and the horn is entered. This maneuver allows orientation of the dissection away from the optic tract. At this point, the incision is carried anteriorly and medially across the anterior fibers of the temporal stem and the junction of the middle and superior third of the amygdala toward the lesser wing of the sphenoid. Dissection is carried medially and inferiorly to the incisura of the tentorium where the uncus of the parahippocampus is identified and an ultrasonic aspirator is used to gently dissect and remove the uncus from the arachnoid overlying the carotid artery, optic and third nerves. The incision along the uncus of the parahippocampus is carried posteriorly over the arachnoid to the anterior midbrain. At this point, the dissection ceases medially and anteriorly and the self-retaining retractor is inserted deeper to gently retract the remaining fibers of the temporal stem, superior temporal gyrus, and the superior aspect of the cut amygdala.

Attention is now turned to the posterior–inferior aspect of the incision where the occipital temporal fasciculus is identified and

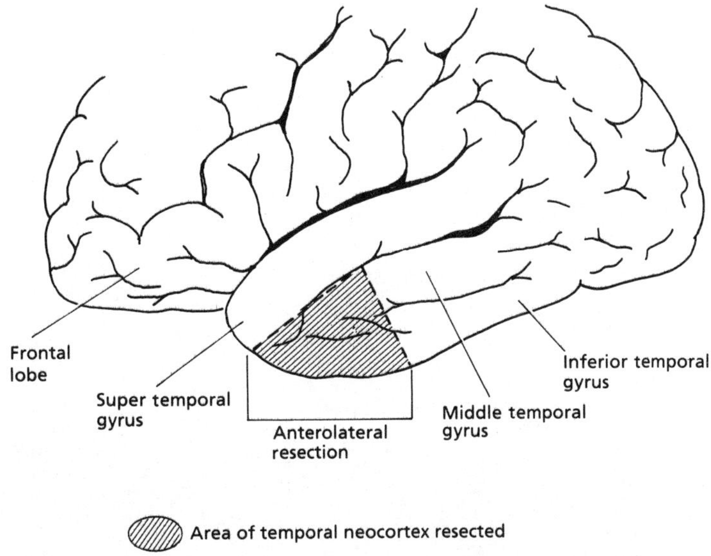

FIGURE 6.25 Saggital view illustrating the 3.5 cm extent of the wedge-shaped neocortical resection.

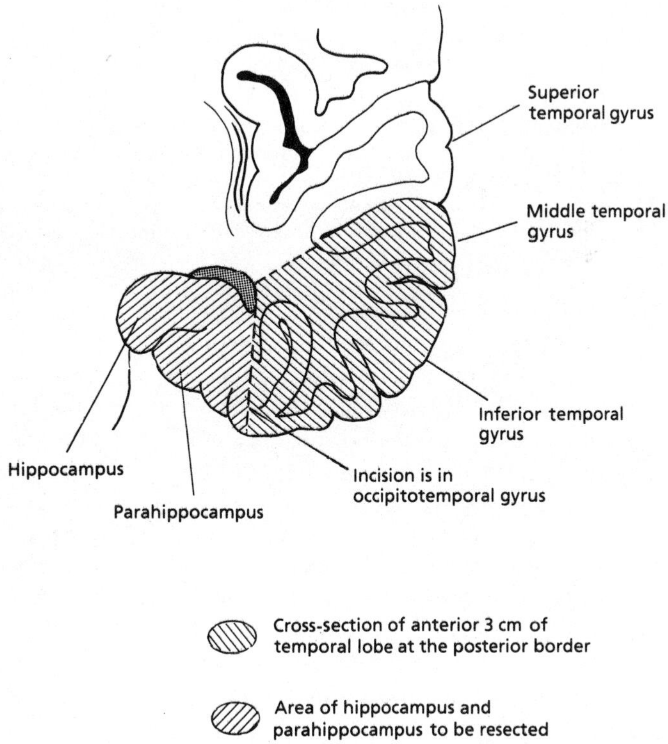

FIGURE 6.26 Coronal cut taken at 3.5 cm from the temporal tip, depicting the incisions along the arachnoid of the superior temporal gyrus to the temporal horn just posterior to the amygdala. The depth of this incision is approximately 3 cm. The next incision is carried to the floor of the middle fossa lateral to the parahippocampus. The volume of this block includes the middle, inferior, and most of the occipitotemporal gyrus.

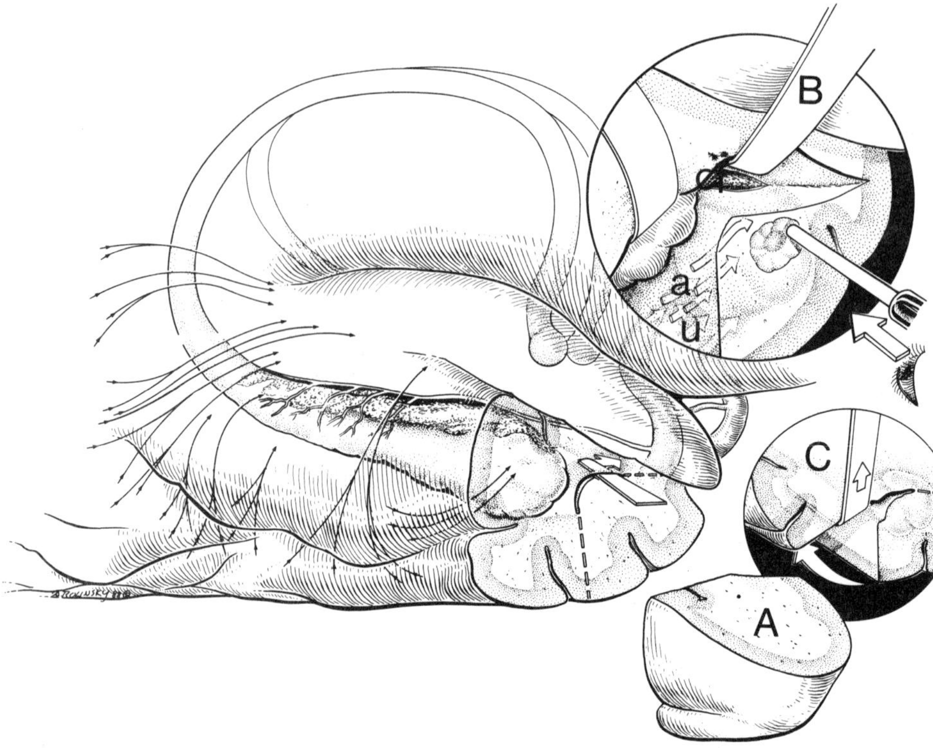

FIGURE 6.27 A, the resected block of temporal pole. B, self-retaining retractor on the superior temporal gyrus and the first medial incision using the ultrasonic aspirator along the arachnoid of the uncus of the parahippocampus. Note that this incision is being directed toward the choroid fissure (cf) and cuts across the amygdala, uncinate fasciculus (u), and the fibers forming the anterior commissure (a). C, elevation of the lateral neocortex as the occipitotemporal fasciculus is incised to the atrium of the lateral ventricle.

incised posteriorly, joining the temporal horn to the floor of the middle fossa. This incision is extended with bipolar coagulation and ultrasonic aspiration following the curve of the hippocampus but not violating it. The posterior dissection is curtailed when the hippocampus begins to curve medially and the arachnoid of the medial occipital temporal gyrus can be identified (Fig. 6.28). As this dissection continues, the neocortical self-retaining retractor is curved and inserted along the line of dissection until the lateral temporal neocortex can be gently elevated exposing the length of the hippocampus, parahippocampus, and the medial aspect of the occipitotemporal gyrus (Fig. 6.29). With the two retractors now in proper position, the microscope is brought into position and the remaining dissection is carried out under microscopic control.

Under the microscope, attention is directed again to the incision along the uncus of the parahippocampus. One can easily identify the thick white bands anterior to the arachnoid of the midbrain which represent the uncinate fasciculus and the anterior commissure (Fig. 6.27). These fibers are divided with the ultrasonic aspirator, again taking care not to violate the arachnoid overlying the midbrain, and this incision is carried posteriorly to join the choroidal fissure and the choroid plexus. At this point, depending upon the bulk of the medial structures present in the middle fossa, one may elect to resect the anterior occipitotemporal gyrus and amygdala using bipolar coagulation and ultrasonic aspiration in a second *en bloc* excision, and this is submitted for histologic examination. Only the hippocampus and parahippocampus remain.

Attention is then directed to the small vessels irrigating the medial parahippocampus and hippocampus emanating from the posterior cerebral artery and the anterior choroidal artery (Fig. 6.30). The vessels from the posterior cerebral artery lie in the arachnoid of the hippocampal fissure and are coagulated in the fissure singly and divided with microscissors. Irrigating vessels from the anterior choroidal artery are coagulated as they supply the hippocampus and are cut sharply. As the dissection continues, the arachnoid posterior to the brain stem and overlying the posteromedial parahippocampus is identified and preserved. The arachnoid just lateral to the incisura of the tentorium is coagulated with bipolar coagulation and incised sharply. The hippocampus can now be gently elevated away from the brain stem. The fimbria is easily identified as it streams from the alveus and it is divided with either a microdissector or with the ultrasonic aspirator.

The dissection continues under microscopic control with further division of smaller perforating vessels from the posterior cerebral artery, which can now easily be seen under the arachnoid. The hippocampus is followed as it approximates the superior colliculus of the midbrain (Fig. 6.31). At this point, the incision from the middle fossa floor is joined to the incision of the posterior body of the hippocampus, and the medial structures including the parahippocampus and hippocampus can be removed *en bloc* (Fig.

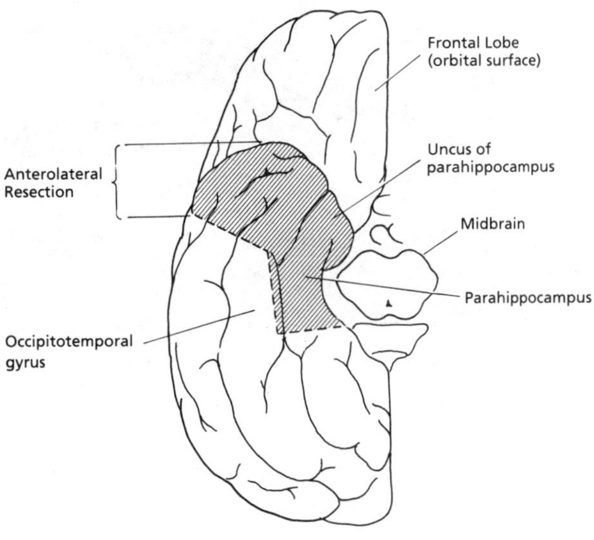

FIGURE 6.28 Basal view depicting how the occipitotemporal fasciculus incision extends along the lateral hippocampus and parahippocampus. The posterior border is the atrium of the lateral ventricle at the level of the superior colliculus.

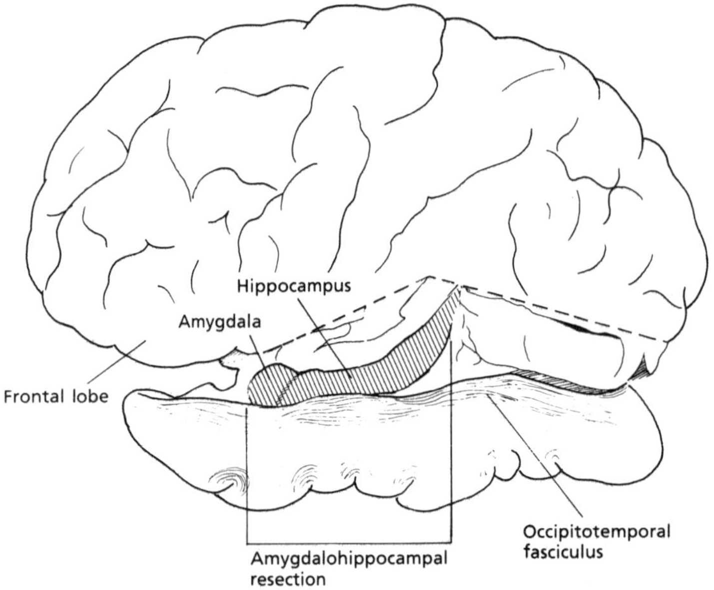

FIGURE 6.29 Sagittal view indicating the occipitotemporal fasciculus incision extending lateral to the hippocampus and into the ventricular atria.

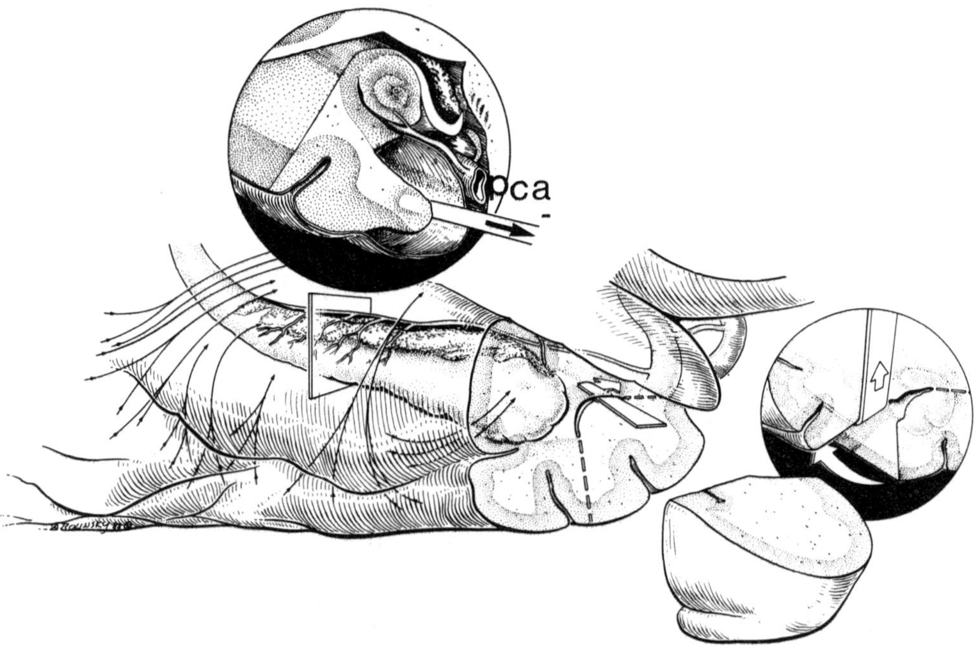

FIGURE 6.30 Subpial dissection of the parahippocampus (the arachnoid over the midbrain should not be violated). The identification of irrigating vessels from the posterior cerebral artery entering the hippocampal fissure is illustrated. Also of note is the fimbria of the fornix which is easily divided, and the choroid plexus which should be retracted but not coagulated.

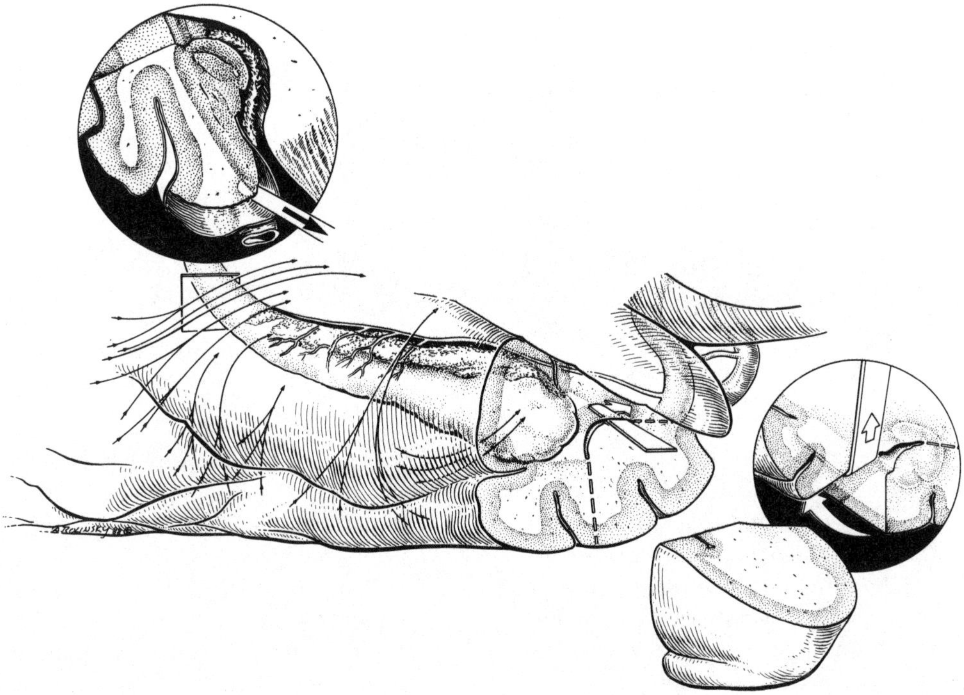

FIGURE 6.31 Continued posterior medial subpial dissection as the hippocampus diminishes in diameter. At the curve of the hippocampus it is cut across joining the occipitotemporal incision.

6.32). At the end of this dissection, one should be able to identify easily, from superior to inferior, the choroid plexus, the arachnoid overlying the inferior aspect of the thalamus and optic tract and the lateral aspect of the midbrain, the coagulated arachnoid and vessels of the hippocampal fissure, the arachnoid overlying the posterior cerebral artery, and the medial edge of the tentorium. The fourth nerve may sometimes be seen running just lateral to the incisural edge, the third nerve is identified anteriorly and medially, again beneath the arachnoid, with the carotid artery in the most anterior position. Meticulous hemostatis is then obtained, retractors are removed allowing the lateral temporal cortex to settle into position, the dura is closed with interrupted sutures, the bone flap is wired into position, and the scalp is closed in layers.

Temporal lobectomy tailored to electrocorticography and functional mapping

George A. Ojemann

Approaches to resective surgery for medically intractable temporal lobe epilepsy are guided by two rather divergent philosophies of temporal lobe organization and its pathophysiology. The approaches that utilize standard

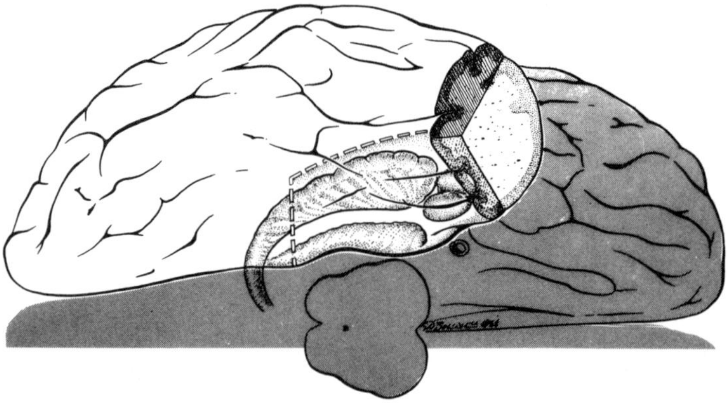

FIGURE 6.32 Basal view showing the relationship of the posterior hippocampal incision to the midbrain. Note that only a small portion of the curving hippocampal formation is not included in the *en block* resection. The remaining medial hippocampus can be easily aspirated if there is strong evidence for posterior hippocampal epileptogenesis.

temporal lobectomies, and the variations that reduce lateral and extend medial resection, are all guided by the view that temporal lobe organization and temporal lobe epilepsy are rather uniform from one patient to the next, and the surgical treatment can be guided by standard anatomy. In the approach described here, temporal lobe organization and temporal lobe epilepsy are considered to vary considerably between patients, so that the surgery must be tailored to mapping of the pathophysiology and eloquent areas in that individual. Rather surprisingly, the extent of variability in the epileptogenic zone in patients with temporal lobe epilepsy is not clear. However, some evidence suggests considerable variability. Epileptiform events in the electrocorticogram (ECoG) were confined to lateral cortex in 46% of 100 cases of temporal lobe epilepsy seizure-free after ECoG-guided resections, while in 28% epileptiform abnormalities were confined to medial structures, and in the remaining 27% were recorded from both [38]. Moreover, temporal resections removing only lateral cortex are reported to be nearly as effective at achieving seizure control as resections confined to medial structures [39,40]. One explanation for this puzzling finding is that cases selected for the different resections represent part of the variability of temporal lobe epilepsy pathophysiology. Indeed, all approaches to the resective surgery of epilepsy individually tailor the extent of the resection for epileptogenic zones outside of temporal lobe; it is only in temporal lobe that some consider the process so uniform that anatomically standardized resections are appropriate.

There is even more evidence for variation in the location of eloquent cortex in temporal lobe. Some degree of individual variation in lateralization and intrahemispheric localization of language is evident in nearly all studies where this has been investigated [41]. Some of those studies suggest that language representation in temporal lobe may occasionally extend into areas traditionally considered "safe" on anatomic criteria [41]. The role of an individual temporal lobe in sustaining recent memory also varies considerably between patients, to the extent that this function is individually evaluated in all approaches to temporal lobe resective surgery.

The different philosophies of temporal lobe organization and pathophysiology affect the approach to preoperative evaluation, as well as the type of resection. In general, the more the resection is tailored to individual localization of epileptogenic zones and eloquent areas, the less extensive the preoperative evaluation. Often this is a matter of when the information is to be obtained, preoperatively or intraoperatively, but it also reflects the greater flexibility of tailored resections. A tailored resection can be easily altered to encompass more extensive neocortical involvement of the epileptogenic zone if that is demonstrated intraoperatively, while an anatomically standard operation requires that the extent of the epileptogenic zone should be fully defined preoperatively, with that zone within the confines of the standard resection. Thus the preoperative evaluation for tailored temporal resections is largely focused on issues of lateralization of the epileptogenic zone and eloquent areas, with the detailed intrahemispheric localization determined intraoperatively. This becomes important in considering the risks and costs of the preoperative evaluation. For many patients, the preoperative evaluation for a tailored resection involves only one invasive procedure, the Sodium Amytal test [42,43]; in some patients the epileptogenic zone may be adequately identified by the location of scalp-EEG recorded interictal discharges supplemented by neuropsychologic assessment [44], obtained on an outpatient basis. Indeed this may be adequate identification of a focus even in the absence of lesions on imaging studies. The investment of health care resources, and the risks to a patient of such an evaluation are much less than a preoperative evaluation that requires intracranial recording of ictal events. As discussed elsewhere, all methods of preoperative identification of the epileptogenic zone depend on a congruence of findings from the clinical ictal features, EEG, imaging studies and neuropsychologic assessment.

The information needed to tailor a resection to the extent of the epileptogenic zone and eloquent areas may be obtained by two different methods. One method uses chronically implanted grids of electrodes placed subdurally or more rarely epidurally [45, 46]. The other method obtains this information intraoperatively. Both methods use EEG findings to identify the epileptogenic zone, and electrical stimulation mapping to delineate eloquent areas. Use of chronic grids allows identification of the epileptogenic zone by recording of ictal as well as interictal events, and allows more time for assessment of location of eloquent areas. Chronic grids are the only option for obtaining the information to plan a tailored resection in some situations, where ictal recordings are needed to identify the epileptogenic zone from multiple interictal foci, or where language cortex must be identified in a patient, such as a child, who cannot tolerate a craniotomy under local anesthesia. However, use of these grids requires a second craniotomy, carries a higher risk of infection, probably provides somewhat less detailed localization of eloquent areas than intraoperative direct cortical stimulation, and requires a substantially larger investment of health care resources than does intraoperative recording and stimulation. Reported outcomes with the two approaches have been similar. Thus for patients who could be managed with either method there seems little to justify the extra risks and costs of chronic grids. The remainder of this chapter discusses intraoperative approaches to tailored temporal lobe resections.

Intraoperative identification of the epileptogenic zone

Interictal epileptiform discharges on the ECoG are used to identify the extent of the epileptogenic zone intraoperatively. This is the classical technique of temporal lobe resection for epilepsy devised by Penfield and Jasper [47]. The essential issue in the use of this technique is how accurately interictal ECoG epileptic discharges can identify tissue that must be removed to control seizures. Scalp interictal discharges are relatively accurate in identifying the side and lobe where resection is likely to control seizures; indeed they are considerably more accurate than scalp-recorded ictal onsets [44,48]. In the chronic animal model of spontaneous epilepsy produced by injecting alumina cream in monkey sensory-motor cortex, excision of the area identified by interictal spikes controls seizures, although excision of only the local pathologic abnormality does not [49]. Moreover, there is the extensive experience from the Montreal Neurological Institute in achieving seizure control with temporal resections guided by excision of tissue identified as epileptic by interictal spikes [38]. In that experience, patients with the more complete removals of interictal epileptiform abnormalities were more likely to ultimately be seizure-free than those with residual discharges after resection [38,50], although the relation between residual spikes on ECoG and ultimate outcome was by no means complete. Moreover, the degree of seizure control achieved with ECoG-guided resections is about the same as that achieved with anatomically standard temporal resections, although the cases selected for surgical therapy by the different techniques are probably not identical. In addition, discrepancies have been identified between side of ictal onset in depth recordings and lateralization of interictal discharges [51]. However, the response to this discrepancy has been either not to proceed with operation, or to operate on the side of ictal onset, so that whether a resection guided by the localization of interictal discharges would have controlled seizures is unknown.

There are a number of different techniques for recording the ECoG intraoperatively. The author's approach, based on Penfield and Jasper [47], has been to obtain these recordings under local anesthesia, if possible. Patients are usually on therapeutic levels of their antiepileptic drugs at the time of operation. Local anesthesia uses a scalp field block of 0.5% lidocaine and 0.25% marcaine, supplemented immediately preoperatively by 0.5–1 cc of Innovar neuroleptanalgesia. Dural anesthesia is induced by injecting a few tenths of a cubic centimetre of the local anesthetic on each side of the middle meningeal artery. The ECoG is recorded from the lateral temporal surface with carbon electrodes, and from the basal and medial surfaces with subdural strip electrodes. Several of these are usually placed, to ascertain the anterior–posterior extent of the medial–basal interictal discharges. Discharges are commonly encountered from basal cortex, both medially and laterally. Subdural electrodes are also often placed over orbital frontal cortex, although these rarely demonstrate discharges. The goal of these recordings is to plan a lateral temporal resection that removes all of the cortex demonstrating interictal discharges, though sparing any eloquent areas identified by functional mapping. After the lateral resection is completed, the temporal horn of the lateral ventricle is opened, and corticography repeated with electrodes on the *surface* of hippocampus, as well as on amygdala and a subdural strip along the PHG. Location of interictal discharges on these recordings are used to plan the medial extent of the resection. This resection is also designed to include any gross pathology, and, based on a retrospective study of the extent of medial resection and degree of seizure control [52], to extend posteriorly to the level of the anterior 1–1.5 cm of pes hippocampus, PHG, and uncus.

Electrocorticography is then repeated, following completion of the initial medial and lateral resections. The appropriate response to interictal discharges on these recordings, especially discharges in new locations, is controversial. Interictal discharges may appear on the margin of the resection in locations where they were absent in the initial recordings — the "activation by partial excision" described by Penfield and Jasper [47]. Those authors recommended further extending the resection to include these "new" spikes, unless limited by the location of eloquent areas. Support for this view is provided by the observation that recurrence of seizures after temporal lobectomy is most often a consequence of "persisting epileptiform abnormalities in areas adjacent to the main excision" [53]. On the other hand, spikes in some locations on the postresection ECoG can be safely ignored. These include discharges from insular cortex [54]. The author's observations suggest that residual discharges in posterior PHG also do not correlate with an adverse outcome, and thus are not an indication for extending the medial resection beyond the line of 1–1.5 cm of the anterior hippocampus. Occasionally interictal epileptiform discharges will be recorded from eloquent cortex based on functional mapping. Usually these areas will not be resected. Up to one-third of patients with good surgical outcomes have some residual interictal discharges on postresection corticography [50], thus trading a functional deficit for complete resection of interictal discharges is usually not worthwhile.

The subpial suction technique is commonly used for tailored resections. The edges of the removal are planned to follow sulci, or, where major gyri must be crossed, the thin crossing sulci usually present. Planning of the resection includes preservation of the blood supply to the remaining gyral bank, and of major arterial vessels providing distal supply to remaining cortex. On the other hand, draining veins from temporal lobe, including the lateral branch of the vein of Labbe, need not be preserved. An intact layer of pia-arachnoid is also maintained medially after resection of the commonly herniated and gliotic uncus, to reduce the risk to the third nerve and the carotid artery and its branches. The ultrasonic aspirator greatly facilitates this subpial resection, especially of firm, gliotic tissue. However, block specimens, for example of anterior hippocampus, can also be taken when they are of value for special studies (with the relation of this tissue to the epileptic process established from corticography). In general, resections tailored to the location of interictal epileptiform discharges have more extensive removals of basal temporal cortex, including inferior temporal and fusiform gyri, than anatomically standard resections. In a recent study of the relation of outcome to the extent of resection as determined from postoperative MRI scans, larger basal and medial removals correlated with more favorable results [55].

Although the author has preferred the spontaneously active ECoG recorded under local anesthesia as the basis for planning a temporal resection, others have used the ECoG recorded under different conditions, including general anesthesia, and with activation by short-acting barbituates [56,57]. When general anesthesia is used during ECoG recording, the patient is frequently paralyzed and the anesthesia lightened considerably for a brief period. Nitrous oxide seems to be more likely to suppress epileptiform events than halogenated anesthetics [58]. In general, little difference in outcome has been reported with resections guided by ECoG recorded under local or general anesthesia [59]. However, there are now relatively few situations where recording under general anesthesia is the only available option, since the use of chronic subdural grids provides a technique for obtaining recordings under awake conditions in patients such as children who cannot tolerate a craniotomy under local anesthesia. Grids also allow for functional mapping.

In the author's experience, nearly all patients have interictal epileptiform discharges at the time of craniotomy, although in some cases they may be confined to medial temporal structures, and thus present only on subdural strip electrodes. This experience is in a setting where antiepileptic drug levels are maintained at therapeutic levels during the operation. However, when discharges are not present, a technique of activation of the ECoG by rapid intravenous injection of 1 mg/kg of methohexital (Brevitol) has been described [57]. During peak activation epileptic discharges will often be present widely in cortex that does not need to be resected; however, the more restricted areas where epileptiform events first appear or linger may indicate the epileptogenic zone. No systematic study comparing results of resections guided by ECoG recorded with Brevitol activation with resections based on the spontaneous ECoG is available. The author has found the after-discharge threshold to cortical electrical stimulation of little value in identifying the epileptogenic zone, although this technique has been reported to be useful in identifying that zone when using multiple intracranial depth electrodes [60].

Intraoperative identification of eloquent areas

Rolandic cortex

Electrical stimulation mapping is used to identify eloquent areas intraoperatively. Application of a current to the cortical surface has both excitatory and inhibitory effects, on both neurons and *en passage* fibers [61]. In a temporal exposure, the only excitatory effects of cortical stimulation that are likely to be encountered are motor and sensory responses from the foot of Rolandic cortex. These often can be evoked at quite small currents under local anesthesia. The author is usually able to evoke tongue and face sensation and movement with stimulation at 2 mA between peaks of biphasic square wave pulses, 1–1.25 ms duration per phase, delivered at 60 Hz through 1 mm bipolar electrodes separated by 5 mm. Throat responses are more variable. Although tongue and face responses are reliably evoked, the more inferior of these responses may be several centimetres above the Sylvian fissure. The anterior–posterior extent of motor and sensory responses is rarely much more than 1 cm with direct cortical stimulation. Motor responses can be evoked under general anesthesia also, though usually at larger currents and without the detail evident with stimulation under local anesthesia. In addition, the inability to discern tongue movement easily under general anesthesia limits the ability to map the foot of motor cortex with its large tongue representation.

Generally, Rolandic cortex can be more conveniently identified by evoked motor responses with electrical stimulation than by recording somatosensory evoked potentials. The one exception may be very young children, who seem to have relatively inexcitable motor cortex. Identification of Rolandic cortex is essential in a temporal resection only if some suprasylvian resection is also planned. However, the author finds the location of the foot of Rolandic cortex a useful landmark in a temporal resection and routinely attempts to identify it.

Language

In the dominant hemisphere, electrical stimulation mapping is also used to identify essential areas for language. Although cortical stimulation hardly ever evokes language, at some sites outside of Rolandic cortex, stimulation will repeatedly disturb ongoing language tasks. Object naming is the language task most often used with stimulation. Stimulation is at the largest current that does not evoke after-discharges in the area of cortex to be sampled. For the author, the other stimulation parameters are the same as those used to evoke motor responses. In the majority of patients, repeated disturbance of object naming is evoked from very localized cortical areas, 1–2 cm^2 in extent, often with sharp margins. There are usually several such areas with repeated evoked anomia, often one frontally and one or more in temporoparietal cortex.

There is evidence that these sites of stimulation evoked repeated naming errors identify the cortex that must be spared to avoid postoperative language deficits. When an anterior temporal resection came within 2 cm of such a site, along a continuous gyrus, there was an increase in language errors of all types on an aphasia battery administered 1 month after the resection. The increase was statistically significantly greater than that observed after resections which had avoided stimulation identified language sites by a wider margin [62]. This difference could not be accounted for by the size of the resection, preoperative verbal abilities, or the degree of postoperative seizure control. The exact location of these areas is highly variable, especially in the temporal lobe. In a series of 117 patients, all with left hemisphere language shown by the Sodium Amytal test, 15% had no identifiable temporal–parietal language sites [41]. Only 65% had language sites anywhere in superior temporal gyrus, with marked variation in the location along that gyrus. Fifteen percent had superior temporal gyrus language sites in front of Rolandic cortex, while 5% had such sites in anterior middle temporal gyrus. Frontal language sites were almost as variable; in 21% no language changes were evoked from posterior–inferior frontal gyrus, the classical Broca area, while some patients had language sites in inferior frontal gyrus as far forward as the pterion.

This combination of discrete localization of essential areas for language in an individual patient, but considerable variation in their location across the patient population, is an indication for individually mapping language in dominant hemisphere temporal resections. No anatomic landmark, whether measurement from the temporal tip, location of Rolandic cortex or the vein of Labbe provides a reliable guide to the location of language. Damage to essential language areas which are unusually far forward in temporal lobe is probably the explanation for aphasias after standard resections [63]. On the other hand, the variability in language localization is such that dominant hemisphere posterior temporal cortex can sometimes be safely resected. Sites of repeated evoked errors in object naming usually provide an adequate indication of the essential areas for all language functions, providing that the resection spares them with a margin of about 2 cm along a continuous gyrus. However, sites essential for other language functions, including naming in second languages [62,64] and reading of simple sentences [62,65], are sometimes separate from those for naming in the primary language. Thus for a resection close to language areas, where there is reason to minimize the risk of any type of language deficit, mapping of other language functions may also be desirable.

The identification of sites essential for language with stimulation mapping is a relatively simple technique. Some care is necessary in selecting the stimulation current, the largest current that does not evoke an after-discharge in the ECoG in the area of cortex to be sampled with stimulation mapping. In the author's experience, this threshold is highly variable between patients, from 1.5 mA, measured between peaks of the biphasic pulses, to >10 mA, although rather uniform in an individual. Failure to determine this threshold is thus likely to lead to the use of a current that is either too weak to block local cortical function, giving false negative results, or too strong, so that a seizure may be evoked. Once the current has been selected, 10–20 cortical stimulation sites are identified by numbered tickets, to include both the resection and areas where language is likely to be located. The goal of the mapping is to indicate both where language is located, as well as where it is not. Only when the location of language is known can sites without errors be resected with maximal safety. An entirely negative mapping does not provided security that the areas are not essential for language.

The patient begins naming a series of common objects. (The author uses slide pictures of objects.) Stimulation is applied during randomly selected objects, separated by several objects named without stimulation. Sites are stimulated consecutively, with stimulation of the entire set repeated several times, so that at least three samples of stimulation effect at each site are obtained. A site is considered essential for language if there are repeated errors, that have a statistically significant difference from the error rate during naming without stimulation. Mapping of a temporal exposure usually requires about 20 minutes.

Memory

It has been suggested that verbal memory deficits after dominant temporal lobe resections represent a major limitation on the use of resective surgery for epilepsy [66]. The usual technique for avoiding this problem is to assess memory preoperatively with the Sodium Amytal test. A major deficit on this test is variously interpreted as either a contraindication to surgery, or an indication for a very limited medial resection, at least minimizing any hippocampal removal. This approach seems to avoid global recent memory deficits, but lesser degrees of recent verbal memory deficits have been reported after dominant temporal resections, whether they were standard resections with exclusion of cases with memory deficits by the Sodium Amytal test [67] or when the medial extent of the resection was modified based on memory deficits on the Sodium Amytal test [68,69].

Stimulation of some sites on dominant hemisphere cortical surface disturbs recent verbal memory [62,70,71] independently of an effect on language [62,70,71]. When the memory measure separated the effects of stimulation during entry of information into memory, from that during the time the memory was stored or when it was retrieved, stimulation of temporoparietal sites was particularly likely to disturb memory when the current was applied during input or storage, but not retrieval [62,68,69,71]. Ojemann and Dodrill [68,69] found that patients with postoperative verbal memory deficits after a dominant hemisphere temporal resection had better preoperative memories, and larger lateral than medial resection than patients without memory deficits. In patients with deficits, those lateral resections were likely to have encroached on a site that had been identified as essential for the input or storage phase of memory by stimulation mapping. Those authors reported two cases where the preoperative Sodium Amytal test suggested that memory was entirely dependent on the dominant hemisphere, but a temporal resection there tailored to avoid lateral cortical sites essential for both language and memory input and storage, as well as minimizing hippocampal removal medially, was associated with no postoperative worsening of verbal memory.

These findings suggest that when the preoperative evaluation suggests that a memory problem may occur with a temporal resection, that deficit may be partly minimized by tailoring the resection to avoid lateral cortical sites identified as essential for memory input or storage by stimulation mapping. The technical details of memory mapping have been discussed elsewhere [68]. Mapping of memory is quite time-consuming, both because of the number of stimulation conditions — sites and input, storage or output memory phases — and also because patients commonly make some memory errors in the absence of stimulation, so that multiple samples of each stimulation condition are needed to establish a statistically significant stimulation effect. As a result usually only three to six sites can be sampled, and memory mapping is restricted to those patients considered to be at risk for verbal memory problems; i.e. left temporal lobectomies in patients with *good* preoperative verbal memories, and those with major memory concerns related to the left hemisphere on the preoperative Sodium Amytal test.

References

1 Gelman S , Newman SW. *Manter and Gate's Essentials of Clinical Neuroanatomy and Neurophysiology.* F.A. Davies, Philadelphia 1987.

2 Nieuwenhuys R, Voogd J, Huijzen C. *The Human Central Nervous System,* 2nd edn. Springer-Verlag, New York, 1981.

3 Carpenter MB, Sutin J. *Human Neuroanatomy,* 8th edn. Williams & Wilkins, Baltimore, 1983.

4 Williams PL, Warwick R. *Gray's Anatomy,* 36th British edn. Churchill Livingstone, New York, 1980.

5 Naidich TP, Daniels DL, Haughton VM, Williams A, Pojunas K, Palacios E. The hippocampal formation and related structures of the limbic lobe: anatomic — MR correlation. I. Surface features and coronal sections. *Radiology* 1987; **162**: 747–754.

6 Naidich TP, Daniels DL, Haughton VM, Pech P, Williams A, Pojunas K, Palacios E. Hippocampal formation and related structures of the limbic lobe: anatomic — MR correlation. II. Sagittal sections. *Radiology* 1987; **162**: 755–761.

7 Lorente de No' R. Studies of the structure of the cerebral cortex. II. *J. Psychol Neurol* 1934; **46**: 113–177.

8 Rose M. Allo cortex bei Tier und Mensch die sog Riechrinde beim Menschen und beim Affen. *J Psychol Neurol, Lpz* 1927; **34**: 261–401.

9 Mettler FA. *Neuroanatomy.* CV Mosby, Baltimore, 1948.

10 Triulzi F, Franceschi M, Ferruccio F, Del Maschio A. Nonrefractory temporal lobe epilepsy: 1. 5-T MR imaging. *Radiology* 1988; **166**: 181–185.

11 Quencer RM, Atlas SW, Batnitzky S, et al. Advances in Neuroradiology. *Am J Neuroradiology* 1989; **10**: 851–866.

12 Kilgore DP, Breger RK, Daniels DL, Pojunas KW, Williams AL, Haughton VM. Cranial tissues: normal MR appearances after intravenous injection of GD-DTPA. *Radiology* 1986; **160**: 757–761.

13 Atlas SW, Zimmerman RA, Bilaniuk LT, Rorke L, Hackney DB, Goldberg HI, Grossman RI. Corpus callosum and limbic system: neuroanatomic MR evaluation of developmental anomalies. *Radiology* 1986; **160**: 355–362.

14 Falconer M, Hill D, Pampliglione G. Discussion on the surgery of temporal lobe epilepsy. *Proc Roy Soc Med* 1953; **46**: 965–976.

15 Falconer MA, Hill D, Meyer A, Mitchell W, Pond DA. Treatment of temporal lobe epilepsy by temporal lobectomy — a survey of findings and results. *Lancet* 1955; **1**: 827–835.

16 Penfield W, Flanigin H. Surgical therapy of

temporal lobe seizures. *Arch Neurol Psychiatr* 1950; **64**: 491–500.
17 Penfield W, Baldwin M. Temporal lobe seizures and the technique of subtotal temporal lobectomy. *Ann Surg* 1952; **136**: 625–634.
18 Gibbs EL, Gibbs FA, Fuster B. Psychomotor epilepsy. *Arch Neurol Psychiatr* **60**: 331–339, 1948.
19 Bailey P, Gibbs FA. The surgical treatment of psychomotor epilepsy. *JAMA* 1951; **145**: 365–370.
20 Falconer, M.A. (1967) Anterior temporal lobectomy for epilepsy. In Rob C, Smith R (eds) *Operative Surgery*, 2nd edn., Vol. 14. Butterworth, London, 1967, pp 142–149.
21 Rhoton AL, Kiyotaka F, Fradd B. Microsurgical anatomy of the anterior choroidal artery. *Surg Neurol* 1979; **12**: 171–187.
22 Wieser HG. *Electroclinical Features of the Psychomotor Seizure.* Butterworth, London, 1983, p 242.
23 Spencer SS, Williamson PD, Spencer DD, Mattson RH. Human hippocampal seizure spread studied by depth and subdural recording: the hippocampal commissure. *Epilepsia* 1987; **28**: 479–489.
24 Engel J, Jr Brown WJ, Kuhl DE, Phelps ME, Mazziotta JC, Crandall PH. Pathological findings underlying focal temporal lobe hypometabolism in partial epilepsy. *Ann Neurol* 1982; **12**: 518–528.
25 Armstrong DD, Bruton CJ. Postscript: What terminology is appropriate for tissue pathology? How does it predict outcome? In Engel J Jr (ed) *Surgical Treatment of the Epilepsies.* Raven Press, New York, 1987, pp 541–552.
26 Babb TL, Brown WJ, Pretorius J, Davenport C, Lieb JP, Crandall PH. Temporal lobe volumetric densities in temporal lobe epilepsy. *Epilepsia* 1984; **25**: 729–740.
27 Dam MA. Hippocampal neuron loss in epilepsy and after experimental seizures. *Acta Neurol Scand* 1982; **66**: 601–542.
28 Spencer DD, Spencer SS, Mattson RH, Williamson PD, Novelly RA. Access to the posterior medial temporal lobe structures in the surgical treatment of temporal lobe epilepsy. *Neurosurgery* 1984; **15**: 667–671.
29 Spencer DD, Spencer SS. Mattson RH, Williamson PD. Intracerebral masses in patients with intractable partial epilepsy. *Neurology* 1984; **34**: 432–436.
30 Babb TL, Wilson CL, Crandall PH. Asymmetry and ventral course of the human geniculostriate pathway as determined by hippocampal visual evoked potentials and subsequent visual field defects after temporal lobectomy. *Exper Brain Res* 1982; **47**: 317–328.
31 Falconer MA, Wilson JL. Visual field changes following anterior temporal lobectomy: their significance in relation to "Meyer's loop" of the optic radiation. *Brain* 1958; **81**: 1–14.
32 Bouchet, Cazauvieilh. De l'épilepsie considérée dans ses rapports avec l'alienation mentale. Recherché sur la nature et le siège de ces deux maladies; memoire qui a remporte le prix au concours établi par M. Esquirol. *Arch Gen Med* 1825; **9**: 510–542.
33 Meynert T. Studien über das pathologisch-anatomische Material der Wiener Irren-Anstalt. *Vierteljahrssch Psychiatr* 1867; **3**: 381–402.
34 Pfleger L. Beobachtungen über Schrumpfung und Sklerose des Ammonshorns bei Epilepsie. *Allgemeine Z Psychiatr* 1880; **36**: 359–365.
35 Stauder KH. Epilepsie und Schlafenlappen *Arch Psychiatr Nervenkr* 1936; **104**: 181–211.
36 Penfield W, Erickson TC. *Epilepsy and Cerebral Localization.* CC Thomas, Springfield, Illinois, 1941.
37 Penfield W, Paine K. Results of surgical therapy for focal epileptic seizures. *Can Med Assoc J* 1955; **73**: 515–531.
38 Rasmussen T. Localizational aspects of epileptic seizure phenomena. In Thompson R, Green J (eds) *New Perspectives in Cerebral Localization.* Raven Press, New York, 1982, pp 177–203.
39 Hardiman O, Coughlan A, O'Moore B, Phillips J, Stanton H. Interictal spike localization with methohexitone; preoperative activation and surgical followup. *Epilepsia* 1987; **28**: 335–339.
40 Yasargil M, Weiser H. Selective amygdalohippocampectomy at the University Hospital, Zurich. In Engel J, Jr (ed) *Surgical Treatment of the Epilepsies.* Raven Press, New York, 1987, pp 653–658.
41 Ojemann G, Ojemann J, Lettich E, Berger M. Cortical language localization in left, dominant hemisphere: an electrical stimulation mapping investigation in 117 patients. *J Neurosurg* 1988; **71**: 316–326.
42 Wada J, Rasmussen T. Intracarotid injection of Sodium Amytal for the lateralization of cerebral speech dominance: experimental and cli-

nical observations. *J Neurosurg* 1960; **17**: 266–282.
43 Woods R, Dodrill C, Ojemann G. Brain injury, handedness and speech lateralization in a series of amobarbital studies. *Ann Neurol* 1988; **23**: 510–518.
44 Dodrill C, Wilkus R, Ojemann G, Ward A, Jr, Wyler A, van Belle G, Tamas L. Multidisciplinary prediction of seizure relief from cortical resection surgery. *Ann Neurol* 1986; **20**: 2–12.
45 Lüders H, Lessr R, Dinner D, Morris H, Hahn J. Friedman L, Skipper G, Wyllie E, Friedman D. Commentary: chronic intracranial recording and stimulation with subdural electrodes. In Engel J, Jr (ed) *Surgical Treatment of the Epilepsies.* Raven Press, New York, 1987, pp 297–322.
46 Goldring, S. Epilepsy surgery. *Clin Neurosurg* 1984; **31**: 369–388.
47 Penfield W, Jasper H. *Epilepsy and the Functional Anatomy of the Human Brain.* Little, Brown, Boston, 1954.
48 Engel J Jr, Crandall PH. Intensive neurodiagnostic monitoring with intracranial electrodes. In Gumnit R (ed) *Intensive Neurodiagnostic Monitoring.* Raven Press, New York, 1986.
49 Harris A, Lockard J. Absence of seizures of mirror foci in experimental epilepsy after excision of alumina and astrogliotic scar. *Epilepsia* 1981; **22**: 107–122.
50 Bengzon A, Rasmussen T, Gloor P, Dassault J, Stephens M. Prognostic factors in the surgical treatment of temporal lobe epileptics. *Neurology* 1968; **18**: 717–731.
51 Bouvier G, Mercier C, St. Hillaire J *et al.* Anterior callosotomy and chronic depth electrode recording in the surgical management of some intractable seizures. *Appl. Neurophysiol.* 1983; **46**: 52–56.
52 Ojemann L, Ojemann G, Baugh-Bookman C. What is the optimal extent of the medical resection in anterior temporal lobe epilepsy? *Epilepsia* 1986; **27**: 636.
53 Ajmone-Marsan C. Depth electrography and electrocorticography. In Aminoff M (ed) *Electrodiagnosis in Clinical Neurology.* Churchill-Livingstone, New York, 1980, pp 167–196.
54 Rasmussen T. Surgical treatment of patients with complex partial seizures. *Adv Neurol* 1975; **11**: 415–449.
55 Awad I, Katz A, Hahn J, Kong A, Ahl J, Lüders H. Extent of resection in temporal lobectomy for epilepsy. *Epilepsia* 1989; **30**: 756–762.
56 Walker A. Temporal lobectomy. *J Neurosurg* 1967; **26**: 641–649.
57 Sypert G. New concepts in the management of epilepsy: medical and surgical. *Clin Neurosurg* 1977; **24**: 600–641.
58 Artru A, Colley P, Ojemann G. Nitrous oxide: suppression of focal epileptiform activity during inhalation and suppression of seizure activity following withdrawal. *J Neurosurg Anesthesiol* 1990; in press.
59 Herman B, Wyler A. Comparative effects of dominant temporal lobectomy under general or local anesthesia: language outcome. *Epilepsia* 1988; **29**: 668.
60 Bernier G, St. Hilaire J-M, Giard N, Bouvier G, Mercier M. Commentary: intracranial electrical stimulation. In Engel J, Jr (ed) *Surgical Treatment of the Epilepsies.* Raven Press, New York, 1987, pp 323–334.
61 Ranck J, Jr. Which elements are excited in electrical stimulation of mammalian central nervous system?: a review. *Brain Res* 1975; **98**: 417–440.
62 Ojemann G. Brain organization for language from the perspective of electrical stimulation mapping. *Behav Brain Sci* 1983; **6**: 189–230.
63 Heilman K, Wilder B, Malzone W. Anomic aphasia following anterior temporal lobecotomy. *Trans Amer Neurol Assoc* 1972; **97**: 291–293.
64 Ojemann G, Whitaker H. The bilingual brain. *Arch Neurol* 1978; **35**: 409–412.
65 Ojemann G. Some brain mechanisms for reading. In von Euler C, Lundberg I, Lennerstrand G (ed) *Brain and Reading.* Macmillan, London, 1988, pp 47–60.
66 Delgado-Escueta A, Treiman D, Walsh G. The treatable epilepsies. Part II. *New Eng J Med* 1983; **308**: 1576–1584.
67 Rausch R and Crandall P. Psychological status related to surgical control of temporal lobe seizures. *Epilepsia* 1983; **23**: 191–202.
68 Ojemann G, Dodrill C. Verbal memory deficits after left temporal lobectomy for epilepsy: Mechanism and intraoperative prediction. *J Neurosurg* 1985; **62**: 101–107.
69 Ojemann G, Dodrill C. Intraoperative techniques for reducing language and memory deficits with left temporal lobectomy. *Adv Epileptol* 1987; **16**: 327–330.
70 Fedio P, Van Buren J. Memory deficits during

electrical stimulation of speech cortex in conscious man. *Brain Lang* 1974; **1**: 29–42.
71 Ojemann G. Organization of short-term verbal memory in language areas of human cortex: evidence from electrical stimulation. *Brain Lang* 1978; **5**: 331–348.

Comment

Allen R. Wyler

Much of the debate surrounding how one should approach temporal lobectomy hinges around where the epileptogenic focus resides within the temporal lobe. With a well-defined lesion, the odds are that the epileptogenic focus resides in the cortex adjacent to the structural abnormality, if not in it. The problem is that our knowledge of where the epileptogenic focus is within temporal lobe in cases of nonlesional temporal lobe epilepsy is very imprecise, although abnormalities can be demonstrated in hippocampus for almost all cases. This is confounded by the knowledge that hippocampal gliosis may be due to seizures, and so gliosis cannot always be assumed to identify the location of the epileptogenic focus. Even if one assumes the hippocampus has the lowest "threshold" for producing seizures of temporal cortex, there is still a debate as to just how much needs to be removed for a satisfactory outcome.

The presently accepted methods of localizing nonlesional epileptogenic foci are: (1) bioelectrical measurements (EEG, EcoG); (2) metabolic measurements (PET scans); and (3) tests of cortical function (neuropsychologic tests). Of these (and other) methods, bioelectrical measurements are the singularly most accurate tests for identifying the cortical region of seizure onset as well as predicting seizure outcome postoperatively [1]. This is especially true if one relies on recording spontaneous seizures using invasive techniques such as depth or subdural electrodes (see Chapter 3). It is particularly important to distinguish between interictal and ictal EEG or ECoG, because both scalp and invasive interictal recordings are particularly inaccurate for localizing foci.

The reason that interictal recordings are inferior to ictal recordings is that interictal recordings primarily identify the location of epileptiform spikes, and epileptiform spikes do not always correlate with the location of the epileptogenic focus. This is because epileptiform spikes are synaptically mediated events that are often propagated and therefore can often be found at sites distant as well as contralateral to the known epileptogenic focus. In addition, epileptiform spikes occur in cortex of animals and humans who do not suffer epileptic seizures [2]. Thus their mere presence does not always indicate seizure-producing cortex. This may relate to the finding that ECoG spikes recorded acutely at the time of surgery, either before or after resection, have little prognostic value regarding eventual seizure outcome.

Taking these factors into account, we shall reexamine the rationales set forth in the preceding chapter. Both Crandall and Spencer state that the vast majority of nonlesional temporal lobe epileptogenic foci reside within mesial temporal structures. Their defence of their view is based on ictal recordings from depth electrodes. On the other hand, Ojemann suggests that temporal lobe foci are quite variable in location and often can include lateral cortex. He supports his thesis on the basis of interictal ECoG recordings done acutely during surgery. Moreover, Ojemann goes on to state that the results from resections of only lateral temporal cortex are as effective as resections involving only medial structures (selective amygdalohippocampectomy). It is unfortunate that the Coughlan series of lateral temporal resections he refers to has been published only as an abstract and the details of that surgical series are not available. The fact is, Coughlan's series is somewhat different from the experience of surgeons in other centers. For example, the experience of Olivier *et al.* [3] suggests the most common cause for failed temporal lobe surgery is inadequate hippocampal resection. Our experience with over 150 cases of temporal lobectomy supports the finding that almost all cases of lateral temporal lobe foci are associated with a structural lesion whereas 95% of nonlesional temporal lobe foci were found to reside in mesial temporal lobe structures and were identified by long-term subdural strip electrode ictal monitoring.

Ojemann is right to point out that speech cortex may involve more anterior superior temporal gyrus than is often suspected based on classical lesional studies. Therefore one is advised to "map" cortical function in cases that involve structural lesions suspected of residing near eloquent cortex. This functional mapping may be done using the techniques Ojemann described, or it can also be accomplished with a large grid of subdural electrodes. However, most cases of nonlesional temporal lobe epilepsy involving either dominant or nondominant temporal lobe can be operated on under general anesthetic using Spencer's approach with excellent seizure and language outcome. Ojemann is probably right in suggesting that the majority of cases will do well with resecting no more than 1.5 cm of hippocampus. Spencer is also right in saying that many patients have posterior hippocampal foci that will continue to cause some seizures (if not complete failure of surgery) if the hippocampus is not resected to a level posterior to the cerebral peduncle. Without evaluating every patient with depth electrodes using the posterior approach that Spencer uses, it is impossible to determine if a patient needs a "radical hippocampectomy." However, from the Zurich experience [4], it would seem that there is little additional morbidity from a complete hippocampectomy. Therefore, we have adopted Spencer's approach to all routine temporal lobectomies and have had excellent results.

References

1 Engel J, Rausch R, Lieb JP, Kuhl DE, Crandall PH. Correlation of criteria used for localizing epileptic foci in patients considered for surgical therapy of epilepsy. *Ann Neurol* 1981; **9**: 215–224.

2 Chatrian GE. Paroxysmal patterns in "normal" subjects. In: Rimond A (ed-in-chief) *Handbook of Electroencephalography and Clinical Neurophysiology*. Elsevier, Amsterdam, Vol. 6A, 1976, pp 114–123.

3 Olivier A, Tanaka T, Andermann F. Reoperations in temporal lobe epilepsy. Am. Epilepsy Soc. Proceedings, 1988 meeting. *Epilepsia* 1988; **29**: 678.

4 Yasargil M, Weiser HG. Selective amygdalohippocampectomy at the University Hospital, Zurich. In Engel J, Jr (ed) *Surgical Treatment of the Epilepsies*. Raven Press, New York, 1987, pp 653–658.

chapter 7

Extratemporal Resections in the Surgical Treatment of Epilepsy

André Olivier

Introduction

Surgery of epilepsy is equated too often with surgery of temporal lobe epilepsy. Indeed, surgical series show that the temporal lobe is by far the most frequent site of surgery for intractable epilepsy. Thus, in the author's series of 525 patients as of March 1987, operations on the temporal lobe represented 74%, while frontal resections represented 11%, central 1.3%, parietal 0.9%, and occipital 0.8%. Multilobe resections (often the equivalent of subtotal hemispherectomies) amounted to 2.5% and callosotomies represented 9.5%. In the experience of the Montreal Neurological Institute, ranging from 1929 to 1980, the resections in 2177 patients were temporal in 56%, frontal in 18%, central in 7%, parietal in 6%, occipital in 1%, and multilobar in 11%.

These differences no doubt reflect the variation in the epileptic threshold of various brain areas. They may, however, reflect two additional factors which must be considered: the difficulty in assessing properly the exact site of origin of seizures outside of the temporal lobe, and the reluctance of the surgeon to venture into some of these often more eloquent or more dangerous extratemporal zones. As stated by Rasmussen [1,2], epileptogenic lesions outside of the temporal lobe are considerably more varied in extent and geographic configuration than the more common temporal lobe epileptogenic lesions.

There is thus an enormous challenge in tackling the extratemporal epilepsies. Nowhere else than in those extratemporal zones are the Rasmussen's triad of localization questions more difficult to answer: (1) where does the seizure start? (2) How much volume must be involved for the seizure to manifest itself? (3) How much tissue should the neurosurgeon remove in order to obtain a good result? The approach consists essentially of identifying as accurately as possible the epileptogenic area and in determining what the optimal cortical removal should be. This paper will deal with these two fundamental problems of extratemporal epilepsy surgery; namely, difficulty of localization and difficulty in resection. They will be covered respectively under the headings "Strategies and techniques of intracranial recording" and "Techniques of cortical resections."

Brain mapping with digital angiography and magnetic resonance imaging

Over the years, methods for determining an epileptogenic focus by intracranial recording and determining the area to be resected have become intimately related and dependent on a comprehensive anatomic approach to pre- and perioperative brain mapping. Frequent referrals to this approach will occur in the descriptions of intracranial recording and actual resection of various extratemporal cortical areas. For this reason it will be described first.

Preoperative anatomic planning

Modern imaging with magnetic resonance imaging (MRI) and digital angiography (DSA) has further defined another modality of presurgical evaluation — the preoperative anatomic planning. This planning is done prior to every surgical procedure for epilepsy, either stereotactic or by craniotomy or following insertion of intracranial strips and grids. It entails the performance of DSA and MRI to obtain a comprehensive appraisal of the patient's cortical topography. Angiography is done, not so much with the idea of detecting a vascular anomaly, but more with the intention of determining the vascular and sulcal anatomy for each individual patient [2]. In order to benefit from this approach, it is essential to master the technique of stereoscopic angiography. Those who cannot do stereoscopy will soon benefit from computerized tridimensional reconstruction of the angiogram. It is now possible to exactly superimpose the optimal arterial and venous phases of the angiogram with digital subtraction angiography. The end result is stereoscopic arterial venous angiography which becomes an important surgical tool in establishing the position of the various sulci. We feel that the risks of angiography are amply compensated by the safety and precision afforded during the craniotomy. When studying the vascular anatomy in contemplation of performing cortical resection, two aspects are considered: (1) the utilization of arteries and veins to visualize the sulcal and gyral topography; and (2) the recognition of crucial venous or arterial territories. The indirect anatomy provided by DSA is then integrated with the direct cerebral anatomy provided by MRI with reference to common landmarks, usually the corpus callosum.

The callosal reference system (Fig. 7.1)

The corpus callosum can be used to establish a system of anatomic planes which are useful to define precisely the location of gyri and sulci and particularly that of the central sulcus and its related convolutions — the pre- and postcentral gyri. A series of lines or planes is first established (Fig. 7.1). The horizontal plane (HP) is represented by a line passing by the inferior border of the splenium and genu of the corpus callosum. This line or plane extends from the occipital to the frontal pole and corresponds to the length of the brain. Three vertical or coronal planes are then established, perpendicular to HP. The anterior callosal (AC) plane passes the anterior border of the genu, and the posterior callosal (PC) plane passes the posterior border of the splenium. A midcallosal (MC) plane, also perpendicular to HP, is drawn at middistance between AC and PC. The MC plane has a close and constant relationship with the central operculum, defined as the continuation of the precen-

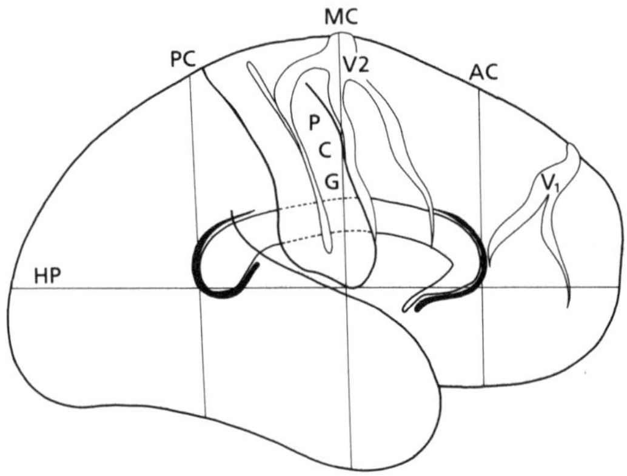

FIGURE 7.1 Diagram to illustrate the callosal reference system. Note position of precentral gyrus in relation to the midcallosal (MC) plane. The black lines around the genu and the splenium of corpus callosum represent the pericallosal artery and the internal cerebral vein, respectively. HP, horizontal plane; AC, anterior callosal plane; PC, posterior callosal plane; MC, midcallosal plane; PCG, precentral gyrus; V1 & V2, veins.

tral gyrus into the postcentral gyrus under the lower end of the central sulcus. Superiorly, the MC plane is related to the precentral sulcus. Secondary planes in coronal and transverse projections can also be established. This callosal grid can be constructed on a lateral angiogram, on the sagittal view of MRI, and on a combination of both. It can be used to identify pertinent vascular or cerebral structures for the placement of depth electrodes and for the identification of the exact position of recording sites when intracranial strips and grids are used. Finally, it is very useful for the identification of sulci and gyri at the time of cortical removal (Fig. 7.2)

Sulcal and gyral anatomy: identification of the central sulcus and central area

Arteries have a tendency to wrap gyri by running on top of them and following them into the depth of sulci. Large venous trunks have a more capricious course in relation to sulci and gyri. The smaller venous afferents to these larger trunks, however, have a definite lamellar disposition within the sulci. By using stereoscopy or tridimensional angiographic reconstruction, a striking representation of most of the principal sulci is obtained.

Whether an extratemporal resection is planned in the frontal, central, or parietal area, the most important step is the identification of the central area. This can be done by topographic or electrophysiologic means, or by both. Identification of the central areas means localization of the central sulcus. Once the central sulcus is identified, it is usually easy to locate the position of the pre- and postcentral gyri. The identification of the inferior frontal sulcus gives the position of the third and second frontal gyri. The positioning of the intraparietal sulcus gives the exact position of the superior and inferior parietal lobules. On the mesial surface, the pericallosal sulci help to divide the cingulate and superior frontal gyri. The parieto-occipital and calcarine sulci provide the position for the lingual, cuneus, and precuneus gyri. Thus the cerebrovascular anatomy can be visualized prior to surgery and at the time of surgery. Depending on the degree of confidence and on the location of the planned resection, only topographic landmarks can be used. If more crucial and func-

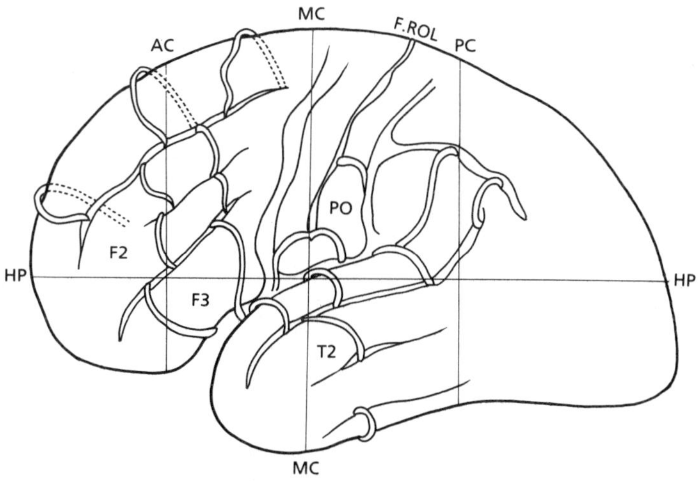

FIGURE 7.2 Diagram showing correlation between vascular, sulcul, and gyral anatomy of the brain. Note position of the callosal grid. HP, horizontal plane; MC, midcallosal plane; AC, anterior callosal plane; PC, posterior callosal plane; PO, postcentral gyrus; F.ROL: central fissure

tional data are needed, additional mapping by stimulation and evoked potentials will be required, preferably under local anesthesia. This preoperative identification of the gyri and sulci is also essential for the precise positioning of epicerebral and intracerebral electrodes in the performance of a stereoelectroencephalography (SEG) study. The technique can also be used to identify the exact gyral position of any recording or stimulating point within a subdural or epidural grid or a subdural strip, by doing a stereoscopic arteriovenous angiogram once the electrodes are in place.

Strategies and techniques of intracranial recording

Intracranial recording can be used to delineate further the area of onset and early propagation of a seizure when this is suspected but not proven by extracranial EEG. It is important to cover the volume of the suspected zone as much as possible, to place the electrodes in strategic areas, and to add specific additional electrodes when the clinical findings strongly suggest a potential focal zone.

The relative value of the various intracranial methods of recording are discussed in Chapter 3. Anyone of these can be used alone or in combination to solve specific problems. Whatever the technique used, the value of the data obtained is totally dependent on the accurate topographic identification of the recording and stimulation points.

In the author's view, the indications for intracranial recording in suspected extratemporal epilepsy are:

1 difficulty with lateralization (usually frontal);

2 determination of a lead of seizure onset in secondary generalized seizures or bilateral synchrony;

3 determination of seizure onset across the central area in the presence of parietocentro frontal discharges;

4 determination of seizure onset across the Sylvian fissure in the presence of frontotemporal discharges.

Epidural and subdural strips

Several recent studies [3,4] have confirmed the usefulness of these methods. Figure 7.3 illustrates how the localization value of strip electrodes can be enhanced by angiographic and MRI mapping. Strips are introduced at specific angles through burr holes and directed at various targets. The final and precise identification of any recording or stimulation site can be established on arteriovenous DSA and MRI (Fig. 7.3).

Intracranial grids

The techniques of subdural and epidural grids have now been used extensively and have been shown to be useful in determining sites of seizure onset over the convexity of one hemisphere [5–7]. Their role in problems of lateralization is limited by the need for bilateral craniotomies. The DSA–MRI correlation technique can be used to determine precisely the gyral and sulcal position of the recording or stimulation points (Fig. 7.4).

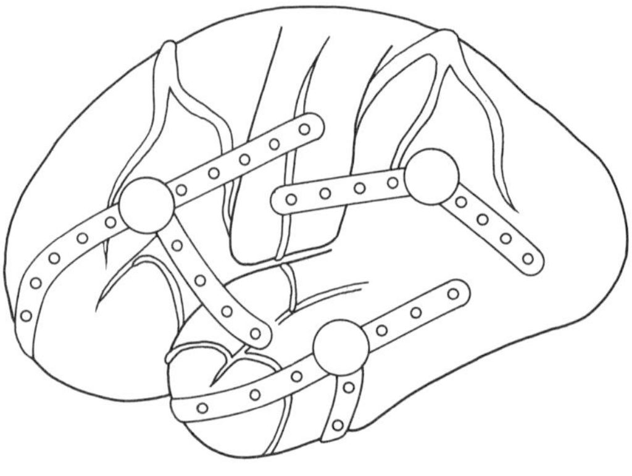

FIGURE 7.3 Subdural strip electrodes. Their exact topographic placement can be inferred by arteriovenous angiographic mapping.

Stereoelectroencephalography

Initially developed by Talairach and Bancaud [8], this technique has now been developed further at the Montreal Neurological Institute by the incorporation of the DSA–MRI stereotactic brain mapping method [9]. As illustrated in Fig. 7.5 electrodes can now be directed precisely on the surface or within a gyrus or toward any deep structure. Intermediate recording sites can also be identified in relationship to neighborhood sulci. "Depth electrodes" is a misnomer for this technique since its purpose is really to provide a tridimensional evaluation of a seizure process, which necessitates placement of electrodes in deep, intermediate, and superficial planes. As for any other intracranial investigation, a well-defined working hypothesis must be developed prior to embarking on such study. The technique can be most useful for solving problems of lateralization and further localization in frontal lobe epilepsy.

Techniques of cortical resections

Anesthesia

Local anesthesia has advantages and inconveniences. Its main disadvantages are the limitation in head fixation, the need for constant supervision by a trained anesthetic team and the time involved. These restrictions aside, local anesthesia remains a most useful technique to approach an epileptic focus in a crucial zone. Electrocorticography (ECoG), stimulation, and evoked potentials can be carried out with greater facility, and verbal, motor, and memory testing can be performed at any time during the procedure. When preoperative EEG studies have clearly demarcated the epileptogenic zone in a non-

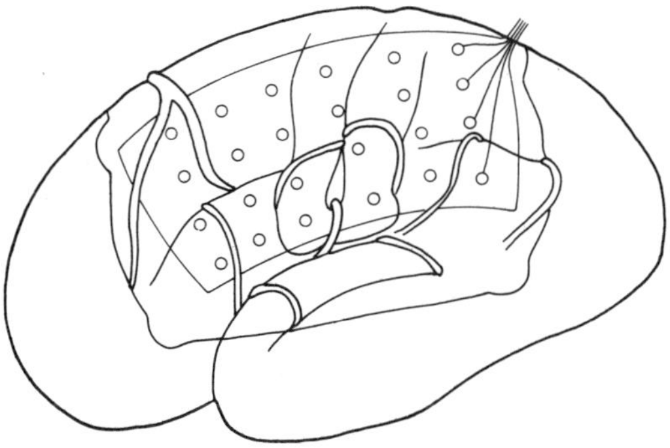

FIGURE 7.4 Epidural and subdural grids. Angiographic mapping of recording sites.

crucial area, general anesthesia can be used quite satisfactorily.

Once the brain is exposed, the study of the surface topography is always carried out whether or not the patient is asleep. Correlations between surface topography and DSA–MRI mapping are particularly useful under general anesthesia.

Electrocorticography

The first condition for a worthwhile ECoG is sufficient brain exposure. The critical areas should be easily recognizable and reachable. A total of 16 electrodes are usually utilized. Their tips are carbon balls supported by flexible wires. They can thus be used to record from the cortical surface and from structures deep within a cavity. The electrodes can be arranged in any montage. Typically, with a large temporofrontal exposure, a row of four electrodes is disposed over the first and second temporal gyri and along the third and second frontal gyrus, with electrodes covering the central area. Flexible subdural electrodes can be used to record from the temporal pole, the undersurface of the temporal lobe, the fronto-orbital area or from cortex covered by dura.

Peroperative stimulation studies of the central area

After preliminary identification of the central sulcus by correlating the angiographic data with the exposed vascular anatomy of the central area, stimulation is carried out over the postcentral gyrus starting at 0.5 V and increasing by increments of 0.5 V up to 5 V. Most of the responses are obtained between 2 and 3 V. It is preferable to stimulate over the postcentral gyrus rather than over the precentral convolution since the stimulation threshold is lower, and undesirable convulsive phenomena can be avoided. In practice, all that is needed is a sequence of sensory responses over the tongue area located at the bottom of the postcentral gyrus (Fig. 7.6) [10].

ECoG provides both diagnostic and prognostic information by further delineating the active zone prior to resection and by indicating the areas of residual discharges after cortical removal.

Study of vascular territories

The study of vascular territories becomes more meaningful when each vessel is recognized in relation to specific structures of various functional significance. In order to minimize morbidity, the surgeon should study the vascular territory of each crucial artery or vein to establish the consequence of their deliberate or inadvertent occlusion before the actual surgery. This approach is absolutely essential when considering surgery in the vicinity of areas such as the motor and speech centers. Special emphasis is placed on studying the pattern of ascending veins to the superior longitudinal sinus since their manipulation and damage at the time of surgery can cause significant morbidity.

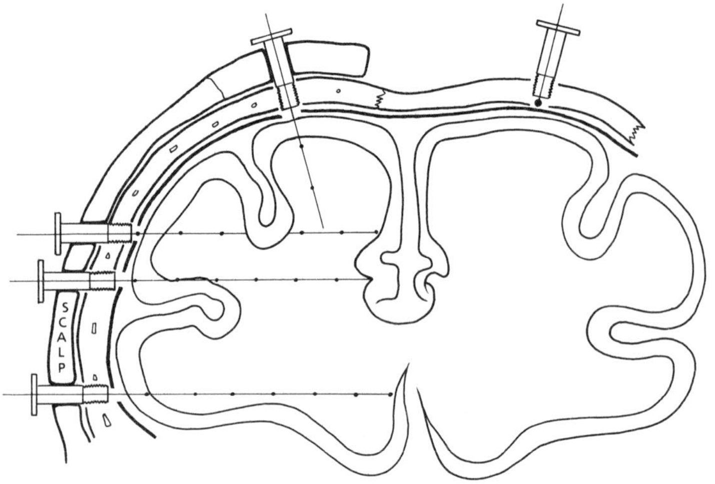

FIGURE 7.5 Stereoelectroencephalography (SEG). Placement of epicerebral and intracerebral electrodes.

Frontal resections

Based on clinical imaging, extracranial and intracranial EEG findings, various types of frontal resections can be considered [11] (Fig. 7.6):

1 Total frontal lobectomy.
2 Paramedian resection.
3 Frontopolar resection.
4 Lateral convexity resection.
5 Central resection.

Total frontal lobectomy (Fig. 7.7)

Large frontal resections in the nondominant hemisphere can be carried out safely in front of the precentral gyrus. Identification of the pre- and postcentral gyrus is accomplished best by stimulation under local anesthesia during electrocorticography. Resection is carried out in two steps (Fig. 7.8). An *en bloc* resection of the three horizontal frontal gyri over the lateral convexity is followed by resection of the anterior cingulate gyrus around the corpus callosum. The posterior orbital cortex is left alone. On the dominant side, the resection is brought down to either the middle of the second frontal gyrus or, preferably, to the inferior frontal sulcus identified by its arteriovenous anatomy. The posterior 2.5 cm of the third frontal gyrus are left alone to avoid speech disturbance. In this region we tend to rely heavily on topographic

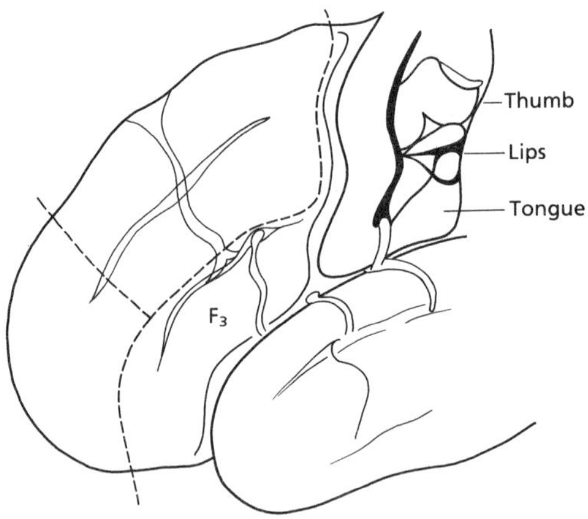

FIGURE 7.6 Frontal resections. Lines of resections as seen from lateral aspect. Identification of the central region is based on both topographic and physiologic data. Note sensory homonculus of postcentral gyrus.

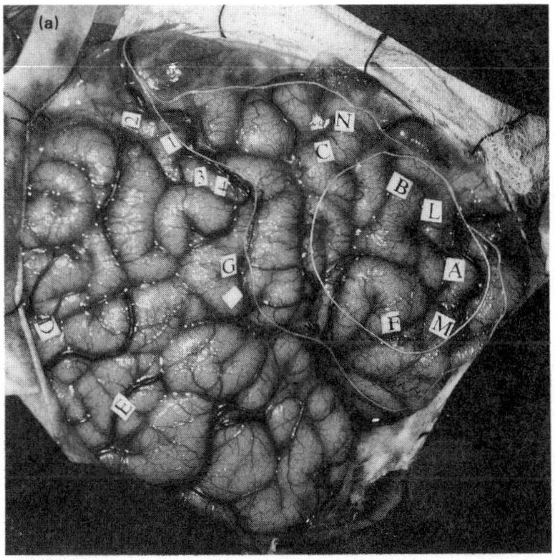

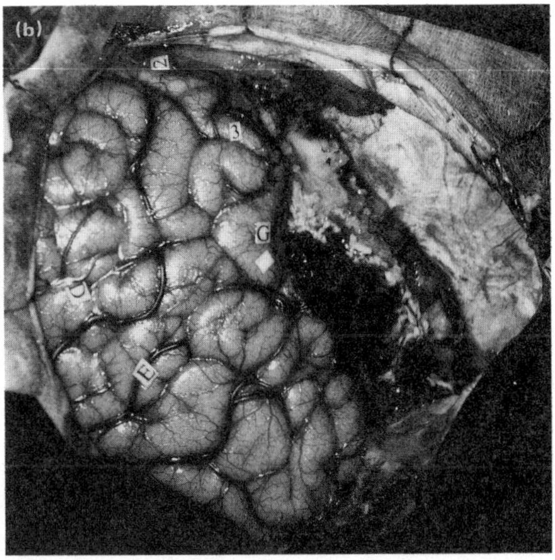

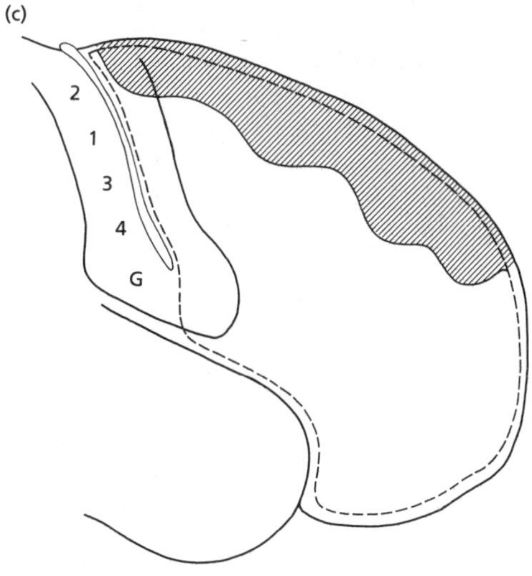

FIGURE 7.7 Example of total frontal lobectomy including precentral gyrus. (a) Exposed frontal, central, and temporal areas showing large parasagittal destructive lesion. Epileptic discharges are indicated by letters and stimulation sensory responses over postcentral gyrus by 1,2,3,4. (b) Diagram showing extent of removal. (c) Orientation diagram for Fig. 7.7a and b.

and anatomic landmarks rather than on response to stimulation. Indeed, speech interference in the so-called "Broca area" is in the author's experience often negative with currents well above sensory and motor thresholds, and a negative response does not always indicate absence of function. Again, of importance is the appraisal of the vascular anatomy. The arterial pattern over the frontal lobe is fairly constant, with a clear watershed zone between the middle and anterior cerebral arteries over the second frontal gyrus. Venous drainage is much more variable. Repercussions of venous occlusion should be

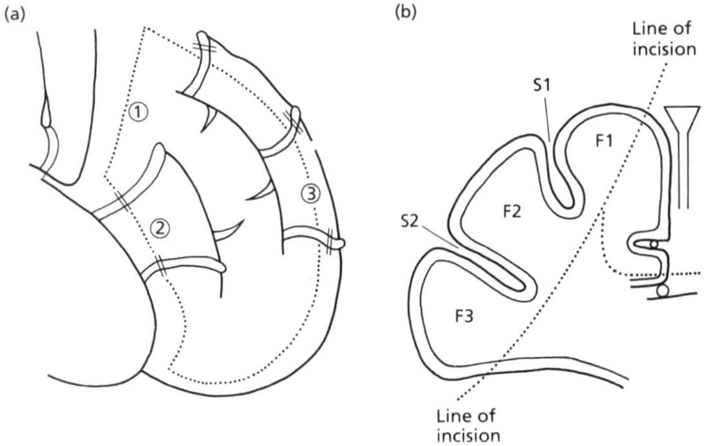

FIGURE 7.8 Staging of resection in frontal removals. (a) Three main stages in the surface cortical removal indicated by 1,2,3. Note how arteries are divided. (b) A lateral block of cortex is first removed followed by residual mesial frontal structures including cingulate gyrus.

assessed. Compensatory downward drainage to the Sylvian veins should be ascertained prior to sacrifice of an ascending frontal vein. In the author's opinion, many instances of transient postoperative dysphasia are not due to actual cortex removal but rather to venous occlusion of ascending frontal veins draining into the superior longitudinal sinus.

Frontal lobectomy: illustrative case

A 15-year-old girl at the time of surgery in 1985 had a past medical history of coarctation of the aorta and cyanosis at birth. Her seizure disorder dated back to shortly after birth with convulsions involving the entire left hemibody. At the time of surgery she had attacks characterized by tonic–clonic movements involving first the hand, then the forearm, and finally the arm. They would last from 5 minutes to 2 hours. There was no loss of consciousness and no incontinence. At the time of admission her seizure frequency was from 0 to 2 focal seizures per day despite medication. Prior EEGs revealed a focal epileptic disturbance in the right posterior temporal and parietal regions. Telemetry revealed generalized epileptic abnormality seen over both hemispheres, with predominance on the right. A computed tomography (CT) scan revealed an area of atrophy in the right frontal lobe corresponding to the distribution of the anterior cerebral artery. Her neurologic examination showed hypodevelopment and diffuse weakness of the left side of the body with marked limping and no useful movements of the hand. The left upper limb was also markedly spastic.

At electrocorticography a well-defined focus was documented, clearly involving the intermediate midfrontal area lateral to the destructive lesion (Fig. 7.7a). A radical frontal lobectomy including the precentral gyrus was carried out after proper identification of the postcentral gyrus by stimulation (Fig. 7.7a and b). With a follow-up of 4 years, the patient has had a remarkable result with only occasional brief stiffening and jerking of the left arm and hand. The function of her left hand was felt to be improved. The postcentral gyrus was left alone to preserve position sense.

Paramedian resection (Fig. 7.9)

The paramedian removal can extend from the frontal pole at the crista galli to the precentral sulcus. Its lateral border should extend at least to the middle of the second frontal gyrus and preferably to the inferior sulcus in order to avoid postoperative edema secondary to vascular occlusions. The cingulate gyrus is usually resected. When the cingulate gyrus is resected it is of even greater importance to remove tissue as far laterally as possible over the convexity since interference with arterial feeders in the depth of the callosomarginal and the pericallosal sulci can occur with subsequent edema. This is especially true if some of the frontal ascending veins have also been divided.

Venous trunks should be divided late in the resection after occlusion of the arterial feeders to maintain an adequate consistency to the block of removal and to prevent venous congestion and oozing. Venous congestion makes bipolar coagulation difficult and lengthens the removal time.

Paramedian resection: illustrative case

A 32-year-old patient had a history of cyanosis at birth and a generalized convulsion shortly after delivery and started having generalized seizures at the age of 5. Later seizures changed to a complex partial type, and increased to a frequency of one per day. The aura was described as a pressure in the head, followed by an ictus lasting for 10 to 15 seconds, with staring, lack of responsiveness, automatic movements with hands grasping things or playing with objects, and urinary incontinence. Electroencephalography revealed an interictal focus in the left frontal area and two electrographic seizures arising from the same area. Six clinical seizures suggested left frontal origin in three. No interictal epileptic activity was recorded from either temporal lobe. The patient underwent a study with three frontal and two temporal intracerebral electrodes bilaterally. Fifty-two seizures arose from the frontal superior electrode, and one cingulate gyrus. One clinical and three electrographic seizures had from the bilateral onset and 20 electrographic seizures had bilateral onset with left-sided predominance.

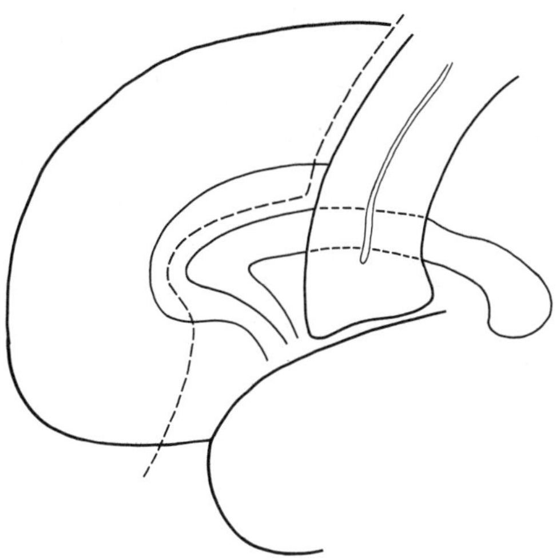

FIGURE 7.9 Paramedian resection.

On 7 April, 1983, the patient underwent a left frontal medial corticectomy. The resection measured 6 cm over the first frontal gyrus and upper part of the second frontal gyrus but did not involve the cingulate gyrus itself. An electrocorticogram showed widespread intermediate frontal epileptiform activity. Postoperatively she continued to have daily complex partial seizures, sometimes with urinary incontinence. She then became seizure-free for 5 months. The attacks returned when she went back to work as a teacher. They were of the same pattern except for the disappearance of the aura. For 1 year there was no urinary incontinence. The husband evaluated the improvement to be of the order of 20%.

The patient again underwent a series of telemetry studies with recording of several seizures with onset in the left parasagittal central area and spread to both frontal and later to both temporal areas. Review of previous depth electrode recordings showed that the majority of seizures began in the superior frontal gyrus, but some began in the cingulate gyrus, with polyspikes spreading to both frontal areas with a 20–30 second delay to both temporal areas.

In January 1984, the patient had a further resection of the anterior cingulate gyrus. Since then, she has had only a single episode of poorly described seizures. One year later her full scale IQ was 113 compared to 111 preoperatively.

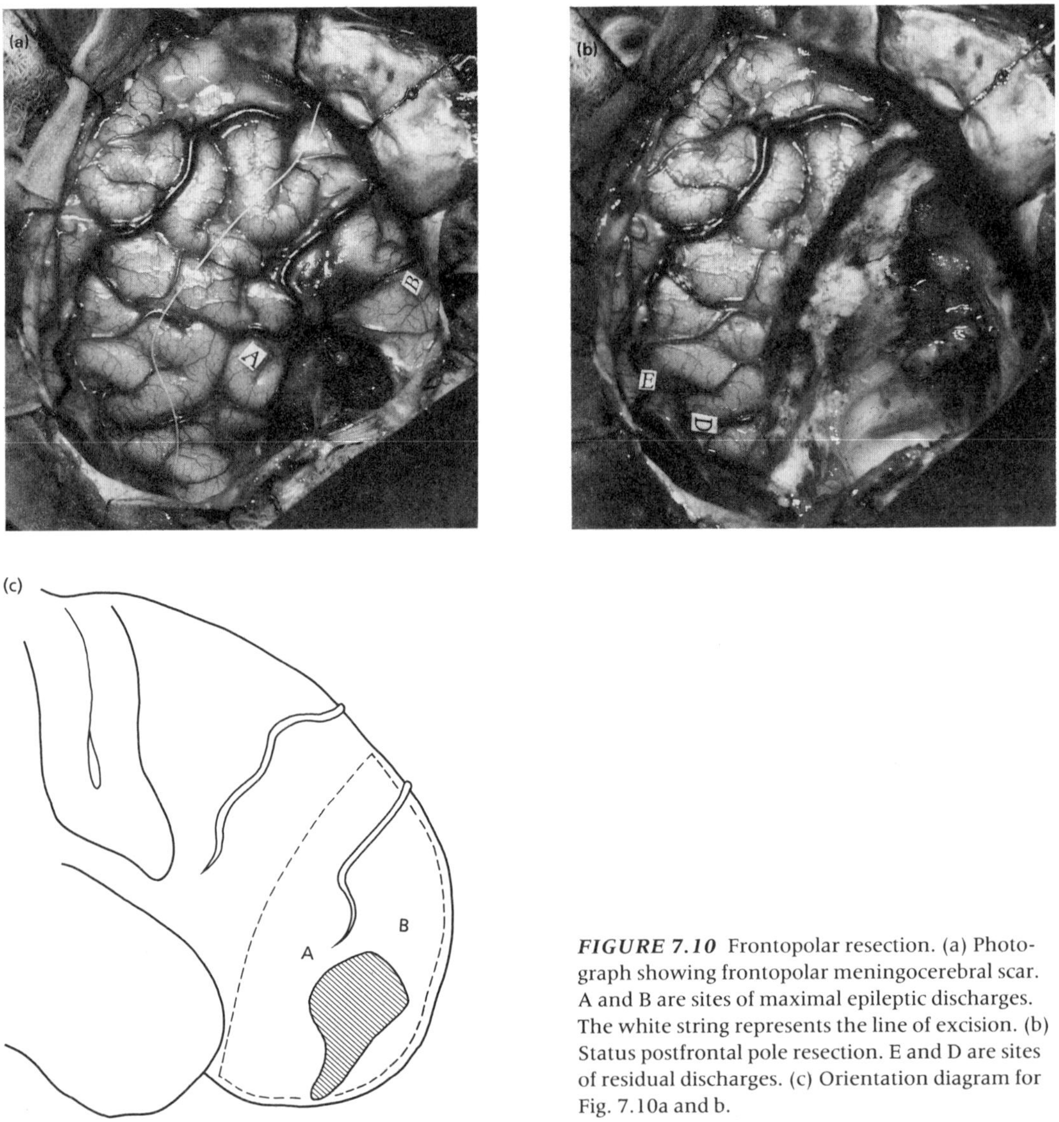

FIGURE 7.10 Frontopolar resection. (a) Photograph showing frontopolar meningocerebral scar. A and B are sites of maximal epileptic discharges. The white string represents the line of excision. (b) Status postfrontal pole resection. E and D are sites of residual discharges. (c) Orientation diagram for Fig. 7.10a and b.

Frontopolar resections (Fig. 7.10)

These resections involve removal of the pole of the frontal lobe as anterior as the crista galli as well as part of the intermediate portion of the frontal lobe.

Frontal polar resection: illustrative case

A 20-year-old man suffered a right frontal depressed fracture at age 12 and developed generalized tonic–clonic seizures at the age of 15. At craniotomy at the age of 20, a porencephalic cyst and severe meningocerebral scar was encountered. A frontopolar resection was carried out and he became seizure-free with follow-up of 10 years.

Lateral convexity resections (Fig. 7.11)

These consist of various resections of the intermediate frontal cortex including the second and third frontal gyri and sometimes the lateral extent of the first, in various combinations.

Lateral convexity: illustrative cases

A patient (D.C.) had postraumatic epilepsy with a single pattern of complex partial seizures consisting of an aura of generalized strange feeling, with chest tightness and occasional fear and familiarity. The ictal phase consisted of turning his head to the left, jumping in bed, and rolling to the left for 1 minute. Occasionally, there was some jumping up and down or running to his bed. Seizures occurred at a frequency of 20 per month. For 2 weeks prior to admission he had had three per day and 10 each night. Numerous preoperative EEGs showed a right frontotemporal abnormality. The site of seizure onset was clarified by electrocorticography, which showed an active circumscribed high-voltage repetitive spike focus over the intermedio-posterior extent of the right third frontal gyrus. A 4×2.5 cm resection of the posterior extent of this gyrus was carried out on May 5 1980 and the patient has remained seizure-free.

A 47-year-old male patient was investigated for seizures presenting as absence and generalized tonic–clonic seizures progressing to severe status. On routine EEG there was ambiguity between a temporal or a frontal focus. Depth electrodes showed electrographic status epilepticus in the right inferior frontal gyrus. A 4.5×3 cm resection of the right F3 gyrus was done after electrocorticography showed epileptic activity in the same area as detected by depth recording, namely F3. He has remained seizure-free for 4 years.

These two cases of lateral convexity removals are particularly instructive, since they show that removal of an identical zone of the third frontal gyrus can completely abolish seizures of different patterns.

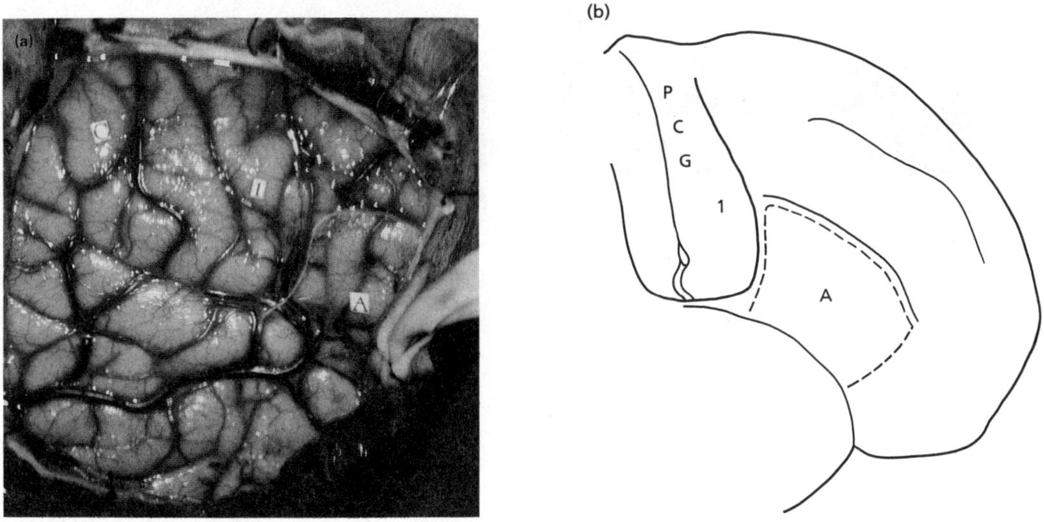

FIGURE 7.11 Frontal resection (lateral convexity). (a) Partial removal of F3 indicated by white string. (b) Orientation diagram for Fig. 7.11a: sites of epileptic discharge and line of excision. PCG, precentral gyrus; A, high-voltage repetitive firing.

Central resection (Fig. 7.12)

Resection of the lower central area, including both the pre- and postcentral gyri, can be done in cases of focal motor or sensory seizures, even in the dominant hemisphere. This is particularly true if the seizure involves the face early in the attack. The removal can extend up to 3 cm above the Sylvian fissure without any deficit as long as the tongue, thumb, and lips area are well identified by stimulation under local anesthesia (Fig. 7.7c). Ascending arteries should be recognized and left absolutely intact, especially the central artery, which is most constant and is usually found looping over the central operculum before penetrating deep within the lower extent of the central sulcus (Fig. 7.2). It is important also to recognize arteries from the pre- and postcentral sulci which vascularize the pre- and postcentral gyri and often penetrate into the central sulcus. The resection is best done by emptying those gyri with an ultrasonic aspirator set at very low parameter of suction and vibration in order to respect the pial banks including the upper bank of the

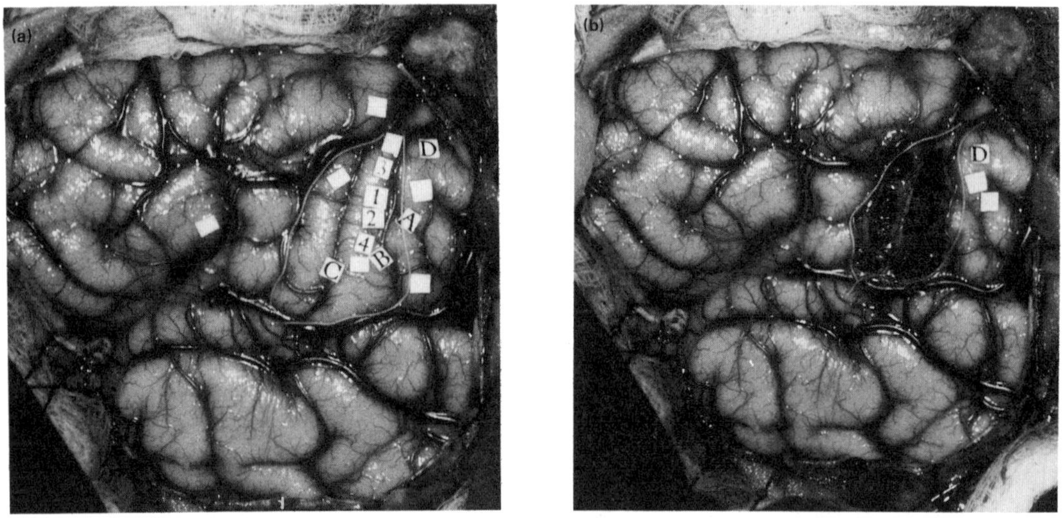

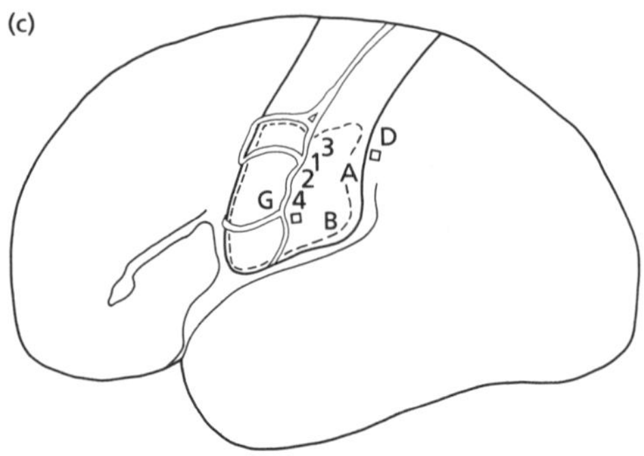

FIGURE 7.12 Central resection. (a) Preresection ECoG and stimulation data. (b) Following resection of both lower pre- and postcentral gyri. (c) Orientation diagram for Fig. 7.12a and b showing ECoG and stimulation data and extent of resection. Letters, epileptic discharges; numbers, tongue responses.

insula. When there is no movement of the hand, absence of position sense and presence of paresis of the lower limb, the whole central area can be removed without additional deficit.

Central resection

Illustrative case

An 11-year-old, right-handed girl had the onset of drop attacks with loss of consciousness at the age of 4. There was a progressive increase in the number of drop attacks with subsequent occurrence of right clonic seizures of the face and arm probably associated with pre- and postictal aphasia.

At the time of hospitalization, there were three predominant seizure patterns: (1) myoclonic movements of the right arm; (2) clonic movements of the right arm and face often preceded by a violent fall forwards or backwards; and (3) nocturnal right focal seizures occurring frequently just before awakening in the morning. Her full-scale IQ was 102, performance 108, and verbal 97. There was also definite progressive worsening of right hand movement.

MRI showed evidence of an enlarged gyrus in the supra-Sylvian motor cortex. At surgery under local anesthesia in October 1985, enlargement of both the pre- and the postcentral gyri was seen. Rhythmic discharges and spontaneous seizures were recorded from the lower postcentral gyrus (Fig. 7.12a). A complete endopial emptying of the lower central area including the pre- and postcentral gyri was carried out, measuring 2 cm in width and 3 cm in height. Pathology showed astrogliosis. In 3 postoperative years, the patient has had only five or six falls without injury. Concentration, speech, and right-hand functions have improved. In this case, lower central resection was useful to decrease seizures including focal motor, drop attacks, and generalized tonic–clonic types.

This case serves to demonstrate that the lower central area including both the lower pre- and postcentral gyri can be removed without causing hemiparesis or dysphasia even if the procedure is done in the dominant hemisphere. Arteries and arterioles should be left intact. The operation should be carried out under local anesthesia with magnification and after accurate identification of the pre- and postcentral gyri.

Parietal resection (Figs 7.13 and 7.14)

Resections in the parietal region are possible only after meticulous identification of the postcentral gyrus. As for the central region proper, it is of the utmost importance to respect and leave intact any ascending vein to the superior sagittal sinus draining from the central or postcentral sulci. On the dominant side, any ascending vein from the inferior parietal lobule should be left intact. The lower 2.5–3 cm of the postcentral gyrus can be resected without significant deficit. Resection of the hand and foot area of the postcentral gyrus will be followed by profound proprioceptive and epicritical deficit. In the nondominant hemisphere the whole parietal lobe posterior to the postcentral sulcus can be removed without sensori-motor deficit as long as the postcentral gyrus is left intact. A partial visual field deficit can be expected. In the dominant hemisphere such resections are entirely confined to the superior parietal lobe. Study of the regional arteriovenous pattern will indicate the position of the intraparietal sulcus which should be the inferior limit of the resection while the anterior limit is the postcentral sulcus.

Indications for operation in the parietal lobe are few and these removals are usually based on strong congruence of clinical, imaging, and EEG data. Intracranial recording may be necessary to establish the participation of the central area in the epileptic discharges.

Parietal resection: illustrative case

A 26-year-old patient, left-handed but with evidence of some speech on the left on Amytal test, had seizure onset at the age of 5, characterized by

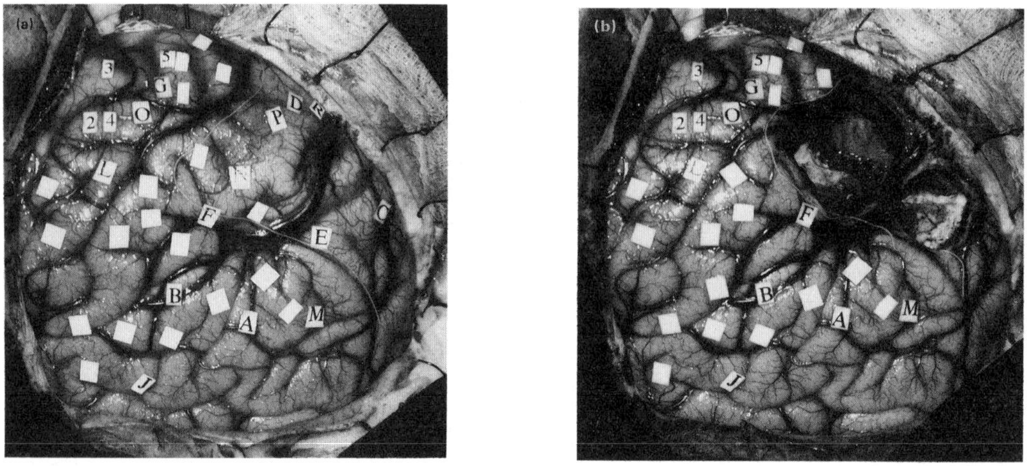

FIGURE 7.13 Parietal resection. (a) Cortical mapping with numbers indicating position of postcentral gyrus and letters indicating sites of epileptic discharges. Blank squares represent negative responses. (b) Following removal of superior parietal lobule. Note ascending parietal veins left intact. See Fig. 7.14 for orientation.

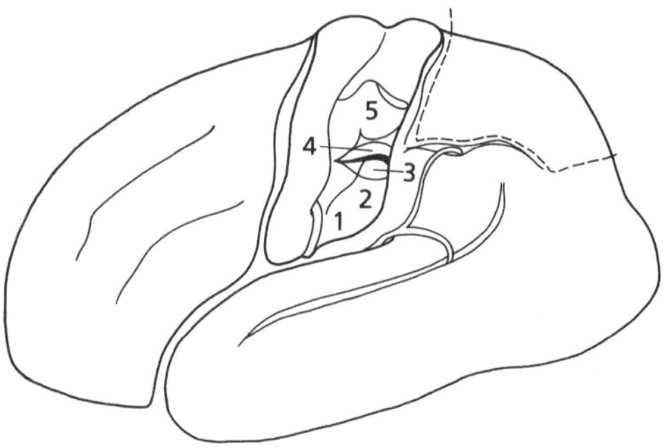

FIGURE 7.14 Line of removal in dominant parietal resection and characteristic sensory sequence of lower postcentral gyrus. Compare with Fig. 7.6. 1 back of tongue; 2 middle of tongue; 3 tip of tongue and lips; 4 lips; 5 thumb.

drop attacks preceded by a scream and sometimes a feeling of numbness in the right foot. A second seizure type consisted of generalized jerking with loss of consciousness sometimes preceded by vertigo. Another seizure type was characterized by right-sided jerking becoming bilateral at times without loss of consciousness. EEG showed an active left parietocentral focus. Computed tomography scan showed a space occupying lesion of the left parietal trigone area which had not progressed over the years (Fig. 7.13a). Following parietal cortex resection and subtotal removal of an hamartoma (Fig. 7.13b) she became seizure-free for 1 year. Her attacks progressively returned although she remained markedly improved compared to her preoperative status. Further posterior parietal resection and subtotal removal of hamartomatous tissue was achieved 4 years later. The patient has remained seizure-free for 1 year.

Occipital resections (Fig. 7.15)

Occipital lobe seizures manifest themselves by visual symptomatology such as transient blindness or visual hallucinations usually characterized by flashes of lights, colored balls, and other geometric patterns which are never fully organized in a complex hallucination. Surgery on the occipital lobe is only done when overwhelming evidence is found for an occipital focus, usually proven by intracerebral electrodes. Since most occipital onset seizures tend to spread to the temporal or parietocentral areas, intracranial recording is recommended to confirm the site of origin of the seizure and to study the direction of its spread. If the seizure only manifests itself when the temporal lobe is invaded, it can sometimes be preferable to proceed with temporal resection first to avoid visual deficit.

Occipital resections: illustrative case

An 11-year-old girl at the time of operation in March 1981 was referred because of a well-documented active right occipital focus. She had two types of seizures: a predominant type characterized by eye and head deviation to the left side with concomitant blindness, and a second type consisting of automatic behavior. Prior to each type of seizure, the patient had a visual warning characterized by diamond-shaped and colored figures. Computed tomography scan showed mild parieto-occipital atrophy. The family was told that surgery would cause a left homonymous hemianopsia without any assurance of seizure cure. At surgery (Fig. 7.15a and b) an extremely active spike focus was found over the lateral surface of the right occipital pole. The occipital pole was resected and the postremoval electrocorticogram showed no residual spiking. The hemianopsia has been difficult to document, even with meticulous visual field examination. She had an episode of three consecutive focal motor seizures 5 years after surgery but otherwise has been seizure-free for 8 years since surgery.

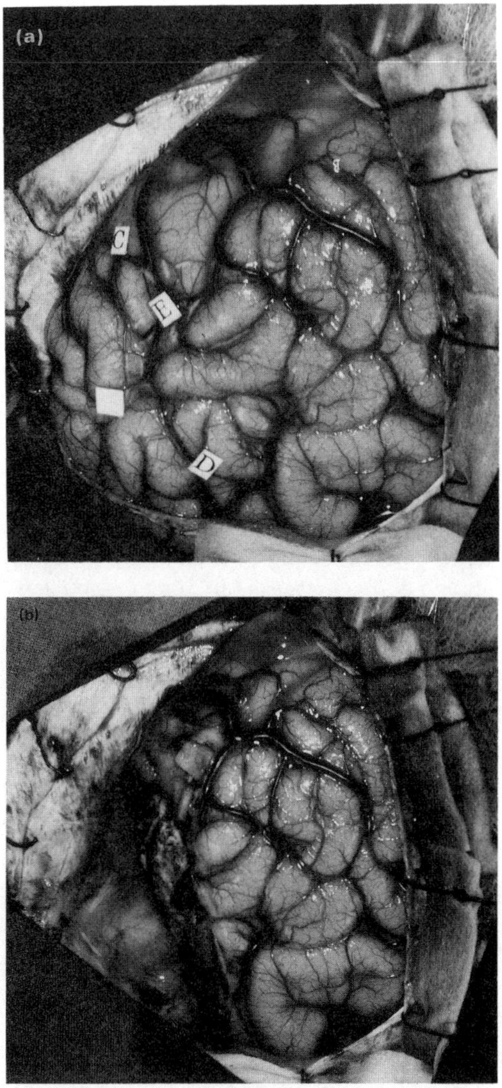

FIGURE 7.15 Occipital resection. (a) Occipital cortex exposed with sites of epileptic discharges marked with letters C,D,E. (b) The occipital pole has been resected including zones of epileptic discharges.

Multilobar resections

Multilobar removals are usually synonymous with subtotal hemispherectomies. They are done for large destructive lesions and epileptic fields clearly affecting more than one lobe of the brain. Rasmussen has frequently noted that even the full battery of recording techniques will fail to demonstrate a focal onset in the damaged hemisphere in many patients. Many of these patients can be further studied by SEG or placement of subdural strips or grids in order to further delineate the predominant epileptogenic zone. Further study by electrocorticography is often indicated. In such instances, various combinations of removal can be performed such as frontotemporal, frontoparietal, and occipitotemporal. Over the last several years we have preferred to proceed in two stages, i.e. limit the resection to one lobar region and proceed, 1 or 2 years later, with extension of the resection and additional removal in another lobar region if seizures persist.

Hemispherectomy

In patients with congenital hemiplegia or chronic encephalitis which has progressed to the stage of hemiplegia, hemispherectomy brings dramatic arrest of focal motor and generalized convulsive seizures. Total hemispherectomy has, however, been associated with a high rate of morbidity and mortality associated with superficial hemosiderosis and hydrocephalus. This led Rasmussen to develop the procedure of central disconnection, the equivalent of an "anatomically incomplete but physiologically complete hemispherectomy" [12,13]. Essentially, this operation consists of a large and deep central resection combined with a temporal removal (Fig. 7.16). All projections, associative and commissural, are thus transected including fibers of the corpus callosum (Fig. 7.16). Classical hemispherectomy is rarely carried out at the Montreal Neurological Institute but subtotal hemispherectomy where one-fifth to one-third of the hemisphere is preserved still has frequent indication and is not associated with delayed hydrocephalus. Of crucial importance in considering such surgery is appraisal of the preoperative manual deficit. There is a continuum in the variety of hand paresis and spasticity. When the hand barely moves, is spastic and kept closed with the elbow flexed, no problem is anticipated. When there is some useful but diminished hand prehension movement without any individual finger movements, the functional deficit after hemispherectomy will be minimal. Patients who have hand prehension are likely to lose this prehension. Patients who have severe limping and no foot tapping movements may develop temporary increased deficit in the lower limb but will not have a permanent added deficit. The potential further loss of function in the hand or foot must be discussed in depth. This is especially true in young patients suffering from Rasmussen's chronic encephalitis, in whom the unilateral weakness is only partial. The occurrence of a complete hemiplegia in trade for arrest of focal seizures is unacceptable. In the Montreal Neurological Institute series of classical hemispherectomies, 84% of patients had a complete or nearly complete control of their attacks and 16% had a moderate or less reduction of their seizure tendency. Following a subtotal hemispherectomy, 68% had a complete or nearly complete control of their attacks and 32% had a moderate or less reduction of the seizure tendency [12].

Outcome of extratemporal resections

Rasmussen has studied the outcome of patients with extratemporal resections carried out at the Montreal Neurological Institute from 1928 through 1980. Among 283 patients with frontal resections, 257 were available for follow-up. With a median follow-up of 16 years, 26% of patients became seizure-free, 30% had a marked but not complete reduction of their seizure tendency, and 40% had a moderate or less reduction. There were four operative deaths, six patients died in the first 2 operative years, and 16 patients had inadequate follow-up [14].

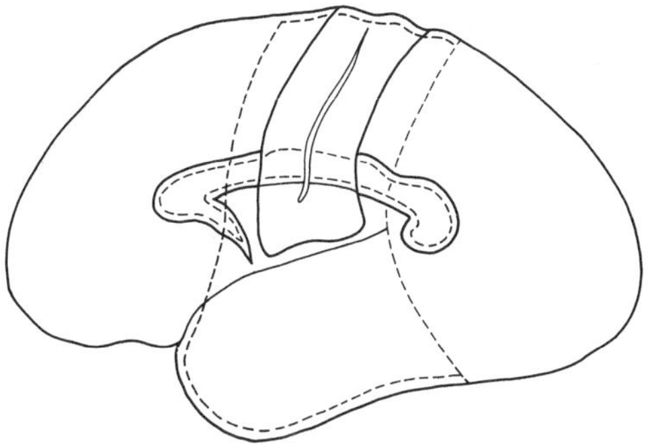

FIGURE 7.16 Modified hemispherectomy after Rasmussen.

Among 203 patients with central, parietal, and occipital epileptogenic lesions, 186 patients were available for follow-up. With a media follow-up of 18 years, 34% became seizure-free, 23% had a marked but not complete reduction of their seizure tendency, and 44% had a moderate decrease. There were four operative deaths, three patients died in the first 2 postoperative years, and the follow-up was inadequate in 10 patients [2]. Long-term follow-up for the era of intensive monitoring, CT and MRI imaging is not yet available.

References

1 Rasmussen T. Commentary: extratemporal cortical excisions and hemispherectomy. In Engel J, Jr (ed) *Surgical Treatment of Epilepsies.* Raven Press, New York, pp 417–424.

2 Rasmussen T. *Esclimont Meeting on Frontal Lobe Epilepsy.* Esclimont, France, 1987.

3 Rosenbaum TJ. Placement of subdural strip electrodes at Good Samaritan Hospital and Medical Center, Portland. In Engel J, Jr (ed) *Surgical Treatment of Epilepsies.* Raven Press, New York, 1987, pp 613–619.

4 Wyler AR, Ojemann GA, Lettich E, Ward AA, Jr. Subdural strip electrodes for localizing epileptogenic foci. *J Neurosurg* 1984; **60**: 1195–1200.

5 Goldring S, Gregorie M. Surgical management of epilepsy using epidural recording to localize the seizure focus. *J Neurosurg* 1984; **60**: 457–466.

6 Lesser RP, J, Lueders H, Rothner AD, Erenberg G. The use of chronic subdural electrodes for cortical mapping of speech. *Epilepsia* 1981; **22**: 240.

7 Lüders H, Hahn J, Lesser RP, Dinners DS, Rothner D, Erenberg G. Localization of epileptogenic spike foci: comparative study of closely spaced scalp electrodes, nasopharyngeal, sphenoidal, subdural and depth electrodes. In Akimoto H, Kazamatsuri H, Sieno M, Ward A (eds) *Advances in Epileptology, Vol. 13, XIIIth Epilepsy International Symposium.* Raven Press, New York, 1982, pp 185–189.

8 Talairach J, Bancaud J. Stereotaxic exploration and therapy in epilepsy. In Vinken PJ, Bruyn GW (eds) *The Epilepsies Handbook of Clinical Neurology,* Vol. 15. North Holland, Amsterdam, 1977, pp 758–782.

9 Olivier A, DeLotbinière A. Stereotactic techniques in epilepsy. *Neuros St Art Rev* 1987; **2**(1).

10 Picard C, Olivier A. Sensory cortical tongue representation in man. *J Neurosurg* 1983; **59**: 781–789.

11 Crandall, PH. Cortical resections. In Engel J, Jr (ed) *Surgical Treatment of the Epilepsies.* Raven Press, New York, 1987, pp 377–404.

12 Rasmussen T. Hemispherectomy for seizures revisited. *Can J Neurol Sci* 1983; **10**: 71–78.

13 Tinuper P, Andermann F, Villemure J-G, Rasmussen TB, Quesney L. Functional hemispherectomy for treatment of epilepsy associated with hemiplegia: rationale, indications, results and comparison with callosotomy. *Ann Neurol* 1988; **24**(1): 27–34.

14 Ramussen T. Focal epilepsies of non-temporal and non-frontal origin. In Weiser HG, Elger CE (eds) *Presurgical Evaluation of Epileptics: Basics, Techniques and Implications.* Springler-Verlag, Berlin, 1987, pp 344–351.

15 Olivier A. Commentary: cortical resections. In Engle J, Jr (ed) *Surgical Treatment of Epilepsies.* Raven Press, New York, 1987, pp 405–415.

16 Szikla G, Bouvier G, Hori T, Petrov V. Angiography of the human brain cortex. Atlas of vascular patterns and stereotactic cortical localization. Springer-Verlag, Heidelberg, 1977.

chapter 8

Corpus Callosum Section

David W. Roberts

In a 1931 paper describing congenital cysts of the cavum septi pellucidi and cavum vergae, Dandy reports the case of a 4½-year-old boy presenting with marked drowsiness and repeated seizures involving the left face, arm, and leg. Following surgical fenestration of a cyst of the cavum septi pellucidi into the lateral ventricles via an approach in which the corpus collosum was divided, the patient did exceedingly well and was free of his seizure disorder [1]. Three years later Van Wagenen and Aird added 15 cases of their own to the literature on cysts of the cavum septi pellucidi and cavum vergae and, having been deterred in at least one patient from operating through the corpus callosum by a large number of veins draining into the sagittal sinus, they express a preference for the transcortical, transventricular approach [2]. This experience and difference of opinion regarding surgical approach takes on particular interest in light of Van Wagenen's subsequent landmark report with Herren of surgical division of the corpus callosum proving efficacious in the control of otherwise intractable seizure disorders [3].

Following Van Wagenen and Herren's 1940 paper on 10 patients undergoing section of the corpus callosum for seizure disorders [3], there were isolated reports of this surgery by Bogen [4–6] and by Luessenhop [7,8] in the 1960s. Sustained appreciation for the benefit of corpus callosum section began with the series of Wilson [9–14]. Since then the number of centers performing commissurotomy surgery and the body of literature reporting that experience have continued to grow. Of note has been the striking consistency of outcome, with infrequent exception, reported by these many centers.

Preoperative evaluation

Selection criteria for corpus callosum section at Dartmouth include: (1) seizure disorders characterized by generalized major motor, tonic, or atonic (drop attack) seizures; (2) absence of an identifiable, resectable seizure focus; and (3) documented medical intractability, including exhaustive anticonvulsant trials with therapeutic levels. Patients whose seizures have been primarily complex partial but without a localizable focus have been operated upon with encouraging results, but the indications in this setting are still being defined [15]. There is some evidence that severe mental retardation is predictive of a poorer response [9,13,16], but this is not at present an absolute contraindication. Concern has been raised by reliable investigators that individuals with mixed or crossed dominance may be at high risk for increased cognitive difficulties following commissurotomy [17]. Such mixed dominance at our institution remains a concern but again not an absolute contraindication.

The typical patient being considered for corpus callosum surgery is seen initially in the outpatient department, and subsequent evaluation is performed during hospitalization on the neurological service. Video EEG monitoring is performed with the goal of capturing at least three of the patient's typical seizures. It is at this stage that the patient with a resectable cortical focus will be identified and resective surgery recommended instead. Computed tomography (CT) and magnetic resonance imaging (MRI) studies are obtained in those who have not in the recent past had those studies. Angiography, performed in the early part of our series, was reinstituted more recently, and Wada Amytal testing is carried out at the time of that study. An extensive battery of neuropsychologic and audiometric testing, including Wechsler Adult Intelligent Scale (WAIS) and an assessment of baseline interhemispheric transfer ability, is administered.

If, at the completion of all these studies, the patient is felt to be a reasonable candidate for commissurotomy, further education of the patient and his or her family through discussion and reading material ensues. In all instances deliberate time to absorb and reflect on the implications of surgery is imposed, and in many the surgery is performed at a later hospitalization.

The extent and staging of commissural section vary among different centers. Of Wilson's 20 patients, the first three underwent what he described as "complete" commissurotomy, with division of the entire corpus callosum, the anterior commissure, and one fornix. The following five patients underwent "frontal" commissurotomy, with division of the anterior half of the corpus callosum, the anterior commissure, and one fornix [14]. In the remaining 12 patients, in whom only the corpus callosum was sectioned, five had a complete, one-stage procedure, and seven had complete section in two stages (the posterior section preceding the anterior section in all but one) [13]. In all patients in whom section included the posterior corpus callosum, the underlying hippocampal commissure was divided as well.

Since 1982 we have limited commissurotomy to the corpus callosum and hippocampal commissure. Whereas previous staging had been performed with the intention of completing the callosal section in all, partial section has been performed in all but four of the last 55 patients with the expectation that at least some patients would not require subsequent completion of the callosal division to obtain satisfactory seizure control. Infrequently, division of the posterior corpus callosum was felt more likely, on the basis of either posteriorly located epileptogenic activity on EEG or occipital pathology on imaging studies, to be efficacious than anterior section; in all others, with either frontal pathology or no localized or regional abnormality, the anterior corpus callosum was divided at initial surgery. Twenty-one patients undergoing either anterior or posterior section subsequently underwent completion of their section. Four patients since 1982 have had complete section at one surgery.

Surgical technique

Anterior corpus callosum section

Following the administration of general anesthesia, the patient is placed supine with the head secured in neutral position in a Gardner, Mayfield, or Sugita head clamp. The anterior scalp is shaved, EEG electrodes are placed in as close approximation to the International 10–20 array as possible, and the skin is prepared, marked, and draped. A 9 cm linear incision just anterior to the coronal suture, with two-thirds of its length to the right of midline, is employed (Fig. 8.1). In patients with right hemisphere dominance or significant left hemisphere damage, a left-sided incision and approach will be used. Hemostasis is achieved using electrocautery, and hemostatic scalp clips or clamps are unnecessary; retraction is achieved using crossed shallow cerebellar retractors (or retraction hooks in the Sugita system). During the opening, 1 g/kg mannitol is administered; dexamethasone will have been given the evening before and prior to induction.

The craniotomy is performed using a 2-inch air-powered trephine. The posterior margin of the opening is approximately at the coronal suture; one-third of its diameter is across the midline. Appropriate care is required over the sagittal sinus, but the more midline opening allows optimal exposure down the interhemispheric fissure with minimal retraction. Gelfoam (Upjohn, Kalamazoo, Minnesota) is laid over the sagittal sinus, and the dura is then opened in a curvilinear fashion with its base on the sinus and secured with a dural retraction suture. It should be noted at this point that any of a number of alternative skin incisions and craniotomy flaps may be employed depending upon individual preference.

Particular attention must now be directed to any veins draining from the exposed cortex into the sagittal sinus. Apuzzo has reported the angiographic findings in 100 patients in whom the pattern of these veins in the region of the coronal suture was studied. In 42 patients, significant bridging veins were

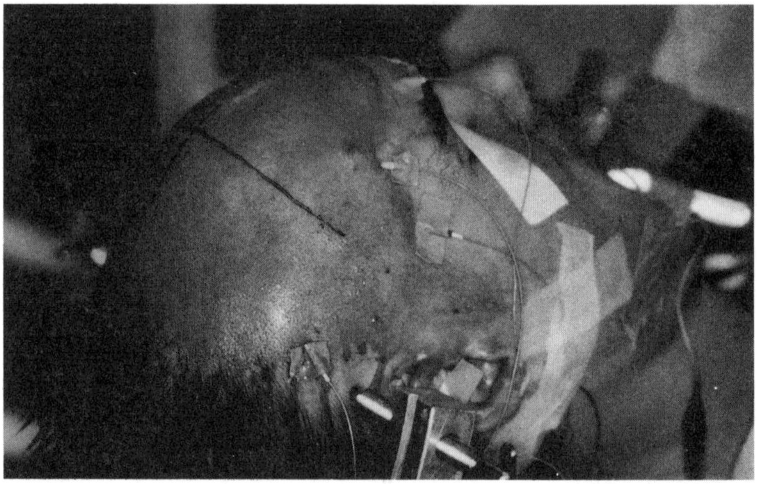

FIGURE 8.1 The anterior corpus callosum procedure utilizes a 9 cm linear incision just anterior to the coronal suture. Two-thirds of its length is to the right of midline.

found within 2 cm of the coronal suture; in 70% of these, the veins were present posteriorly [18]. If a vein is encountered, it should be preserved, and recognition of the frequently oblique course toward the sinus and of adhesions to the sinus prior to actual drainage into it may enable one to obtain working room around such a structure. In the worst case of a vein bisecting the exposure, one may still comfortably complete the section using present microsurgical technique. More common than bridging veins are arachnoidal adhesions, and these are easily taken down with microscissors or an arachnoid knife. Compressed Gelfoam is now placed over the entire exposed cortex for its protection throughout the remainder of the procedure.

Initial examination of the exposure along the falx and medial hemispheric surface is aided with a hand-held retractor. At the first encounter with deeper adhesions, Gelfoam is laid over the medial cortical surface and a medium width self-retaining retractor blade placed. Using the operating microscope, adhesions between the cingulate gyri may divide easily with gentle manipulation or sharp dissection, but the adhesions often, particularly if there is a history of earlier trauma or infection, render separation of the hemispheres without cortical injury difficult. Should this prove troublesome, one may work more posteriorly and take advantage of the deeper falx to obtain the necessary exposure.

Many have described the distinct whiteness of the dorsal aspect of the exposed corpus callosum and the importance of recognizing this identifying color in distinguishing the structure from the potentially mistaken cingulate gyrus. Protecting the callosomarginal and pericallosal arteries from excessive pressure, the retractor blade is repositioned to allow good visualization of the corpus callosum. In some patients an additional retractor blade on the opposite cingulate gyrus may prove advantageous, though care should be exercised to avoid compression of the sagittal sinus. Minor adhesions between the pericallosal arteries may need to be divided, and occasionally small vessels serving only the corpus callosum are coagulated with bipolar forceps. Subsequent callosal section may be most easily accomplished between the pericallosal arteries, but should division appear to be easier lateral to the vessels, or more commonly both medial and lateral to one artery, that is of little consequence.

Earlier in the series the next step would involve exposing the entire length of corpus callosum to be divided, but for the sake of efficiency in retractor positioning that is no longer done. For reasons to be elaborated upon division is begun at the level of the posterior genu and anterior body. The commissural fibers are divided using a gentle lengthwise sweeping of a blunt microinstrument, such as a Rhoton #8 microdissector, along the approximate midline for a length of about 1 cm. The field is kept dry using regulated microsuction on a micropatty at the dependent portion of the exposure just posteriorly.

Wilson and others have described carrying this division ventrally until one comes to the bluish appearance of the ventricular ependyma [11,12]. One may use such a strategy, following that limiting ependymal layer as one subsequently proceeds anteriorly and posteriorly, but fortuitous entry into a cavum septi pellucidi early in the series has modified our technique [19–21]. In nearly all of our last 55 patients, a cavum or its remnant has been found, and the advantages which accompany its recognition and utilization are well worth the little extra effort at this point in the procedure required to find the anatomic midline. To do this one continues the callosal division until one does note a darker hue to the ventral fibers. At this point, a side-to-side sweeping of a broader dissector will show either a whiter line following the midline, representing the apposed leaves of the septum pellucidum as they attach to the undersurface of the corpus callosum, or an opening into a cavum which may be distinguished from a lateral ventricle by the absence of recognizable vessels and choroid plexus. The cavum septi pellucidi is normally present in prematures and newborns, and after 6 months of age remains greater than 1 mm in width in approximately 12% of individuals [22]. A range of incidence figures for the cavum can be found in the literature, depending primarily on the criteria used for defining its presence, but even in those patients in whom a cavum has not been demonstrable preoperatively by CT or MRI, and in whom initial surgical exposure does not suggest a grossly apparent cavum, the lamella of the septum pellucidum will usually fall apart leaving a useful space. At the depth of this space will be a deep midline cleft separating the frontal horns of the lateral ventricles (Fig. 8.2). Shaw points out in his anatomic study of the cavum and its involution that the cavity closes last in the region of the posterior genu and anterior body [22], and our experience would confirm this. It is for this reason that section is begun at that portion of the corpus callosum.

The advantages of using the midline include greater ease in subsequent performance of the section and assurance of the section's completeness. Proceeding anteriorly, one may lift up from the midline cleft and join the division from the dorsal and anterior aspects of the genu (Fig. 8.3). The thinner rostrum is divided as far as can be comfortably visualized, and as previously noted, the anterior commissure is not divided. Proceeding posteriorly the retractors are repositioned as necessary, and continuing section performed by lifting up from the midline cleft with a blunt microdissector. Orientation along the corpus callosum may be aided by actual measurement with an adapted paper ruler or instrument of known dimension and then comparing that measurement with the preoperative midsagittal MRI study. Alternatively, identifiable features of the corpus callosum in a given individual, such as thinning in the posterior body, may be seen on the MRI and serve as useful landmarks in the surgical field. The extent of planned resection in a typical patient will be approximately two-thirds of the corpus callosum, although this may be extended as far as the junction of the body and the splenium if temporal pathology has been suggested during the preoperative evaluation.

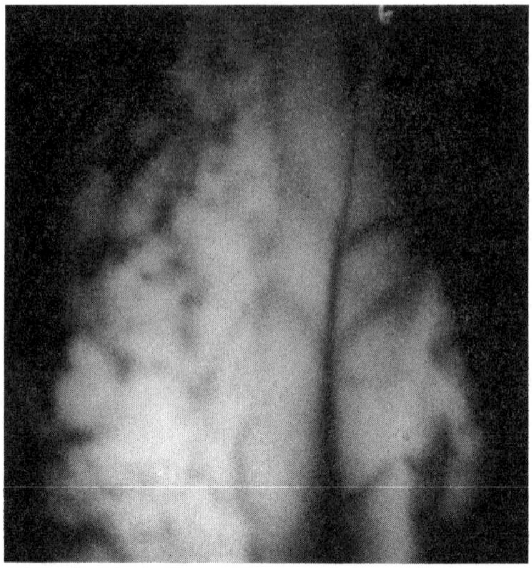

FIGURE 8.2 Division of the anterior body and posterior portion of the genu in the midline allows the lamellae of the septum pellucidum to fall away from each other. The midline cleft between the lateral ventricles is well visualized and serves as a convenient guide in the subsequent division anteriorly and posteriorly.

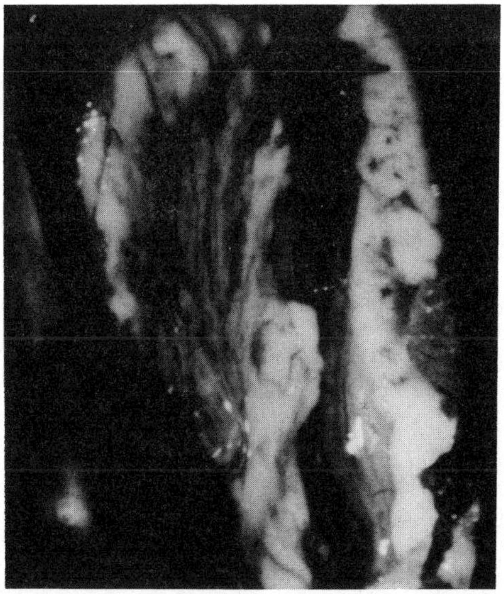

FIGURE 8.3 Between the cut surface of the divided genu, one can see the course of the anterior cerebral arteries sweeping forward, up, and then backward.

When the division has been extended to its desired length, hemostasis is assured and a Ligaclip (Ethicon, Somerville, New Jersey) attached to a small piece of Gelfoam is placed at the posterior limit of resection. This will best identify the extent of section on postoperative imaging studies (the MRI artefact of this clip has been minimal) and will facilitate subsequent surgery should that be necessary.

The Gelfoam on the medial and convexity cortical surfaces is now irrigated off, the dura is closed over Gelfilm (Upjohn, Kalamazoo, Minnesota) using 4–0 Vicryl suture (Ethicon, Somerville, New Jersey), and Gelfoam is laid over the suture line. The bone plug is secured with 2–0 Nurolon suture (Ethicon, Somerville, New Jersey), the galea aponeurosis reapproximated with inverted 2–0 Vicryl suture, and the skin reapproximated with a running 4–0 Prolene suture (Ethicon, Somerville, New Jersey) or staples. A sterile head dressing is applied, and particular, attention is given to protection of the wound from the patient's own hands.

Posterior corpus callosum section

In positioning the patient for posterior callosal section, the patient is again placed supine with the table slightly flexed. The head is secured in pin fixation, but the neck is now slightly flexed such that the scalp incision, at the level of the biparietal eminence, lies at approximately the same position relative to the operating room as the anterior incision had previously been (Fig. 8.4). Lack of attention to positioning for either stage will cause awkward angulation of the surgical trajectory at either the anterior or posterior extreme of the section.

As in the anterior section, the skin incision and trephination are placed with one-third of their length or diameter extending across midline. The general principles of cortical and vascular protection are similarly observed. The exposure of the posterior portion of the corpus callosum is considerably easier than the anterior on account of the deeper falx, which prevents adhesions between the two cingulate gyri. The self-retaining retractor may usually be placed with immediate exposure of the splenium.

Whether or not an anterior corpus callosum section has been previously performed, the posterior division is usually begun at the posterior margin of the splenium. The principal overlying vascular structure is a vein draining posteriorly and this is always preserved. Smaller vessels supplying only the splenium may be coagulated with bipolar cautery and divided sharply. The section is again performed using a blunt microinstrument, sweeping from posterior to anterior. The underlying hippocampal commissure bridging the more lateral crura of the fornices

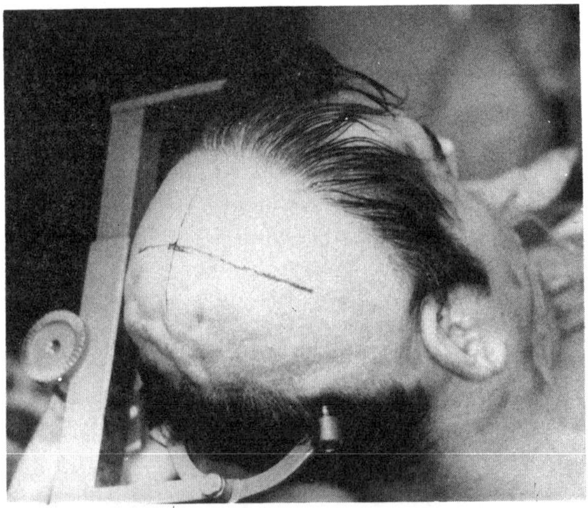

FIGURE 8.4 For the posterior corpus callosum procedure, the neck is slightly flexed, and a 9 cm linear incision at the level of the parietal eminence is employed.

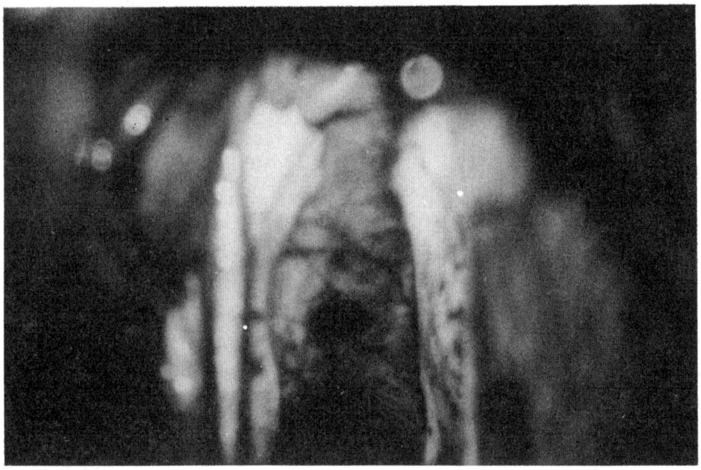

FIGURE 8.5 As the splenium is divided, the easily visualized underlying arachnoid assures the completeness of the section.

is without any distinguishing midline landmark, but one may be confident of the midline orientation aided by the inferior edge of the deeper falx. The incidence of a cavum vergae, which would separate the posterior corpus callosum from the hippocampal commissure, has been estimated at approximately 2% [23] and is certainly far lower than that of a cavum septi pellucidi. When the hippocampal commissure is apposed to the ventral surface of the posterior corpus callosum, division of the latter will include the former. One may follow the underlying arachnoid as one proceeds anteriorly, and inadvertent sparing of commissural fibers would be difficult (Fig. 8.5).

As the fornices approach one another, care to stay midline is warranted to protect against unintentional damage to one of them. If the anterior corpus callosum has been sectioned earlier, the Ligaclip placed at the posterior extent of that section will be most appreciated now. Gliotic reapposition of earlier divided corpus callosum may render determination of what was previously sectioned uncertain; finding a deposited Ligaclip will obviate unnecessary exposure and repeat division. After retrieval of this clip, the closure is the same as for the anterior section.

Acute postoperative management

Postcommissurotomy patients are observed in the recovery room or intensive care unit until the following morning, and then transferred to the general neurosurgical floor. A nasogastric tube may be necessary during the immediate postoperative period if anticonvulsant administration so requires. The patient is mobilized immediately, and physical therapy instituted early with anticipated discharge from hospital in 1–2 weeks.

The acute effects of anterior, posterior, and complete corpus callosotomy have been well described [24,25]. The decreased spontaneity of speech, urge incontinence, and mild nondominant leg weakness variably seen following anterior section generally clear within days or occasionally a few weeks. The sensory disconnection effects seen following posterior section, such as the inability to respond verbally to tachistoscopically presented stimuli in the nondominant hemisphere's (contralateral) visual field, are demonstrable from the time of surgery but are not behaviorally evident during normal activity when both hemispheres may access both hemifields by strategies such as scanning. Following completion of the commissurotomy, there may be an inability to execute verbally given commands with the nondominant hand, but as with the sensory disconnection this has not been disabling in daily activities. A transient increase in seizure activity during the immediate postoperative period has been occasionally seen and may reflect either an acute disconnection effect or a fluctuation in anticonvulsant levels perioperatively; as with patients who are entirely seizure-free during the first few weeks, correlation of such seizure frequency with long-term outcome is not apparent.

Electroencephalography and neuropsychological testing may be performed during the postoperative stay, but more practically useful information may be derived after a longer follow-up interval. Magnetic resonance imaging is now usually obtained prior to discharge [26]. The patient and his or her family are instructed to continue their previous seizure precautions, and anticonvulsant medications are continued unchanged. Both may be modified if significant response is evident at follow-up in 1–2 months. Should a less than satisfactory response — in terms of continued generalized seizures — follow the initial procedure, consideration is given to completion of the corpus callosum section. This is done at a minimum of 2 months and more often at 6 months.

Results

The experiences of a number of institutions now performing surgery of the corpus callosum for seizure disorders have been reported [3–17,20,24,25,27–47]. Although the extent of surgery and the selection of patients vary, the results have been fairly consistent and may be summarized with respect to seizure type. Spencer [24] recently summarized the results with 160 patients reported from various institutions and notes that generalized seizures of all types were eliminated or markedly decreased in 80–90% following complete section; similar benefit was obtained in significantly fewer patients following partial section. With regard to partial seizures of all types, less than 50% of patients experienced elimination or marked reduction in those seizures, and approximately 25% of patients had an increase or new onset of focal seizures [24].

Of patients undergoing either partial or complete callosal section at Dartmouth and followed a minimum of 1 year, approximately two-thirds of those with major motor seizures and a similar number of those with absence seizures preoperatively experienced either elimination or greater than 80% reduction of those seizures. The same response was obtained in three quarters of patients with atonic or akinetic seizures. With both major motor and atonic/akinetic groups, reduction in the severity of remaining seizures was frequently an important benefit. Simple partial seizures when present preoperatively were helped to the same degree in only one-third of patients. Two patients had an increase in the frequency of this seizure type, and 12 patients (24%) experienced new simple partial seizures. In nearly all instances, these new seizures were the attenuated expression of previously generalized seizures, an observation also made by Gates and colleagues [32].

An interesting subgroup of patients are those with complex partial seizures, approximately 50% of whom in our experience have had the above degree of improvement [15]. While commissurotomy has not been advocated as an alternative to temporal resection in patients who are candidates for resective surgery, the response is provocative both with regard to patients in whom a resectable focus cannot be identified and to our understanding of the behavioral expression of this seizure type.

Conclusions

Section of the corpus callosum for the treatment of medically intractable seizure disorders in patients in whom a resectable seizure focus cannot be identified is being performed in increasing numbers. Modern microsurgical technique allows this surgery to be performed safely and with assurance of complete division of commissural fibers. A midline approach utilizing the cavum septi pellucidi or its remnant has been most useful in our experience, although it is recognized that alternative techniques are also satisfactory. Results from a large number of institutions have been generally consistent and demonstrate reasonable success in patients with atonic (drop), tonic, and tonic–clonic generalized seizures. Neuropsychological effects of commissurotomy can be demonstrated but are generally outweighed by the improvement in seizures.

References

1 Dandy WE. Congenital cerebral cysts of the cavum septi pellucidi (fifth ventricle) and cavum vergae (sixth ventricle): diagnosis and treatment. *Arch Neurol Psychiatr* 1931; **25**: 44–66.

2 Van Wagenen WP, Aird RB. Dilatations of the cavity of the septum pellucidum and cavum vergae: report of cases. *Am J Cancer* 1934; **20**(3) : 539–557.

3 Van Wagenen WP, Herren RY. Surgical division of the commissural pathways in the corpus callosum: relation to spread of an epileptic attack. *Arch Neurol Psychiatr* 1940; **44**: 740–759.

4 Bogen, JE, Fisher ED, Vogel PJ. Cerebral commissurotomy: a second case report. *JAMA* 1965; **194**(12): 1328–1329.

5 Bogen JE, Sperry RW, Vogel PJ. Addendum: commissural section and propagation of seizures. In Jasper HH, Ward AA, Pope A (eds) *Basic Mechanisms of the Epilepsies*. Little, Brown, Boston, 1969, p 439.

6 Bogen JE, Vogel PJ. Cerebral commissurotomy in man: preliminary case report. *Bull Los Ang Neurol Soc* 1962; **27**: 169–172.

7 Luessenhop AJ. Interhemispheric commissurotomy (the split brain operation) as an alternative to hemispherectomy for control of intractable seizures. *Am Surg* 1970; **36**: 265–268.

8 Luessenhop AJ, dela Cruz TC, Fenichel GM. Surgical disconnection of the cerebral hemispheres for intractable seizures. *JAMA* 1970; **213**(10): 1630–1636.

9 Harbaugh RE, Wilson DH, Reeves AG, Gazzaniga MS. Forebrain commissurotomy for epilepsy: review of 20 consecutive cases. *Acta Neurochir (Wien)* 1983; **68**: 263–275.

10 Wilson DH, Culver C, Waddington M, Gazzaniga M. Disconnection of the cerebral hemispheres: an alternative to hemispherectomy for the control of intractable seizures. *Neurology* 1975; **25**(12): 1149–1153.

11 Wilson DH, Reeves, A, Gazzaniga M. Division of the corpus callosum for uncontrollable epilepsy. *Neurology* 1978; **28**: 649–653.

12 Wilson DH, Reeves A, Gazzaniga M. Corpus callosotomy for control of intractable seizures. In Wada JA, Penry JK (eds) *Advances in Epileptology: The Xth Epilepsy International Symposium.* Raven Press, New York, 1980, pp 205–213.

13 Wilson DH, Reeves AG, Gazzaniga MS. "Central" commissurotomy for intractable generalized epilepsy: series two. *Neurology* 1982; **32**: 687–697.

14 Wilson DH, Reeves AG, Gazzaniga MS, Culver C. Cerebral commissurotomy for control of intractable seizures. *Neurology* 1977; **27**(8): 708–715.

15 Roberts DW, Reeves AG. Effect of commissurotomy on complex partial epilepsy in patients without a resectable seizure focus. *Appl Neurophysiol* 1987; **50**: 398–400.

16 Spencer SS, Spencer DD, Williamson PD, Sass K, Novelly RA, Mattson RH. Corpus callosotomy for epilepsy. I. Seizure effects. *Neurology* 1988; **38**: 19–24.

17 Sass KJ, Spencer DD, Spencer SS, Novelly RA, Williamson PD, Mattson RH. Corpus callosotomy for epilepsy. II. Neurologic and neuropsychological outcome. *Neurology* 1988; **38**: 24–28.

18 Apuzzo MLJ, Chikovani OK, Gott PS. Transcallosal, interfornicial approaches for lesions affecting the third ventricle: surgical considerations and consequences. *Neurosurgery* 1982; **10**: 547–554.

19 Roberts DW. Corpus callosotomy: surgical technique. In Reeves AG (ed) *Epilepsy and the Corpus Callosum.* Plenum Press, New York, 1985, pp 259–267.

20 Roberts DW. Section of the corpus callosum for epilepsy. In Schmidek HH, Sweet WH (eds) *Operative Neurosurgical Techniques: Indications, Methods and Results.* 2nd edn. Grune & Stratton, Orlando, 1988, pp 1243–1250.

21 Roberts DW. Cava septi pellucidi et vergae: recognition and utilization in callosal surgery. Submitted, 1989.

22 Shaw C-M, Alvord, EC., Jr. Cava septi pellucidi et vergae: their normal and pathological states. *Brain* 1969; **92**: 213–224.

23 Schwidde JT. Incidence of cavum septi pellucidi and cavum vergae in 1,032 human brains. *Arch Neurol Psychiatr* 1952; **67**: 625–632.

24 Spencer SS. Corpus callosum section and other disconnection procedures for medically intractable epilepsy. *Epilepsia* 1988; **29**(Suppl 2): S85–S99.

25 Spencer SS, Gates JR, Reeves AG, Spencer DD, Maxwell RE, Roberts D. Corpus callosum section for uncontrolled epilepsy. In Engel J (ed) *Surgical Treatment of Epilepsy.* Raven Press, New York, 1987, pp 425–444.

26 Harris RD, Roberts DW, Cromwell LD. Magnetic resonance imaging of corpus callosotomy. *AJNR* 1989; **10**: 677–680.

27 Amacher AL. Midline commissurotomy for the treatment of some cases of intractable epilepsy. *Child Brain* 1976; **2**: 54–58.

28 Avila JO, Radvany J, Huck FR, Pires de Camargo CH, Marino R, Jr, Ragazzo PC, Riva D. Anterior callosotomy as a substitute for hemispherectomy. *Acta Neurochir (Wien)* 1980; (Suppl 30): 137–143.

29 Bouvier G, Mercier C, St Hilaire JM, Giard N, Labrecque R, Beique RA. Anterior callosotomy and chronic depth electrode recording in the surgical management of some intractable seizures. *Appl Neurophysiol* 1983; **46**: 52–56.

30 Gates JR, Leppik IE, Yap J, Gumnit RJ. Corpus callosotomy: clinical and electroencephalographic effects. *Epilepsia* 1984; **25**: 308–316.

31 Gates JR, Maxwell R, Leppik IE, Gumnit RJ. Electroencephalographic and clinical effects of total corpus callosotomy. In Reeves AG (ed) *Epilepsy and the Corpus Callosum.* Plenum Press, New York, 1985, pp 315–328.

32 Gates JR, Rosenfeld WE, Maxwell RE, Lyons RE. Response of multiple seizure types to corpus callosum section. *Epilepsia* 1987; **28**(1): 28–34.

33 Garcia-Flores E. Corpus callosum section for

patients with intractable epilepsy. *Appl Neurophysiol* 1987; **50**: 390–397.

34 Geoffroy G, Lassonde M, Delisle F, Decarie M. Corpus callosotomy for control of intractable epilepsy in children. *Neurology* 1983; **33**: 891–897.

35 Huck FR, Radvany J, Avila JO, Pires de Camargo CH, Marino R, Jr, Ragazzo PC, Riva D, Arlant P. Anterior callosotomy in epileptics with multiform seizures and bilateral synchronous spike and wave EEG pattern. *Acta Neurochir (Wien)* 1980; (Suppl 30): 127–135.

36 Marino R, Jr, Ragazzo PC. Selective criteria and results of selective partial callosotomy. In Reeves AG (ed) *Epilepsy and the Corpus Callosum*. Plenum Press, New York, 1985, pp 281–301.

37 Murro AM, Flanigin HF, Gallagher BB, King DW, Smith JR. Corpus callosotomy for the treatment of intractable epilepsy. *Epilepsy Rev* 1988; **2**: 44–50.

38 Purves SJ, Wada JA, Woodhurst WB, Moyes PD, Strauss E, Kosaka B, Li D. Results of anterior corpus callosum section in 24 patients with medically intractable seizures. *Neurology* 1988; **38**: 1194–1201.

39 Rappaport ZH, Lerman P. Corpus callosotomy in the treatment of secondary generalizing intractable epilepsy. Acta Neurochir 1988; **94**: 10–14.

40 Rayport M, Corrie WS, Freguson SM. Corpus callosum section for control of clinically and electroencephalographically classified seizures. In: Reeves AG (ed) *Epilepsy and the Corpus Callosum*. Plenum Press, New York, 1985, pp 329–337.

41 Rayport M, Ferguson SM, Corrie WS. Outcomes and indications of corpus callosum section for intractable seizure control. *Appl Neurophysiol* 1983; **46**: 47–51.

42 Reeves AG, O'Leary PM. Total corpus callosotomy for control of medically intractable epilepsy. In: Reeves AG (ed) *Epilepsy and the Corpus Callosum*. Plenum Press, New York, 1985, pp. 269–280.

43 Sainte-Hilaire JM, Giard N, Bouvier G, Labrecque R. Anterior callosotomy in frontal lobe epilepsies. In: Reeves AG (ed) *Epilepsy and the Corpus Callosum*. Plenum Press, New York, 1985, pp 303–314.

44 Spencer DD, Spencer SS. Corpus callosotomy in the treatment of medically intractable secondarily generalized seizures of children. *Cleve Clin J Med* 1988; **56**(Suppl 1): S69–S77.

45 Spencer SS, Spencer DD, Glaser GH, Williamson PD, Mattson RH. More intense focal seizure types after callosal section: the role of inhibition. *Ann Neurol* 1984; **16**: 686–693.

46 Spencer SS, Spencer DD, Williamson PD, Mattson RH. Effect of corpus callosum section on secondary bilaterally synchronous interictal EEG discharges. *Neurology* 1985; **35**: 1689–1694.

47 Williamson PD. Corpus callosum section for intractable epilepsy: criteria for patient selection. In Reeves AG (ed) *Epilepsy and the Corpus Callosum*. Plenum Press, New York, 1985, pp 243–257.

part *III*

Outcome

chapter 9

Dogma, Data, and Directions

Susan S. Spencer and Dennis D. Spencer

Introduction

Reversing a chronic disease by surgery is nowhere as dramatic as in the epileptic population. Understandably, as publicity enhances public and professional awareness of this possibility, more patients, their families, and their physicians, are seeking such a "cure." Some perspective is required.

Surgery does not always stop seizures. Furthermore, epilepsy surgery cannot reverse a lifetime of disability, social alienation, disease-provoked behavioral patterns, drug-induced cognitive impairments, delayed achievement, and family turmoil. Epilepsy surgery will not reverse the initial neurologic insult causing the uncontrolled seizures, nor will it erase the possible effects of injuries and repeated seizures. Epilepsy surgery cannot do all of these things for any patient, but it can certainly help.

Although many of the expert contributions to this volume have reported, or alluded to, the outcome of various surgical procedures for uncontrolled epilepsy and the determination of successful outcome, they have reported the literature in a limited way, in the context of their chapter, and with respect to only some of the variables. Before concluding the volume we feel, as editors, the need to provide a more general review of outcome from epilepsy surgery, along with the indicated caveats for interpreting the applicable literature.

Interpretation of the literature

Standards

Although proposals have been made to do so, epilepsy surgery centers presently do not adhere to uniform criteria for assessing outcome in any sphere. Excellent results may include only patients with no seizures at all after surgery, or may include those with auras or occasional seizures. Good, fair, and poor categories are similarly variable. Categorization of results as "worthwhile" or "not worthwhile" improvements are additional ways to confound comparison or tabulation of results at various centers. Reported results of corpus callosum section carry these ambiguities to greater heights, judging best results with respect to social outcome, seizure reduction, or (usually) some arbitrary and variable combination of these two factors.

An outcome scale cannot be mandated, however, and many previously reported results bear scrutiny because they represent years of follow-up in a substantial number of patients to whom new ways of tabulating outcome cannot be applied. The differences and difficulties with interpretation of reported results must therefore be accepted and recognized while we attempt to improve the situation in the future.

Types of outcome

It is the uncontrolled seizures which prompt surgery, but many epileptic patients also have a psychiatric history of variably significant proportions [1]. Often, they have also been underemployed, underschooled, or undersocialized. The effects of surgery on the separate variables of psychiatric, psychosocial, and seizure status, and their obvious interdependence upon one another (and many other factors), are important and have been relatively neglected. If surgery worsens any one of these, overall functional status may not be improved despite dramatic improvement in another sphere of function. Taylor has rightly noted that the question of whether patients are "better" after epilepsy surgery still begs an answer [2].

On an anecdotal basis, however, most physicians who participate in an epilepsy surgery program can substantiate widespread claims of dramatic improvement in lifestyle, accomplishments, and level of function after epilepsy surgery, usually linked to control of seizures. It seems appropriate, therefore, to make our primary concern interpretation of the available information on change of seizures after surgery, with the caveat that seizure control does not necessarily imply psychosocial or psychiatric improvement, and with the suggestion that in the future the dependent and independent variables of psychiatric and psychosocial status be analyzed as well.

Patient perceptions

Related to the aspects of psychosocial and psychiatric outcome of epilepsy surgery are the patient's and family's perceptions of outcome. An improved self-image promotes improved psychological status. In our experience, this variable is not necessarily related to seizure outcome. After resective procedures which aim to stop seizures, persistence of auras or partial seizures are often ignored by the patient who has a markedly improved self-image, with accompanying functional advancement. After corpus callosum section, despite counselling as to its expected effects on only generalized seizures, persistence of partial seizures is often viewed by the family as failure and accompanied by persistent psychosocial retardation (despite normal IQ). The messages here are clear: reports of improvement are another variable with some, but not total, dependence on seizure response, and ways to promote positive perception of outcome, or its prediction, should be sought.

Variable operations

Epilepsy surgery is not an operation, but a group of operations. Most commonly, these include resective procedures of variable extent in variable cerebral locations (from topectomy through lobectomy) and corpus callosum section, also of variable extent (anterior, posterior, total). Even within the specific groups, subgroups can be identified. Thus, anterior corpus callosum section may include anterior one-third, one-half, two-thirds; temporal lobectomy may include total hippocampal resection, partial hippocampectomy, no hippocampal resection. When possible, results should be compared for the same operation, but sometimes the extent of surgery is not quantified or known. A given center may also vary the resection, based on peculiar criteria. To obtain reasonable numbers of patients for analysis we must group patients, but we have no *a priori* basis upon which to compare them. Recent developments in magnetic resonance imaging (MRI) may enable more valid comparisons of surgical groups. Still, the comments above apply: large numbers of reported patients in the present literature have much to convey, despite the difficulties with interpretation, and this information must be utilized as it stands, with recognition of its nature and hope for better documentation and standardization in the future.

Goals

Corpus callosum section aims only to prevent generalized seizures, while resective procedures aim to stop all seizures [3]. The term "success" needs to be qualified with respect to the operation and its particular goals.

In some instances, when all factors are not ideal, patients may be offered a certain operation with more limited expectations that are acceptable to the patient and the family because of the severity of the disability. Thus, at times, the same operations may be done with different goals [4]. Interpretation of collected or individual results at different centers may reflect the degree to which patients with lower expectation of good results are reported in the candidates selected for surgery.

Follow-up

Much happens between the day of surgery and the day outcome is assessed. Occasional seizures may occur early or late; they may be related to emotional factors, hormonal changes, or intercurrent illnesses. New medications, adjustment of existing antiepileptic medications, or change in patient compliance may alter the dynamics of cerebral excitability. Improved self-image, change in timing of seizures, improved mobility due to driving, change in domicile or work environment, or change in psychiatric or neurologic status, may impact positively or negatively on the reliability of patient reporting of seizure-like events. We cannot hope to hospitalize all patients pre- and postoperatively for enough time to obtain consistent and comparable information, and we must recognize these deficiencies in our ability to judge what has happened to an individual's seizures.

Duration of follow-up

Surgical outcome is usually judged at present, i.e. latest follow-up. This date is variably distant from surgery. At centers established more than two decades ago, most patients have more than 5 years follow-up and a substantial number have 10 or 15 years follow-up. Can such patients be compared to those with shorter follow-up at the same or other centers?

Evolving patient selection criteria over decades may independently change criteria for surgery over such a span of time, and few surgical centers have reported changing results over the years. Crandall showed, after new criteria were adopted for patient selection at UCLA, improved results from temporal lobectomy [5]. At Yale, good to excellent results after temporal lobectomy went from 75% in the first 50 patients to 90% in the next 50 patients. Even then, such changes over time, at a single center, are reported for latest follow-up, producing bias toward good results in more recent patients. The suggestion that all follow-up be reported at a fixed date from operation is difficult to implement in older series, but is one possible solution to this ambiguity in reporting results [4].

Future

With so many caveats, we can still interpret the literature to some degree and have made progress in defining criteria for good surgical outcome after resective or corpus callosum section procedures. These conclusions are discussed below. They appear to have enabled improved patient selection. Yet, our conclusions could be better if deficiencies in reporting were corrected. Comprehensive and prospective data storage at all centers who perform epilepsy surgery is encouraged.

Resective procedures

Seizure outcome

Reported The most recent overall data available for worthwhile results after resective procedures is presented in the monograph resulting from the first International Conference on Surgical Treatment of the Epilepsies in 1987 [4]. At that time, centers throughout the world were asked to report the results of resective procedures according to fixed categories, enabling the first set of intercenter data of a comparable nature. Despite the standardization, results were widely discrepant. Twenty-six to 80% of the patients reported were seizure-free after temporal lobectomy, 0–73% after extratemporal resection, and 0–100% after hemispherectomy. Figures for "worthwhile improvement" and "not improved" were similarly variable. On an average, 55% of patients were seizure-free after temporal lobectomy, 43% after extratemporal resection, and 77% after hemispherectomy. These figures compare roughly with results reported by Jensen, who reviewed the literature on temporal lobectomy between 1928 and 1973 [6]. They are thus representative of the collective experience around the world for many decades.

More recent reports suggest improved outcome, with 90% of patients in the seizure-free category after resective procedures (usually temporal) [4,5]. Whether these reflect improved selection criteria, shorter follow-up, more rigorous evaluation, more extensive resections, or more expertise at established centers is open to question. Nevertheless, it can be firmly stated, on the basis of multiple reports, that more than one-half of the patients selected for temporal lobectomy by various criteria undergoing variable operations with variable but at least 1 year follow-up have no seizures, and perhaps three-quarters of such patients experience worthwhile improvement, with a slightly lower percentage of successful outcome for extratemporal resections, and slightly higher for hemispherectomy.

Determinants of success It is widely held that accurate identification of the epileptogenic zone and complete resection are the two critical factors predictive of successful seizure control after resective procedures [7–9]. These are theoretical concepts which bear close scrutiny.

The first accepted determinant of successful resective surgery for epilepsy, accurate localization of the focus, is an ambiguous concept. How can we judge accurate localization? Using seizure control after surgery is difficult because of its dependence on patient reports, medications, and mechanisms by which surgery may be effective (see below). Pathologic analysis of the tissue for deviations from the expected normal seems a reasonable approach, but normal depends on the techniques with which the tissue is studied, which may not be adequate. Furthermore, the critical tissue may not be available for analysis, depending on the technique of operation. If abnormalities are found, are they incidental? Against this thought is the observation, repeatedly confirmed, that positive pathology correlates with good seizure control after resective surgery [10,11]. Are abnormalities, therefore, the cause, or effect, of the seizures? This is difficult to answer, but the extent of abnormality in resected temporal lobe associated with tumors in patients with epilepsy is less than the extent in temporal lobe epilepsy without tumors, and is not correlated with seizure duration, suggesting that not all of the abnormalities we are presently able to analyze are an effect of epilepsy (personal observations). Nevertheless, pathologic analysis is a critical approach to understanding the reasons why epilepsy surgery works and has important implications in patient selection.

Logic dictates that total removal of the area causing seizures should stop them. The reports of Olivier *et al.* [12], indicating that seizure control was successful after more temporal lobe was removed in some patients who failed their initial temporal lobe resection, and of Babb *et al.* [13] indicating inferior results if abnormalities persist in posterior hippocampus, support this concept. Perhaps merely debulking this zone of epileptogenicity is sufficient. Some reports indicate a "wearing down" phenomenon of gradual diminution and eventual cessation of seizures after resective procedures, which supports this theory [14]. We have no evidence, however, that epilepsy emanates from a zone at all. Perhaps a small focal area is critical to generate the seizures, and the likelihood of its removal is merely increased with the increasingly large resections required in the theoretical zone concept.

Alternatively, the area, region, point, or zone of origin may be only as important as its anatomic connections. In this concept, disconnection of the discharging abnormality from other cerebral regions could be solely responsible for cure of seizures [15]. Some support for this disconnection concept is supplied by the partly satisfactory results in seizure control obtained from any of multiple operations done for temporal lobe epilepsy (removal of only temporal neocortex, only hippocampus, or varying portions of both) [5], despite singular pathologic abnormalities in the hippocampus in most patients with temporal lobe epilepsy (in whom the hippocampus is available for analysis) [10]. The persistence of auras without seizures in many patients is also consistent with the disconnection concept as an explanation for response to these varying degrees of temporal lobectomy. Although theoretical, the above discussion emphasizes our lack of understanding of the pathologic, anatomic, and physiologic basis for an operative procedure that "works" in many patients.

Psychiatric outcome

Reported Whether by virtue of their lifelong disability and its effects, or of the anatomic substrate or pathogenesis of their seizures, epileptic patients often have psychiatric disease. The incidence of preoperative psychosis was estimated by Jensen and Larsen at 15% in one series, and almost all these patients had some psychiatric disorder [16]. Other estimates suggest one-third of epilepsy patients have required psychiatric admission, preoperatively, with 5–10% incidence of preoperative psychosis [17].

Upon this rather discrepant information documenting preoperative psychiatric status in epilepsy surgery patients, is superimposed an additional set of data concerning the response of psychiatric disease to epilepsy surgery. Some literature suggests improvement in neurotic, aggressive, and personality traits after resective procedures [18–21]. Preoperative psychosis, however, was generally unchanged regardless of the effects of surgery on seizures [2,22].

Of greatest concern is the reported high rate of postoperative suicide [23] and of development of significant postoperative psychosis, which is estimated to occur in 5–15% of patients after temporal lobectomy [1, 16,17]. The issues here are confused further by exclusion of patients with significant preoperative psychiatric disorder from resective procedures at certain centers [1].

Determinants of psychiatric outcome If psychosis and other psychiatric disorders are common in epilepsy patients, and if only improvement or lack of change were reported, psychiatric disease could be considered an independent entity from the seizures which prompt surgery, constituting neither an indication nor a contraindication for surgery. But, since about 10% of patients also *develop* psychosis after epilepsy surgery, the question remains as to whether surgery is etiologic in these individuals. Therefore, the major issue in the psychiatric realm is predicting which patients are at risk for postoperative psychosis.

At least some attempts to answer this question have concluded that left-handed female patients with dominant hemisphere temporal lobe foci associated with alien tissue are at greatest risk for postoperative psychosis [2,24–26]. However, others have failed to confirm these findings [16]. Even so, the chances of a patient meeting all these risk factors are inordinately slim [2]. Finally, since patients with or without psychiatric pathology have equal chances of seizure control [2], no strong recommendation can be made for denying epilepsy surgery to any patient on the basis of at least pre-existing psychiatric illness, unless the psychosis prevents cooperation, puts the patient at undue risk to life during the preoperative evaluation, or is felt to unequivocally prevent successful rehabilitation or benefit, even if seizure control is achieved.

Psychosocial outcome

Probably the most global outcome measure of any therapeutic intervention is the subsequent psychosocial function of the individual: are they now able to resume or improve their level of work, school, or daily function in society? This complex variable presupposes adequate compensation in the psychiatric realm and improvement in the disease (here, seizures) which was presumably disabling before therapy was undertaken. Measuring psychosocial change is difficult, and in the uncontrolled epilepsy patient, after surgery, assumes the vagaries inherent in the psychiatric and seizure assessments. Very few investigators have even tried.

Those who have accepted this challenge gave unimpressive results. Only 17 of 100 patients studied by Taylor and Falconer [27] improved to normal in psychosocial level. Augustine *et al.* showed that patients improved by elevating their work status, while those who had been unemployed remained so after surgery, regardless of seizure effects [28]. These observers were consistent in their implication that preoperative level of function was an important variable in determining psychosocial rehabilitation after resective surgery for uncontrolled epilepsy: presence of low IQ, low social class, and implied minimal support systems, were implicated as negative criteria for psychosocial improvement.

Neurologic and neuropsychologic outcome

Neurologic deficits are obviously dependent on the area or the lobe involved in the resective procedure, are addressed in detail in the context of discussions about particular surgical approaches, and are in general of minimal clinical significance, provided unexpected complications do not occur and due respect to functional areas is paid. These particular issues will, therefore, not be readdressed.

Of some importance, however, is the predictable deficit involved with certain proposed resections involving functional cortex, and the advisability of surgical procedures in these areas. This is most often an issue when the location of the seizure focus is in the occipital lobe or adjacent to motor, sensory, or language areas. No guidelines exist here except careful and repeated discussions and estimates of risk, so that an informed decision can be made regarding acceptable losses in neurologic function in exchange for the possibility of seizure control.

Corpus callosum section

Seizure outcome

Reported Response to corpus callosum section has been categorized on the basis of worthwhile improvement, response of particular seizure types or syndromes, percentage reduction in seizure frequency combined with psychosocial improvement, and other scales. Collectively, the impression emerges that this operation is beneficial when generalized seizures (tonic, atonic, tonic–clonic, but not necessarily absence or myoclonic) and/or falls, and/or episodes of status epilepticus, are the major impediment to a safe or functional life, and that is because the operation has been most successful in these respects. More than 80% of patients respond with decrease or cessation of generalized seizures, falls, and episodes of status [29]. Partial seizures may also be diminished, but this occurs much less predictably (approximately 40%) and cannot be considered an indication for corpus callosum section, especially since partial seizures may also worsen in frequency or intensity (approximately 25%) [30].

Determinants of success As for resective procedures, correlates can be drawn to the concept that accurate localization and extent of surgery determine success, but these are much more loosely applied to this population of patients and this particular operation. Spencer *et al.* showed that improved localization (positive CT lesion, unilateral disease) is correlated with improved response of generalized and partial seizures to corpus callosum section [31]. Conversely, low IQ and diffuse cerebral involvement were correlated with decreased success. But localization in this context takes on the meaning of restricted, rather than focal. Similarly, extent of surgery is also a determinant of success for corpus callosum section, since partial section produces beneficial responses one-half as often as total section [32]. But, extent here takes on the meaning of amount disconnected, rather than amount removed.

The latter comment raises an important differential between the resective procedures and corpus callosum section. Corpus callosum section is a disconnection procedure. As such, no tissue is removed and no pathologic analysis is possible. The study and subsequent refinement of determinants of success in such procedures, therefore, is dependent entirely on clinical studies of patient characteristics and electrophysiologic analysis of seizure origin and spread in the individual patient — at best difficult analyses requiring years of experience and large numbers of patients.

Psychiatric outcome

Psychiatric issues, before and after corpus callosum section, have been ignored. Besides the science fiction and popular literature on divided brains, only one report comments on changing behavior. Spencer observed an increase in aggressive and violent tendencies in some patients — all of these patients had preoperative behavioral difficulties [29]. In a recent review of our patients, 35% had behavioral worsening at 1 year and 30% continued to worsen over 5 years, while only 15% had improved behavior at 1 year with no improvement thereafter. The determinants of such poor behavioral outcome are unknown: in this group, seizure change, IQ, and other neurologic complications were not related. Such observations underline the need, in patients undergoing corpus callosum section as well as resective procedures, to ask whether they are, indeed, better. We require long-term follow-up of multiple variables besides those which are traditionally studied.

Psychosocial outcome

On the surface, the reported results after corpus callosum section would appear to pay significant attention to psychosocial and functional rehabilitation as a result of the procedure, since most reports have incorporated functional improvement into the seizure outcome rating. Partly, this is because corpus callosum section is a palliative procedure, after which seizures, often frequent, are expected to continue. Improved functional status, then, assumes a different connotation, one of improved life circumstances more than lifestyle. Removal of the helmet is as important as resuming full-time employment to certain individuals. In this context, psychosocial improvement after corpus callosum section is more closely tied to control of (generalized) seizures than it is to control of seizures after resective procedures, where many other factors operate in enabling an individual who is *free* of seizures to undertake what is essentially a normal lifestyle.

Neurologic and neuropsychologic outcome

Twenty percent of carefully analyzed patients have neurologic or neuropsychologic deficits after corpus callosum section, including weakness or apraxia (usually nondominant leg), language disturbance (usually expressive), cognitive impairments (usually memory decline), or disconnection syndromes (sensory, motor, or both) [29,33]. Some investigators have suggested that severe, early, unilateral, cerebral damage prevents such deficits because function is then assumed by a single hemisphere and unaffected by disconnection, while early damage of only moderate degree (or later damage) requires hemispheric cooperation in functional recovery, which is then susceptible to disruption by disconnection [33]. The variably precise methods for determining extent of prior injury include Amytal testing, neurologic examination, neuropsychologic evaluation, and imaging studies. None is known to predict disconnection syndrome, and no mechanism exists to judge extent of expected deficit before the fact. Much work remains to be done in this area.

Summary

Epilepsy surgery is a proven modality which works to diminish (corpus callosum section) or stop (resective procedures) seizures in the great majority of patients. An unknown but substantial number have improved psychosocial and functional status too. Psychiatric status may worsen in a small number of patients, but is generally an independent variable. Analysis of comparable groups, improved data collection and reporting, and more sophisticated pathologic and electrophysiologic assessments are the most likely means for advancing successful outcome in all spheres and for understanding the mechanisms by which these procedures effect improvement.

References

1 Fenwick PBC. Postscript: what should be included in a standard psychiatric assessment? In Engel J, Jr (ed) *Surgical Treatment of the Epilepsies.* Raven Press, New York, 1987, pp 505–510.

2 Taylor DC. Psychiatric and social issues in measuring the input and outcome of epilepsy surgery. In Engel J, Jr (ed) *Surgical Treatment of the Epilepsies.* Raven Press, New York, 1987, pp 485–503.

3 Spencer SS. Surgical options for uncontrolled epilepsy. In RJ Porter, Theodore WH (eds) *Epilepsy.* Neurological Clinics of North America, Vol 4, No. 3. WB Saunders, Philadelphia, 1986, pp 669–695.

4 Engel J, Jr. Outcome with respect to epileptic seizures. In Engel J, Jr (ed) *Surgical Treatment of the Epilepsies.* Raven Press, New York, 1987, pp 553–571.

5 Crandall PH. Cortical resections. In Engel J, Jr (ed) *Surgical Treatment of the Epilepsies.* Raven Press, New York, 1987, pp 377–404.

6 Jensen I. Temporal lobe surgery around the world. *Acta Neurol Scand* 1975; **52**: 354–373.

7 Rossi GF. Considerations on the principles of surgical treatment of partial epilepsy. *Brain Res* 1975; **95**: 395–402.

8 Rasmussen T. The place of surgery in the treatment of epilepsy. In Morley TP (ed) *Current Controversies in Neurosurgery.* WB Saunders, Philadelphia, 1976, pp 463–477.

9 Spencer SS. Depth electroencephalography in selection of refractory epilepsy for surgery. *Ann Neurol* 1981; 9: 207–214.

10 Babb TL, Brown WJ. Pathological findings in epilepsy. In Engel J, Jr (ed) *Surgical Treatment of the Epilepsies.* Raven Press, New York, 1987, pp 511–540.

11 Engel J, Driver MV, Falconer MA. Electrophysiological correlates of pathology and surgical results in temporal lobe epilepsy. *Brain,* 1975; **98**: 129–156.

12 Olivier A, Tanaka T, Andermann F. Reoperations in temporal lobe epilepsy. *Epilepsia* 1988; **29**: 678.

13 Babb TL, Brown WJ, Pretorius J, Davenport C, Lieb JP, Crandall PH. Temporal lobe volumetric cell densities in temporal lobe epilepsy. *Epilepsia* 1984; **25**: 729–740.

14 Rasmussen T. Surgical treatment of complex partial seizures: results, lessons, and problems. *Epilepsia* 1983; **24** (Suppl 1): 65–76.

15 Falconer MA, Serafetinides EA, Corsellis JAN. Etiology and pathogenesis of temporal lobe epilepsy. *Arch Neurol* 1964; **10**: 233–248.

16 Jensen I, Larsen K. Mental aspects of temporal lobe epilepsy. *J Neurol Neurosurg Psychiatr* 1979; **42**: 256–265.

17 Walker AE, Blumer D. Behavioral effects of temporal lobectomy for temporal lobe epilepsy. In Blumer D (ed) *Psychiatric Aspects of Epilepsy.* American Psychiatry Press, Washington DC, 1985, pp 294–323.

18 Taylor DC. Aggression and epilepsy. *J Psychosom Res* 1969; **13**: 229–236.

19 Lindsay J, Ounsted C, Richards P. Long-term outcome in children with temporal lobe seizures. V. Indications and contraindications for neurosurgery. *Dev Med Child Neurol* 1984; **26**: 25–32.

20 Polkey CE. Effects of anterior temporal lobectomy apart from the relief of seizures: a study of 40 patients. *J R Soc Med* 1983; **76**: 354–358.

21 Rausch R. Crandall PH. Psychological status related to surgical control of temporal lobe seizures. *Epilepsia* 1982; **23**: 191–202.

22 Bruens JH. Psychoses in epilepsy. In Vinken PJ, Bruyn GW (eds) *Handbook of Clinical Neurology*

Vol 15. North-Holland Publishing Co., Amsterdam, 1974, pp 593–610.

23 Taylor DC, Marsh SM. The influence of sex and side of operation on personality questionnaire responses after temporal lobectomy. In Gruzelier J, Flor-Henry P (eds) *Hemisphere Asymmetries of Function in Psychopathology*. Elsevier/North-Holland, Amsterdam, 1979, pp 391–400.

24 Taylor DC. Factors influencing the occurrence of schizophrenia-like psychosis in patients with temporal lobe epilepsy. *Psychol Med* 1975; **5**: 249–254.

25 Sherwin I. Psychosis associated with epilepsy: significance of the laterality of the epileptogenic lesion. *J Neurol Neurosurg Psychiatr* 1981; **44**: 83–85.

26 Sherwin I, Person-Magnan P, Bancaud J *et al.* Prevalence of psychosis in epilepsy as a function of the laterality of the epileptogenic lesion. *Arch Neurol* 1982; **39**: 621–625.

27 Taylor DC, Falconer MA. Clinical socioeconomic and psychological changes after temporal lobectomy for epilepsy. *Br J Psychiatr* 1968; **114**: 1247–1261.

28 Augustine EA, Novelly RA, Mattson RH, Glaser GH, Williamson PD, Spencer DD, Spencer SS. Occupational adjustment following neurosurgical treatment of epilepsy for seizure control. *Ann Neurol* 1984; **15**: 68–72.

29 Spencer SS. Corpus callosotomy in the treatment of intractable seizures. In Pedley TA, Meldrum BS (eds) *Recent Advances in Epilepsy* Vol 4. Churchill Livingstone, New York, 1988, pp 181–204.

30 Spencer SS, Spencer DD, Glaser GH, Williamson PD, Mattson RH. More intense focal seizure types after callosal section: the role of inhibition. *Ann Neurol* 1984; **16**: 686–693.

31 Spencer SS, Spencer DD, Williamson PD, Sass K, Novelly RA, Mattson RH. Corpus callosotomy for epilepsy I: seizure effects. *Neurology* 1988; **38**: 19–24.

32 Spencer SS, Spencer DD, Williamson PD, Sass KJ, Novelly RA, Mattson RH. Partial vs. total corpus callosotomy for epilepsy. In *Advances in Epileptology* Vol 16. The 16th Epilepsy International Symposium. Raven Press, New York, 1987, pp 323–325.

33 Sass KJ, Spencer DD, Spencer SS, Novelly RA, Williamson PD, Mattson RH. Corpus callosotomy for epilepsy II: neurological and neuropsychological outcome. *Neurology* 1988; **38**: 24–28.

Index

Page references in *italics* refer to tables or figures.